T0348493

2012
YEAR BOOK OF
**DIAGNOSTIC
RADIOLOGY**®

The 2012 Year Book Series

Year Book of Anesthesiology and Pain Management™: Drs Chestnut, Abram, Black, Gravlee, Lien, Mathru, and Roizen

Year Book of Cardiology®: Drs Gersh, Cheitlin, Elliott, Gold, Graham, and Thourani

Year Book of Critical Care Medicine®: Drs Dries, Zanotti-Cavazzoni, Latenser, Martinez, Rincon, and Zwank

Year Book of Dermatology and Dermatologic Surgery™: Dr Del Rosso

Year Book of Diagnostic Radiology®: Drs Elster, Abbara, Oestreich, Offiah, Rosado de Christenson, Stephens, and Strickland

Year Book of Emergency Medicine®: Drs Hamilton, Bruno, Handly, Minczak, Mullin, Quintana, and Ramoska

Year Book of Endocrinology®: Drs Schott, Apovian, Clarke, Eugster, Ludlam, Meikle, Oetgen, Ovalle, Schteingart, and Toth

Year Book of Hand and Upper Limb Surgery®: Drs Yao, Adams, Isaacs, Lee, and Rizzo

Year Book of Medicine®: Drs Barker, Garrick, Gersh, Khardori, LeRoith, Panush, Talley, and Thigpen

Year Book of Neonatal and Perinatal Medicine®: Drs Fanaroff, Benitz, Donn, Neu, Papile, Polin, and Van Marter

Year Book of Neurology and Neurosurgery®: Drs Klimo, Minagar, Gandhi, House, Kevill, Liu, Mazia, Panagariya, Ragel, Riesenburger, Robottom, Schwendimann, Shafazand, Uhm, and Yang

Year Book of Obstetrics, Gynecology, and Women's Health®: Drs Dungan and Shulman

Year Book of Oncology®: Drs Arceci, Bauer, Chiorean, Gordon, Lawton, Murphy, Thigpen, and Tsao

Year Book of Ophthalmology®: Drs Rapuano, Cohen, Flanders, Hammersmith, Milman, Myers, Nagra, Nelson, Penne, Pyfer, Sergott, Shields, Talekar, and Vander

Year Book of Orthopedics®: Drs Morrey, Huddleston, Rose, Swiontkowski, and Trigg

Year Book of Otolaryngology-Head and Neck Surgery®: Drs Sindwani, Balough, Franco, Gapany, and Mitchell

Year Book of Pathology and Laboratory Medicine®: Drs Raab and Bissell

Year Book of Pediatrics®: Dr Stockman

Year Book of Plastic and Aesthetic Surgery™: Drs Miller, Gosman, Gurtner, Gutowski, Ruberg, Salisbury, and Smith

Year Book of Psychiatry and Applied Mental Health®: Drs Talbott, Ballenger, Buckley, Frances, Krupnick, and Mack

Year Book of Pulmonary Disease®: Drs Barker, Jones, Maurer, Spradley, Tanoue, and Willsie

Year Book of Sports Medicine®: Drs Shephard, Cantu, Feldman, Galea, Jankowski, Janssen, Lebrun, and Nieman

Year Book of Surgery®: Drs Copeland, Behrns, Daly, Eberlein, Fahey, Huber, Klodell, Mozingo, and Pruett

Year Book of Urology®: Drs Andriole and Coplen

Year Book of Vascular Surgery®: Drs Moneta, Gillespie, Starnes, and Watkins

2012

The Year Book of DIAGNOSTIC RADIOLOGY®

Editor-in-Chief

Allen D. Elster, MD, FACR

Professor and Chair, Division of Radiologic Sciences, Director of Radiologic Sciences, Wake Forest University Health Sciences, Winston-Salem, North Carolina

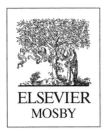

ELSEVIER
MOSBY

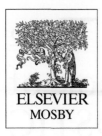

ELSEVIER
MOSBY

Vice President, Continuity: Kimberly Murphy
Editor: Teia Stone
Supervisor, Electronic Year Books: Donna M. Skelton
Electronic Article Manager: Mike Sheets
Illustrations and Permissions Coordinator: Dawn Vohsen

Printed and bound by CPI Group (UK) Ltd, Croydon, CR0 4YY
Transferred to Digital Print 2012

Composition by TNQ Books and Journals Pvt Ltd, India

Editorial Office:
Elsevier
Suite 1800
1600 John F. Kennedy Blvd.
Philadelphia, PA 19103-2899

International Standard Serial Number: 0098-1672
International Standard Book Number: 978-0-323-08877-0

Associate Editors

Suhny Abbara, MD
Associate Professor, Harvard Medical School; Director, Cardiac Imaging Fellowship, Massachusetts General Hospital; Director of Education Cardiac MR/CT Program, Boston, Massachusetts

Alan E. Oestreich, MD
Professor Emeritus of Radiology, University of Cincinnati College of Medicine; Pediatric Radiologist Emeritus, Cincinnati Children's Hospital Medical Center, Cincinnati, Ohio; Professor of Radiology and Pediatrics, University of Kentucky, Lexington, Kentucky

Amaka C. Offiah, BSc, MBBS, MRCP, FRCR, PhD
HEFCE Clinical Senior Lecturer, Academic Unit of Child Health, Sheffield Children's NHS Foundation Trust, Western Bank, Sheffield, United Kingdom

Melissa L. Rosado de Christenson, MD, FACR
Section Chief, Thoracic Imaging, St. Luke's Hospital of Kansas City; Professor of Radiology, University of Missouri–Kansas City, Kansas City, Missouri

Tanya W. Stephens, MD
Associate Professor, Department of Diagnostic Radiology, Division of Diagnostic Imaging, The University of Texas M.D. Anderson Cancer Center, Houston, Texas

Colin Strickland, MD
Assistant Professor, Division of Musculoskeletal Radiology, Department of Radiology, University of Colorado School of Medicine, Aurora, Colorado

Contributors

Russell Chapin, MD
Musculoskeletal Radiology Division, Medical University of South Carolina, Charleston, South Carolina

Deanna L. Lane, MD
Assistant Professor, Department of Diagnostic Radiology, Division of Diagnostic Imaging, The University of Texas M.D. Anderson Cancer Center, Houston, Texas

Huong Le-Petross, MD
Associate Professor, Department of Diagnostic Radiology, Division of Diagnostic Imaging, The University of Texas M.D. Anderson Cancer Center, Houston, Texas

Table of Contents

JOURNALS REPRESENTED   xiii

INTRODUCTION   xv

1. Thoracic Radiology   1

    Introduction   1

    Lung Cancer   2

    Nodules   8

    Malignant Neoplasia   13

    Radiography   17

    Computed Tomography   23

    Interstitial Lung Disease   29

    Infection   31

    Pulmonary Thromboembolic Disease   36

2. Breast Imaging   43

    Introduction   43

    Anatomy   43

    The Augmented Breast   44

    Breast MRI   47

    Follow-up Care   50

    Image Quality   53

    Screening Mammography   55

    Patient Perceptions   60

    Postneoadjuvant Pathologic Tumor Response   61

    Post-Surgical Breast   62

    Pregnant and Lactating Women   64

    Ultrasound   65

    Miscellaneous   71

3. Musculoskeletal   75

    Introduction   75

    Tumors   76

    Trauma   78

    Systemic   79

Arthritis 88
Joints/Sports Injuries 94
Other 113
4. Pediatric Radiology 115
Introduction 115
Gastrointestinal 116
Genitourinary 129
Musculoskeletal 143
Neurologic/Vertebral 158
Thoracic/Airway/Vascular 172
Miscellaneous 187
5. Economics, Research, Education, and Quality 191
Introduction 191
Appropriate Criteria and Cost Effectiveness 192
Clinical Practice 196
Medical Economics 209
Radiation Safety 211
Contrast Agents 218
Quality 224
6. Cardiac Imaging 229
Introduction 229

ARTICLE INDEX 241
AUTHOR INDEX 249

Journals Represented

Journals represented in this YEAR BOOK are listed below.

Academic Emergency Medicine
Academic Radiology
Acta Paediatrica
Aesthetic Plastic Surgery
AJNR American Journal of Neuroradiology
AJR American Journal of Roentgenology
American Journal of Obstetrics and Gynecology
American Journal of Respiratory and Critical Care Medicine
Annals of Saudi Medicine
Annals of Surgical Oncology
Archives of Internal Medicine
British Journal of Radiology
Circulation
Circulation Cardiovascular Imaging
Clinical Orthopaedics and Related Research
Clinical Radiology
European Heart Journal
European Journal of Radiology
International Journal of Cancer
Journal of Cardiovascular Computed Tomography
Journal of Clinical Rheumatology
Journal of Computer Assisted Tomography
Journal of Pediatric Orthopedics
Journal of Pediatric Surgery
Journal of Pediatric Urology
Journal of Pediatrics
Journal of the American College of Cardiology
Journal of the American College of Radiology
Journal of Thoracic Imaging
Journal of Thoracic Oncology
Journal of Ultrasound in Medicine
Lancet
Musculoskeletal Surgery
New England Journal of Medicine
Pediatric Emergency Care
Pediatric Neurology
Pediatric Radiology
Pediatrics
Pediatrics & Neonatology
Radiographics
Radiology
Respiratory Medicine

Skeletal Radiology
Spine
Ultrasound in Obstetrics & Gynecology

STANDARD ABBREVIATIONS

The following terms are abbreviated in this edition: acquired immunodeficiency syndrome (AIDS), cardiopulmonary resuscitation (CPR), central nervous system (CNS), cerebrospinal fluid (CSF), computed tomography (CT), deoxyribonucleic acid (DNA), electrocardiography (ECG), health maintenance organization (HMO), human immunodeficiency virus (HIV), intensive care unit (ICU), intramuscular (IM), intravenous (IV), magnetic resonance (MR) imaging (MRI), ultrasound (US), and ribonucleic acid (RNA).

NOTE

The YEAR BOOK OF DIAGNOSTIC RADIOLOGY® is a literature survey service providing abstracts of articles published in the professional literature. Every effort is made to assure the accuracy of the information presented in these pages. Neither the editors nor the publisher of the YEAR BOOK OF DIAGNOSTIC RADIOLOGY® can be responsible for errors in the original materials. The editors' comments are their own opinions. Mention of specific products within this publication does not constitute endorsement.

To facilitate the use of the YEAR BOOK OF DIAGNOSTIC RADIOLOGY® as a reference tool, all illustrations and tables included in this publication are now identified as they appear in the original article. This change is meant to help the reader recognize that any illustration or table appearing in the YEAR BOOK OF DIAGNOSTIC RADIOLOGY® may be only one of many in the original article. For this reason, figure and table numbers will often appear to be out of sequence within the YEAR BOOK OF DIAGNOSTIC RADIOLOGY®.

Introduction

The year 2012 marks a time of historic transition for the YEAR BOOK OF DIAGNOSTIC RADIOLOGY. After 12 years of dedicated service, Dr Anne Osborn has decided to step down as Editor-in-Chief and I have been selected to assume her role.

I take this new position with all humility and respect, knowing that I indeed have the proverbial "big shoes" to fill. Anne, my mentor and friend, is truly an icon in the world of radiology—a brilliant and inspiring woman who has reshaped not only her own subspecialty of neuroradiology but the entire domain of radiology education. In her role as Editor-in-Chief, she has assembled a world-class team of Associate Editors who each year scour hundreds of imaging and clinical journals to identify the most significant papers advancing the field of Diagnostic Radiology.

This year's edition contains slightly fewer articles than in the past, but they are as interesting and informative as ever. I won't ruin the story by revealing the key highlights you will find in the following pages, but I can assure you that you will be surprised and delighted along how many dimensions our field has advanced during the last year. As many of the selected articles come from clinical (not radiologic) journals, understanding the perspectives of the role of imaging in various diseases held by our clinical colleagues is among the most valuable insights you may gain.

I sincerely appreciate your continued support and readership during this transition, and please give your thanks to Anne Osborn for bringing the YEAR BOOK OF DIAGNOSTIC RADIOLOGY to the high level of quality it now enjoys.

Allen D. Elster, MD, FACR

1   Thoracic Radiology

Introduction

It is my pleasure to present the final selection of thoracic imaging articles from the 2011 literature. This was indeed a landmark year for thoracic imaging. While the featured articles are mostly representative of the US diagnostic radiology literature, important articles from the oncology, pathology, and medical literature are also included.

I call the reader's attention to a few critical articles featured in this years' selections. The National Lung Screening Trial Research Team presented data supporting reduced lung cancer mortality with low-dose CT screening. The article by Travis and colleagues presents a new international multidisciplinary classification for lung adenocarcinoma and recommends discontinuation of the term "bronchioloalveolar carcinoma" (BAC). Thus, the tumor formerly known as BAC has undergone a major reclassification in which radiologists play a crucial role. The article by Leung and colleagues (sponsored by the American Thoracic Society and the Society of Thoracic Radiology) presents a new official clinical practice guideline that is likely to impact clinicians' ordering practices for the evaluation of suspected pulmonary thromboembolic disease in pregnant patients. The article by Tang and colleagues published in the *Archives of Internal Medicine* challenges the traditional management of radiographically detected pneumonia, suggesting that follow-up to complete radiographic resolution is not always necessary. Finally, the article by Raghu and colleagues provides international evidence-based guidelines for the diagnosis of idiopathic pulmonary fibrosis in which the radiologist plays a crucial role. While some of these articles represent major departures from traditional clinical practice, it remains to be seen how well they will be received by the medical community and to what extent they will impact practice patterns.

Additional important topics addressed by this year's selections include: the morphologic features of lung cancers detected at screening, FDA-approved software for improved detection of lung nodules on chest radiography, and techniques for reducing dose, improving diagnostic yield, and optimizing image quality on CT, among several others.

I hope that YEAR BOOK readers find this year's selections useful in addressing the challenges of the daily practice of thoracic imaging.

Melissa L. Rosado de Christenson, MD, FACR

Lung Cancer

International Association for the Study of Lung Cancer/American Thoracic Society/European Respiratory Society International Multidisciplinary Classification of Lung Adenocarcinoma

Travis WD, Brambilla E, Noguchi M, et al (Memorial Sloan-Kettering Cancer Ctr, NY)
J Thorac Oncol 6:244-285, 2011

Introduction.—Adenocarcinoma is the most common histologic type of lung cancer. To address advances in oncology, molecular biology, pathology, radiology, and surgery of lung adenocarcinoma, an international multidisciplinary classification was sponsored by the International Association for the Study of Lung Cancer, American Thoracic Society, and European Respiratory Society. This new adenocarcinoma classification is needed to provide uniform terminology and diagnostic criteria, especially for bronchioloalveolar carcinoma (BAC), the overall approach to small nonresection cancer specimens, and for multidisciplinary strategic management of tissue for molecular and immunohistochemical studies.

Methods.—An international core panel of experts representing all three societies was formed with oncologists/pulmonologists, pathologists, radiologists, molecular biologists, and thoracic surgeons. A systematic review was performed under the guidance of the American Thoracic Society Documents Development and Implementation Committee. The search strategy identified 11,368 citations of which 312 articles met specified eligibility criteria and were retrieved for full text review. A series of meetings were held to discuss the development of the new classification, to develop the recommendations, and to write the current document. Recommendations for key questions were graded by strength and quality of the evidence according to the Grades of Recommendation, Assessment, Development, and Evaluation approach.

Results.—The classification addresses both resection specimens, and small biopsies and cytology. The terms BAC and mixed subtype adenocarcinoma are no longer used. For resection specimens, new concepts are introduced such as adenocarcinoma in situ (AIS) and minimally invasive adenocarcinoma (MIA) for small solitary adenocarcinomas with either pure lepidic growth (AIS) or predominant lepidic growth with ≤5 mm invasion (MIA) to define patients who, if they undergo complete resection, will have 100% or near 100% disease-specific survival, respectively. AIS and MIA are usually nonmucinous but rarely may be mucinous. Invasive adenocarcinomas are classified by predominant pattern after using comprehensive histologic subtyping with lepidic (formerly most mixed subtype tumors with nonmucinous BAC), acinar, papillary, and solid patterns; micropapillary is added as a new histologic subtype. Variants include invasive mucinous adenocarcinoma (formerly mucinous BAC), colloid, fetal, and enteric adenocarcinoma. This classification provides guidance for small biopsies and cytology specimens, as approximately 70% of lung cancers are diagnosed in such samples. Non-small cell lung carcinomas (NSCLCs), in patients with advanced-stage disease, are to be classified into more specific types such as adenocarcinoma or squamous cell carcinoma, whenever possible for several reasons: (1) adenocarcinoma or NSCLC not otherwise specified should be tested for epidermal growth factor receptor (*EGFR*) mutations as the presence of these mutations is predictive of responsiveness to EGFR tyrosine kinase inhibitors, (2) adenocarcinoma histology is a strong predictor for improved outcome with pemetrexed therapy compared with squamous cell carcinoma, and (3) potential life-threatening hemorrhage may occur in patients with squamous cell carcinoma who receive bevacizumab. If the tumor cannot be classified based on light microscopy alone, special studies such as immunohistochemistry and/or mucin stains should be applied to classify the tumor further. Use of the term NSCLC not otherwise specified should be minimized.

Conclusions.—This new classification strategy is based on a multidisciplinary approach to diagnosis of lung adenocarcinoma that incorporates clinical, molecular, radiologic, and surgical issues, but it is primarily based on histology. This classification is intended to support clinical practice, and research investigation and clinical trials. As *EGFR* mutation is a validated predictive marker for response and progression-free survival with EGFR tyrosine kinase inhibitors in advanced lung adenocarcinoma, we recommend that patients with advanced adenocarcinomas be tested for *EGFR* mutation. This has implications for strategic management of tissue, particularly for small biopsies and cytology samples, to maximize high-quality tissue available for molecular studies. Potential impact for tumor, node, and metastasis staging include adjustment of the size T factor according to only the invasive component (1) pathologically in invasive tumors with lepidic areas or (2) radiologically by measuring the solid component of part-solid nodules.

▶ This article, sponsored by the International Association for the Study of Lung Cancer, the American Thoracic Society, and the European Respiratory Society, introduces a new classification for primary adenocarcinoma of the lung. The new classification outlines a multidisciplinary approach to the diagnosis of lung adenocarcinoma and aims to address advances in medical science with regard to the diagnosis and management of affected patients and to provide uniform terminology and diagnostic criteria for the various subtypes of adenocarcinoma, including those diagnosed via small biopsy specimens.

One of the most salient changes in the new classification is the recommendation to discontinue the use of the term "bronchioloalveolar carcinoma," a term that is embedded in the body of radiologic literature. The new classification divides adenocarcinomas into preinvasive lesions that include atypical adenomatous hyperplasia and adenocarcinoma in situ (AIS), minimally invasive adenocarcinoma, invasive adenocarcinoma, and variants of invasive adenocarcinoma. Some of these lesions are further classified as mucinous or nonmucinous. Atypical adenomatous hyperplasia (AAH) is defined as a proliferation of mildly to moderately atypical type II pneumocytes and/or Clara cells lining alveolar walls and at times respiratory bronchioles measuring less than 0.5 cm. AIS is defined as a small solitary adenocarcinoma measuring less than 3 cm with pure lepidic growth. The authors further state that patients with AIS should have nearly 100% disease-specific survival if the lesion is completely resected.

Minimally invasive adenocarcinoma is defined as a solitary adenocarcinoma with a predominantly lepidic pattern of growth and less than 5 mm of invasion in any 1 focus. Invasive adenocarcinomas and their variants constitute more than 70% of resected adenocarcinomas and should be subject to histologic subtyping with the pathologist describing the various histologic patterns within the tumor, identifying the predominant pattern, and estimating the percentage of the different subtypes. The authors also recommend that biopsy samples previously characterized as non–small cell lung cancer be further classified into more specific cell types whenever possible and that the term "non–small cell lung cancer—not otherwise specified" be used as little as possible.

Because the new classification embraces a multidisciplinary approach to adenocarcinoma, sections of the article address issues relevant to the clinical, molecular, radiologic, and surgical diagnosis and management of patients with such lesions. Of particular interest is the radiology section of the article, which includes the following:

- Definitions of the terminology used to describe lung cancers (including solid and subsolid lung nodules)
- CT appearances of the new categories of atypical adenomatous hyperplasia, adenocarcinoma in situ, and minimally invasive adenocarcinoma
- Description of imaging appearances of invasive adenocarcinoma
- Imaging features of invasive behavior, including lesion spiculation, pleural retraction, and lobular contours
- Guidelines for measuring subsolid nodules with separate measurements for solid and nonsolid components of the lesions

The new classification discourages the use of the term "bronchioloalveolar carcinoma" by radiologists and describes pulmonary lesions formerly designated by that term. In addition, radiology considerations for good practice are provided including the following:

- Obtaining tissue (during image-guided biopsies) not just for diagnosis but for immunohistochemical and molecular analysis
- Using thin-section CT to record lesion size and analyze subsolid lesions
- Describing changes in size, shape, and attenuation in lesions to determine their malignant potential
- Recommendations for areas of future research

The new classification of adenocarcinoma is complex and requires a multidisciplinary approach to the diagnosis and management of affected patients. It remains to be seen whether the classification is reproducible and to what extent it is accepted and followed by the medical community outside academic centers. In addition, prospective studies correlating the various morphologic features of adenocarcinoma with patient outcomes and survival will have to be performed to validate the new classification.

M. L. Rosado de Christenson, MD

Reduced Lung-Cancer Mortality with Low-Dose Computed Tomographic Screening
The National Lung Screening Trial Research Team (Univ of California at Los Angeles; Brown Univ, Providence, RI; Natl Cancer Inst, Bethesda, MD; et al)
N Engl J Med 365:395-409, 2011

Background.—The aggressive and heterogeneous nature of lung cancer has thwarted efforts to reduce mortality from this cancer through the use of screening. The advent of low-dose helical computed tomography (CT) altered the landscape of lung-cancer screening, with studies indicating that low-dose CT detects many tumors at early stages. The National Lung Screening Trial (NLST) was conducted to determine whether screening with low-dose CT could reduce mortality from lung cancer.

Methods.—From August 2002 through April 2004, we enrolled 53,454 persons at high risk for lung cancer at 33 U.S. medical centers. Participants were randomly assigned to undergo three annual screenings with either low-dose CT (26,722 participants) or single-view posteroanterior chest radiography (26,732). Data were collected on cases of lung cancer and deaths from lung cancer that occurred through December 31, 2009.

Results.—The rate of adherence to screening was more than 90%. The rate of positive screening tests was 24.2% with low-dose CT and 6.9% with radiography over all three rounds. A total of 96.4% of the positive screening results in the low-dose CT group and 94.5% in the radiography group were false positive results. The incidence of lung cancer was 645 cases per 100,000 person-years (1060 cancers) in the low-dose CT group, as compared with 572 cases per 100,000 person-years (941 cancers) in the radiography group (rate ratio, 1.13; 95% confidence interval [CI], 1.03 to 1.23). There were 247 deaths from lung cancer per 100,000 person-years in the low-dose CT group and 309 deaths per 100,000 person-years in the radiography group, representing a relative reduction in mortality from lung cancer with low-dose CT screening of 20.0% (95% CI, 6.8 to 26.7; $P = 0.004$). The rate of death from any cause was reduced in the low-dose CT group, as compared with the radiography group, by 6.7% (95% CI, 1.2 to 13.6; $P = 0.02$).

Conclusions.—Screening with the use of low-dose CT reduces mortality from lung cancer. (Funded by the National Cancer Institute; National Lung Screening Trial ClinicalTrials.gov number, NCT00047385.)

▶ The National Lung Screening Trial (NLST) is a randomized trial that investigated lung cancer screening with low-dose chest computed tomography (CT) compared with the use of chest radiography. This was a collaborative effort of the Lung Screening Study administered by the National Cancer Institute (NCI) Division of Cancer Prevention and the American College of Radiology Imaging

Network sponsored by the NCI Division of Cancer Treatment and Diagnosis, Cancer Imaging Program. There were 33 participating medical institutions, and participants were enrolled from August 2002 through September 2007. Participants eligible for the study were between 55 and 74 years of age with a history of smoking at least 30 pack-years and, if former smokers, had a history of smoking cessation within the 15 years prior to enrollment. A total of 53 454 persons were enrolled with 26 722 randomly assigned to the low-dose CT group and 26 732 to the radiography group. Participants underwent 3 screenings at 1-year intervals. All low-dose CT scans were acquired with a variety of multidetector CT scanners with a minimum of 4 channels. Exposure parameters were selected to deliver an average effective dose of 1.5 mSv (as opposed to the approximately 8 mSv delivered by diagnostic chest CT). Positive results in the low-dose CT group were any noncalcified nodule measuring at least 4 mm in any dimension. Additional abnormalities classified as positive results included lymphadenopathy and pleural effusion. If abnormalities suspicious for lung cancer were stable across the 3 rounds of imaging, they were reclassified as minor abnormalities rather than as positive results.

On October 20, 2010, the independent Data and Safety Monitoring Board charged with reviewing the study data determined that a definitive result had been reached for the primary endpoint of the trial and recommended that the results be reported.

The NLST found a 20.0% decrease in mortality rate from lung cancer in the low-dose CT arm of the study compared with that of the radiography arm. They also found that the false-positive results in the low-dose CT arm of the study were higher than those in the radiography arm by a factor of more than 3. However, the authors add that the majority of such results were nodules determined to represent minor findings on follow-up studies. Complications or death from invasive procedures were uncommon according to the authors. The authors also observed a high rate of adherence to the screening protocol by the population enrolled.

The authors report a series of limitations including the "healthy volunteer" effect that may characterize some of the patients enrolled and the fact that current CT technology is more advanced than that used during the trial and could potentially decrease mortality even more or result in higher false-positive rates. The trial was conducted at institutions with immense expertise in the diagnosis and management of lung cancer, and the results, particularly the low rate of complications, might not translate to screening performed in the community. Low-dose chest CT was only compared with radiography and not to community care.

Potentially harmful effects of screening, such as overdiagnosis, cannot be determined at this time. In addition, ionizing radiation from screening could in turn result in the development of malignancy.

M. L. Rosado de Christenson, MD

Screen-detected Lung Cancer: A Retrospective Analysis of CT Appearance

Dhopeshwarkar MR, Roberts HC, Paul NS, et al (Univ Health Network, Toronto, Ontario, Canada)

Acad Radiol 18:1270-1276, 2011

Rationale and Objectives.—The aim of this study was to retrospectively evaluate characteristics of lung cancers diagnosed in a low-dose computed tomographic lung cancer screening study.

Materials and Methods.—As part of the International Early Lung Cancer Action Program, a cohort of 4782 at-risk participants were screened. A total of 86 cancers in 84 individuals were detected and evaluated for location, morphology (density, border), size, histology, stage at diagnosis, treatment, and survival. Follow-up imaging for computation of growth rates was available in 41 cases.

Results.—Eighty-six cancers were detected in 84 individuals (60 women, 24 men). Of these, seven (8%) were incidence cancers. Most cancers were radiologically described as solid ($n = 52$ [61%]). The median tumor size was 18×13 mm (range, 6−56 mm). Histopathologic diagnoses revealed 10 (11.6%) bronchoalveolar carcinomas, 55 (64%) adenocarcinomas, 11 (12.8%) squamous-cell carcinomas, two (2.3%) large-cell carcinomas, three (3.5%) carcinoids, and five (5.8%) small-cell lung cancers. Of the 41 cases with follow-up computed tomographic scans, 36 nodules had increased in size. The mean doubling time for all cancers was 259 days (median, 154 days). In women ($n = 25$), the mean doubling time was 313 days (median, 156 days), while in men ($n = 11$), the mean doubling time was 137 days (median, 92 days). Overall, 55 lung cancers (68%) were stage I. Most cancers ($n = 62$ [73%]) were surgically resected.

Conclusions. In this cohort, screening detected lung cancer in early treatable stages, and women had more slow-growing adenocarcinomas than men. Most screen-detected lung cancers were surgically resectable.

▶ This retrospective study analyzed the morphologic and biologic characteristics of a large number of screen-detected lung cancers found as part of the multicenter International Early Lung Cancer Action Program (I-ELCAP). Inclusion criteria are described as age of 50 years or more, smoking history of 10 pack-years or more, and general good health. The enrolled population included 4782 individuals who met the inclusion criteria and were screened with low-dose multidetector chest computed tomography (CT). The authors found a total of 86 lung cancers in 84 individuals with an overall lung cancer detection rate of 1.79%. There were 2 non−small cell cancers not further specified and 3 atypical carcinoids. The remaining 81 non−small cell lung cancers included 10 "bronchioloalveolar carcinomas" (although the use of this term is no longer recommended, the authors do not provide a more current classification of these neoplasms), 53 adenocarcinomas, 11 squamous-cell carcinomas, and 2 large-cell carcinomas. There were also 5 small cell carcinomas.

The authors report that most lung cancers were found on the first round of screening and were therefore characterized as prevalence cancers, and only

0.20% were found on subsequent screening rounds and were therefore characterized as incidence cancers. Sixty-three percent of cancers occurred in the upper lobes. Thirty-nine percent of nodules were characterized as subsolid with 23% of the total nodules being part solid. However, most cancers (63%) were of solid attenuation on CT. Forty percent of the lesions had smooth and spiculated margins, respectively.

The authors remark that the majority of the cancers were peripheral and that most were diagnosed in women. It is unknown how many of these screen-detected lung cancers represented overdiagnosis (that is, diagnosis of a lung cancer that may never become lethal even if untreated).

This article gives us an idea of the morphologic and histologic features of cancers diagnosed with lung cancer screening and may be useful to radiologists who are entering into the lung cancer screening field.

M. L. Rosado de Christenson, MD

Nodules

Lung Nodules: Improved Detection with Software That Suppresses the Rib and Clavicle on Chest Radiographs

Freedman MT, Lo S-CB, Seibel JC, et al (Georgetown Univ Med Ctr, Washington, DC; Georgetown Univ, Washington, DC; BioStat Solutions, Mt Airy, MD)
Radiology 260:265-273, 2011

Purpose.—To demonstrate possible superiority in the performance of a radiologist who is tasked with detecting actionable nodules and aided by the bone suppression and soft-tissue visualization algorithm of a new software program that produces a modified image by suppressing the ribs and clavicles, filtering noise, and equalizing the contrast in the area of the lungs.

Materials and Methods.—The study and use of anonymized and deidentified data received approval from the MedStar—Georgetown University Oncology Institutional Review Board. Informed consent was obtained from 15 study radiologists. The study radiologists participated as observers in a reader study of 368 patients in an approximately 2:1 cancer-free—to-cancer ratio. The localized receiver operating characteristic (LROC) method was used for analyses. Images were rerandomized for each radiologist. Each patient image was sequentially read, first with the standard radiograph and then with the software-aided image. Normal studies were confirmed with computed tomography (CT), follow-up, and/or panel consensus.

Results.—Each reader and the combined scores of the 15 readers showed improvement. The area under the combined LROC curve increased significantly from 0.460 unaided to 0.558 aided by visualization software ($P =.0001$). When measured according to the reader's indication that a case should be sent or not sent for CT or biopsy, sensitivity for cancer detection increased from 49.5% unaided to 66.3% aided by software ($P < .0001$); specificity decreased from 96.1% to 91.8% ($P =.004$).

Seventy-four percent of the aided detections occurred in cancers with 70% or greater overlap of the bone and the nodule.

Conclusion.—The radiologists using visualization software significantly increased their detection of lung cancers and benign nodules.

▶ The earliest imaging manifestation of primary lung cancer may be a pulmonary nodule. Such nodules may exhibit great variability in border characteristics on radiography. The authors state that overlying skeletal structures are a common cause of missed lung cancer. They cite studies of missed lung cancer that report that osseous structures obscured the lesions in anywhere from 22% to 95% of cases.

New software is now available that allows suppression of ribs and clavicles while at the same time filtering noise and equalizing contrast in the lungs (Fig 3 in the original article). This is designed to help radiologists identify lung nodules that may be an early manifestation of lung cancer. The authors state that the software works as an add-on to the picture-archiving and communication system by processing digital images (including digitized films) so they can be evaluated at the time the clinical image is being evaluated. The images produced are similar to those achieved with dual-energy subtraction equipment. The authors set out to determine whether this technology helped radiologists identify actionable pulmonary nodules.

The authors selected 351 patients as the sample size that with a 2:1 ratio of nodule absent to nodule present would provide 80% power to detect a difference in areas under the curve of 0.10 or greater. This retrospective study included chest radiographic images from 368 patients and consisted of 266 digitized screen film images, 66 computed radiography images, and 19 digital radiographic images. There were 122 patients with nodules documented to represent primary lung cancer and 246 patients with documentation of absence of cancer in the chest.

There were 15 participating radiologists who were tasked with reviewing the original images and marking actionable nodules. Subsequently, the radiologists reviewed the software-enhanced image presented on a second monitor and the radiologist again marked any actionable nodules. Radiologists were also asked to record their confidence levels and any decisions to recommend further imaging on the basis of each of the images reviewed. The radiologists recorded a combined interpretation based on both images.

The authors found that radiologist sensitivity increased by approximately 34% above their performance on the conventional images. In addition, specificity decreased by 4.3% because of additional false-positive findings on the software-enhanced images. In 2% of cases, correct location marks were removed on the software-enhanced images, and either a different location was not selected or an incorrect location was selected.

The authors acknowledge the following limitations to the study:

- The testing environment did not mimic the interruptions and distractors that exist in clinical practice.

- A very large proportion of the images were acquired with film-screen systems, which is not representative of today's practice.

The authors point out the relatively low cost of the software and the fact that it works with any picture-archiving and communication system so that a single unit can serve multiple chest radiograph acquisition units. They conclude that addition of this software "should be of important clinical utility."

M. L. Rosado de Christenson, MD

A Comparison of Follow-Up Recommendations by Chest Radiologists, General Radiologists, and Pulmonologists Using Computer-Aided Detection to Assess Radiographs for Actionable Pulmonary Nodules

Meziane M, Obuchowski NA, Lababede O, et al (Cleveland Clinic Foundation, OH)

AJR Am J Roentgenol 196:W542-W549, 2011

Objective.—The primary objective of our study was to compare the effect of a chest radiography computer-aided detection (CAD) system on the follow-up recommendations of chest radiologists, general radiologists, and pulmonologists.

Materials and Methods.—A chest radiography CAD system (Rapid-Screen 1.1) that has been approved by the U.S. Food and Drug Administration (FDA) and a second-generation version of the system (OnGuard 3.0) not yet approved by the FDA were applied to single frontal radiographs of 200 patients at high risk for lung cancer. One hundred patients had actionable nodules (mean size, 16.9 mm) and 100 patients did not. Six chest radiologists, six general radiologists, and six pulmonologists independently interpreted each image first without CAD and then with CAD during blinded reading sessions. The frequency with which readers correctly referred patients for follow-up tests was measured. Differential effects based on nodule size, shape, location, density, and subtlety were tested with multiple-variable logistic regression.

Results.—For patients without actionable lesions, pulmonologists showed an increase in their recommendations for follow-up from 0.46 unaided to 0.52 with CAD ($p = 0.001$), whereas chest and general radiologists had much lower average rates and were not affected by CAD's false marks (0.26 without CAD vs 0.25 with RapidScreen 1.1 and 0.26 with OnGuard 3.0, $p \geq 0.734$). CAD improved all readers' detection of moderately subtle lesions ($p = 0.013$) but did not significantly increase follow-up rates overall for patients with actionable nodules (0.63 unaided vs 0.63 with RapidScreen 1.1, $p = 0.795$; and 0.63 unaided vs 0.64 with OnGuard 3.0, $p = 0.187$).

Conclusion.—The effect of CAD on readers' clinical decisions varies depending on the training of the reader. CAD did not improve the performance of chest or general radiologists. Nonradiologists are particularly vulnerable to CAD's false-positive marks (Fig 3).

▶ Detection of early-stage lung cancer on chest radiography is one of the most challenging tasks in thoracic imaging. Computer-aided detection (CAD) of suspicious lesions is commonly used in mammography. Food and Drug

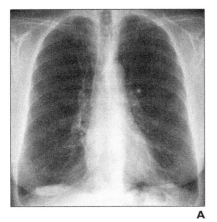 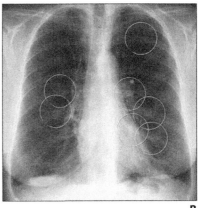

A   **B**

FIGURE 3.—68-year-old woman with pulmonary emphysema. **A,** Posteroanterior chest radiograph shows multiple focal areas of fibrosis (i.e., no actionable nodule). **B,** When radiograph is processed with RapidScreen 1.1 (Riverain Medical), multiple areas of focal fibrosis (*circles*) are identified as regions of interest. (Reprinted from Meziane M, Obuchowski NA, Lababede O, et al. A comparison of follow-up recommendations by chest radiologists, general radiologists, and pulmonologists using computer-aided detection to assess radiographs for actionable pulmonary nodules. *AJR Am J Roentgenol.* 2011;196:W542-W549, with permission from the American Journal of Roentgenology.)

Administration—approved CAD systems are also available for chest radiography. The authors report that several studies have shown that CAD may improve diagnostic accuracy for readers, particularly those who are less experienced. The authors state that these studies did not assess the performance of pulmonary medicine specialists who (depending on the practice) may perform and interpret chest radiographs in their patients.

The authors designed a retrospective study to assess the affect of CAD on 3 groups of readers, which included thoracic radiologists, general radiologists, and pulmonary medicine specialists. They evaluated 2 CAD systems and measured the resultant change in readers' clinical decisions based on the use of CAD and attempted to identify the characteristics of the lesions that CAD helped detect.

The patient population was selected by collecting CT images and pathology results of patients aged 45 years or older who were undergoing surgery or biopsy and had also undergone chest radiography between August 2003 and April 2007. An expert reader selected the radiographs that had actionable malignant nodules and was blinded to the CAD marks. Images from several vendors were included but most were performed on Siemens Healthcare (n = 125) or Canon (n = 68) equipment.

The readers (6 thoracic radiologists, 6 general radiologists, and 6 pulmonologists) were asked to review the images and score them before and after CAD. Readers were asked to determine lesion size and location. Lesions had to be scored on a 10-point confidence scale (10 = a definite nodule) and on a 10-point scale to determine whether the nodule was actionable (10 = definitely actionable). After CAD, the readers were asked to record lesion size and location, score for confidence level and actionable nodule, and indicate whether further follow-up was indicated. All readers reviewed the 200 images, but the images were randomized to 1 or the other CAD system.

The authors found the following:

- Thoracic and general radiologists recommended unnecessary follow-up in approximately one-quarter of cases, but pulmonologists recommended about twice as many unnecessary follow-up studies.
- Pulmonologists were negatively affected by CAD with a significant increase in follow-up rates. The authors explain that this may relate to a high rate of additional abnormalities in the study sample (Fig 3).
- Radiologists did not have difficulty dismissing false-negative marks and maintaining an unaided follow-up rate.
- Thoracic and general radiologists had similar follow-up rates for patients with lung cancer with no significant improvement on CAD. Approximately 10% of cancers missed by thoracic imagers were detected by CAD, and approximately 14% of cancers missed by general radiologists were detected by CAD.
- Reader performance was not improved by CAD, unlike in other published studies. This may have related to the study design in which chest radiographs with and without CAD were scored separately, with readers having no access to their pre-CAD markings.
- CAD did not improve performance in detecting inconspicuous lesions nor did it affect high performance in detecting conspicuous lesions. CAD did improve all performances in detection of moderately subtle lesions, especially for thoracic radiologists.
- Pulmonary medicine specialists had more difficulty ignoring false-positive findings highlighted by CAD than did radiologists.

Limitations include the following:

- The study did not use a consecutive patient sample because it was designed to see how nodule characteristics affected CAD readings and to compare the effects of CAD readings among specialties.
- Two versions of CAD were used, one with a significantly higher sensitivity and lower false-positive rate.
- Selection bias was introduced because only patients with CT or pathology confirmation were included.
- Readers' recommendations were the primary endpoint.
- Only malignant nodules were included.
- One chest radiologist selected all the cases for the study.

The authors conclude that there is potential for increase in inappropriate follow-up testing using CAD for nonradiologist clinicians. There was no improvement in lung cancer detection for general and chest radiologists. The authors recommend that CAD not be universally adopted until it reaches a high level of accuracy with a minimum number of false positives.

M. L. Rosado de Christenson, MD

Malignant Neoplasia

CT Features of Peripheral Pulmonary Carcinoid Tumors

Meisinger QC, Klein JS, Butnor KJ, et al (Univ of Vermont College of Medicine, Burlington)
AJR Am J Roentgenol 197:1073-1080, 2011

Objective.—Pulmonary carcinoid tumors are low-grade malignant neoplasms thought to arise primarily within the central airways in 85% of cases. The CT features of pulmonary carcinoid tumors that arise as solitary pulmonary nodules (SPNs) have not been well elucidated. We reviewed our experience with primary pulmonary carcinoid tumors to determine the distribution of lesions within the lung at diagnosis and to identify CT features that might aid in distinguishing these neoplasms from benign pulmonary nodules.

Materials and Methods.—CT scans, if available, of all patients with a primary pulmonary carcinoid tumor diagnosed by biopsy or surgical resection over the previous 15 years were reviewed. The CT scans were reviewed for the following features: lesion location; order of bronchus involved; lesion size, contour, and density; contrast enhancement; and the presence of peripheral atelectasis, hyperlucency, and bronchiectasis. We defined central lesions as those involved with a segmental or larger bronchus. Subsegmental bronchial involvement and tumors surrounded by lung parenchyma without direct airway involvement were defined as peripheral lesions. The final pathologic diagnosis for all cases was confirmed by review of cytologic or histologic specimens.

Results.—Twenty-eight carcinoid tumors were identified in 28 patients: 24 typical carcinoids and four atypical carcinoids. The study group was composed of 23 females and five males with a mean age of 52.4 years (range, 14–83 years). Twelve of the 28 lesions (43%) were central (i.e., involved a segmental or larger bronchus), and the remaining 16 lesions (57%) were peripheral. The mean tumor diameter for the 16 peripheral tumors was 14 mm (range, 9–28 mm); the majority (14/16, 88%) had a lobulated contour. Of six peripheral lesions with unenhanced and contrast-enhanced CT nodule enhancement studies, the mean maximal enhancement was 55.2 HU (range, 34–73 HU). Thirteen of the 16 peripheral carcinoid tumors (81%) involved a subsegmental bronchus, with 10 (63%) showing peripheral hyperlucency, bronchiectasis, or atelectasis.

Conclusion.—In our series, primary pulmonary carcinoid tumors presenting as peripheral SPNs were more common than central endobronchial lesions in contrast to the published literature. The CT features of peripheral carcinoid tumors presenting as SPNs that suggest the diagnosis include lobulated nodules of high attenuation on contrast-enhanced CT; nodules that densely enhance with contrast administration; the presence of calcification; subsegmental airway involvement on thin-section analysis; and

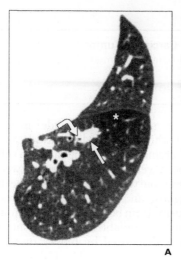
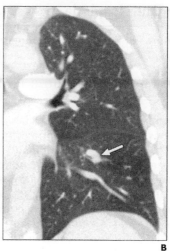

A B

FIGURE 3.—53-year-old man with subsegmental bronchus carcinoid tumor and peripheral hyperlucency. **A,** Axial CT scan obtained at lung windows shows lobulated nodule (*straight arrow*) is obstructing subsegmental branch of anteromedial basal segmental bronchus (*curved arrow*). Hyperlucency (*asterisk*) is seen peripheral to lesion. **B,** Coronal CT reconstruction at lung windows shows tumor (*arrow*) with peripheral subsegmental hyperlucency. Lobectomy showed 14 × 8 × 8 mm typical carcinoid tumor. (Reprinted from Meisinger QC, Klein JS, Butnor KJ, et al. CT features of peripheral pulmonary carcinoid tumors. *AJR Am J Roentgenol.* 2011;197:1073-1080, with permission from the American Journal of Roentgenology.)

nodules associated with distal hyperlucency, bronchiectasis, or atelectasis (Fig 3).

▶ The authors performed a retrospective review of carcinoid tumors diagnosed in their institution from 1996 to April 2010. Although they describe these lesions as the second most common primary malignant pulmonary neoplasms in adults, they constitute only 1.57 cases per 100 000 patients in the United States. Carcinoid tumors are categorized as typical or atypical based on histologic findings.

Twenty-eight cases met the inclusion criteria for the study based on availability of CT imaging studies and pathologic diagnosis of carcinoid tumor. As expected from prior studies, the majority of lesions (86%) were typical carcinoid tumors. The authors defined the tumors as peripheral when they arose from a subsegmental or more distal bronchial branch or when there was no discernable bronchial connection. Based on this definition, the majority of the lesions in the study (57%) were peripheral. In addition, the majority of peripheral carcinoids (82%) were incidentally discovered pulmonary nodules ranging in size from 9 to 28 mm. Most lesions (85%) had lobular contours and 11% demonstrated calcification. Eighty-nine percent exhibited airway involvement, with significant postobstructive effects including bronchiectasis, distal hyperlucency (Fig 3), and distal opacity or atelectasis. Seventy-nine percent exhibited lobular margins, and most lesions imaged with contrast exhibited high attenuation. Because many lesions manifested as peripheral lung nodules, many patients underwent transthoracic needle biopsy, which the authors found valuable for preoperative diagnosis. As some of the lesions were prospectively suspected to represent carcinoid tumors, many underwent octreotide imaging, which was positive in 42% of 12 lesions.

M. L. Rosado de Christenson, MD

Computed Tomography Findings Predicting Invasiveness of Thymoma
Marom EM, Milito MA, Moran CA, et al (The Univ of Texas MD Anderson Cancer Ctr, Houston)
J Thorac Oncol 6:1274-1281, 2011

Purpose.—To identify preoperative computed tomography (CT) findings associated with thymoma invasiveness before surgical resection and with clinical outcome.

Methods.—We retrospectively reviewed CT scans of 99 patients with thymoma surgically treated at our institution between September 1999 and April 2010. Chest CT findings documented were size, volume, and heterogeneity of primary tumor; abutment of mediastinal vessels; and presence of calcifications, lobulation, infiltration of fat surrounding tumor, adjacent pulmonary changes, adenopathy, and pleural nodularity.

Results.—Our study group consisted of 53 (54%) men and 46 (46%) women, age 18–79 years (mean: 53.2 years). Masaoka pathologic stages were stage I for 10 (10%), stage II for 48 (48%), stage III for 21 (21%), and stage IV for 20 (20%). The median radiologic tumor size was 7 cm (range: 2.5–21 cm). A multivariable logistic regression model showed that primary tumors with prechemotherapy radiologic tumor size ≥ 7 cm (odds ratio [OR]: 3.18, 95% confidence interval [CI]: 1.16–8.67, $p = 0.02$), a lobulated tumor contour (OR: 8.20, 95% CI: 1.63– 41.35, $p = 0.01$), and infiltration of surrounding fat (OR: 3.76, 95% CI: 1.45–9.78, $p = 0.007$) were more likely to have stage III or IV disease. Cox's proportional hazard model showed that the presence of pulmonary nodules on staging CT was the only imaging parameter associated with shorter progression-free survival (hazard ratio: 4.93, 95% CI: 1.60 –15.17, $p = 0.005$) and overall survival ($p = 0.03$).

Conclusion.—The primary tumor CT imaging features can differentiate between stage I/II and stage III/IV disease and, thus, help identify patients more likely to benefit from neoadjuvant therapy (Fig 3).

▶ The authors performed a retrospective review of imaging findings of thymoma for patients diagnosed at their institution between September 1, 1999, and April 5, 2010, with the purpose of identifying CT features associated with invasive behavior. The authors state that patients with locally invasive thymoma at the time of presentation may benefit from neoadjuvant chemotherapy to enable successful resection given that complete resection, even in patients with advanced disease, is associated with improved survival. The study population

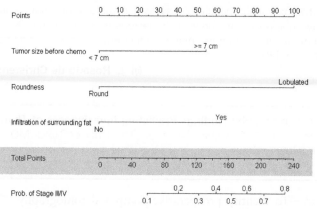

FIGURE 3.—Nomogram to predict stage III/IV thymoma using computed tomography (CT) findings at presentation. The nomogram consists of six rows. Row 1 (points row) is the point assignment for each variable. Rows 2 to 4 correspond to the variables included in the model. For an individual patient, each variable in rows 2 to 4 is assigned a point value, which is determined by drawing a vertical line from the appropriate position on the variable row to the points row. The assigned points for all three variables are added, and the total is marked on row 5 (shaded row called: total points). Then, the probability of having stage III/IV disease is calculated by drawing a vertical line from the appropriate position on the total points row to the row 6, which shows the probability of stage III or IV disease. Thus, for a patient with a lobular, larger than 7 cm tumor, which infiltrates the surrounding fat, the points added would be 100, 55, and 63 points, respectively, which adds to 218 total points or a 75% probability of having stage III/IV disease. The concordance index of this nomogram is 0.804. After internal validation using 200 bootstrap samples, the bias-corrected concordance index was 0.795 with an optimism of 0.009. Using this point system, total points ≥164 predict a ≥50% probability of having stage III/IV disease. (Reprinted from Marom EM, Milito MA, Moran CA, et al. Computed tomography findings predicting invasiveness of thymoma. *J Thorac Oncol.* 2011;6:1274-1281, with permission from the International Association for the Study of Lung Cancer.)

included 99 patients who were treated surgically for thymoma and had preoperative CT imaging studies available for review.

The authors describe the Masaoka staging system for thymoma as follows:

Stage I—Completely encapsulated thymoma

Stage IIa—Microscopic invasion of the tumor capsule

Stage IIb—Macroscopic invasion of adjacent fat or mediastinal pleura

Stage III—Macroscopic invasion of a neighboring organ

Stage IVa—Pleural or pericardial dissemination

Stage IVb—Lymphatic or hematogenous metastatic disease

They also reviewed the cases to identify imaging features consistent with stage III or stage IV thymoma. They concluded that larger tumor size, lobulated tumor contour, and infiltration of the adjacent mediastinal fat are findings that suggest a high probability of Masaoka stage III or IV disease. In patients with normal-appearing pleura, tumor heterogeneity and infiltration of the adjacent mediastinal fat were most associated with Masaoka stage III disease. Based on their findings, the authors constructed a nomogram for predicting stage III or stage IV thymoma based on CT features (Fig 3). The nomogram uses tumor size, tumor roundness versus lobulation, and presence of infiltration of surrounding fat to assign points to a lesion, which when added together may yield a percentage probability of the tumor being stage III or IV. The authors acknowledge the limitations of their study, including its retrospective design and small sample size, but hope that their findings may be validated by larger studies.

M. L. Rosado de Christenson, MD

Radiography

Incidence, Correlates, and Chest Radiographic Yield of New Lung Cancer Diagnosis in 3398 Patients With Pneumonia

Tang KL, Eurich DT, Minhas-Sandhu JK, et al (Univ of Alberta, Edmonton, Canada; et al)
Arch Intern Med 171:1193-1198, 2011

Background.—One reason chest radiographs are recommended after pneumonia is to exclude underlying lung cancer. Our aims were to determine the incidence and correlates of new lung cancer and the diagnostic yield of new lung cancer by chest radiography in patients with pneumonia.

Methods.—We conducted a population-based cohort study of patients with chest radiography—confirmed pneumonia, who were discharged alive from hospitals and emergency departments in Edmonton, Alberta, Canada. Patients were enrolled from 2000 through 2002 and followed up for 5 years. We determined incidence of new lung cancer and receipt of chest radiographs within 90 days, 1 year, and 5 years. Multivariable proportional hazards analyses were used to determine independent correlates of lung cancer.

Results.—There were 3398 patients; 59% were 50 years or older, 52% were male, and 17% were smokers. Half (49%) were admitted to hospital. At 90 days, 36 patients (1.1%) had new lung cancer; at 1 year, 57 patients (1.7%); and over 5 years, 79 patients (2.3%). The median time to diagnosis was 109 days (interquartile range, 27-423 days). Characteristics independently associated with lung cancer included age 50 years or older (adjusted hazard ratio [aHR], 19.0; 95% confidence interval [CI], 5.7-63.6), male sex (aHR, 1.8; 95% CI, 1.1-2.9), and smoking (aHR, 1.7; 95% CI, 1.0-3.0). Of the patients, 1354 (40%) had follow-up chest radiographs within 90 days, and the diagnostic yield of lung cancer was 2.5%; if radiographs were restricted to patients 50 years or older, the yield would have been 2.8%.

Conclusions.—The incidence of new lung cancer after pneumonia is low: approximately 1% within 90 days and 2% over 5 years. Routine chest radiographs after pneumonia for detecting lung cancer are not warranted, although our study suggests that patients 50 years or older should be targeted for radiographic follow-up.

▶ The authors state that community-acquired pneumonia is common with an approximate annual incidence of 12 cases per 1000 persons. Management of radiographically evident community-acquired pneumonia has traditionally called for follow-up chest radiography 6 weeks (4—8 weeks) following treatment to document resolution and exclude underlying malignancy. The authors point out that the most recent Infectious Disease Society of America—American Thoracic Society consensus guidelines are "(for the first time) silent on the topic." The authors cite a recent study by Mortensen et al that showed a 9.2% incidence of new lung cancer after pneumonia over 5 years of follow-up but that all other previous studies have indicated a much lower incidence of approximately 3% or less.

This Canadian study was performed to determine the short- and longer-term incidence of new lung cancer after treatment for pneumonia, clarify the independent correlates associated with new lung cancer diagnosis, and determine the diagnostic yield of routine chest radiography within 90 days of pneumonia.

To this end, 6874 patients with pneumonia evaluated in all 7 emergency departments and 6 hospitals in Edmonton, Alberta, Canada were enrolled in a population-based clinical registry and followed for up to 5 years. The authors state that the area serves a population of more than 1 million people with universal health care coverage who are cared for by more than 1000 family physicians with an annual health care budget of almost $2 billion. The current study identified 4261 potentially eligible adults with signs and symptoms of pneumonia and chest radiography confirming the diagnosis. Patients with tuberculosis, cystic fibrosis, immunocompromise, or pregnancy were not included. Patients who died in the hospital, those with documented cancer, and those who could not be linked to provincial databases for follow-up were also excluded. Because patients with cancer were excluded, all new lung cancers diagnosed were considered incident. Cumulative incidence of new lung cancer at 90 days, 1 year, and the entire duration of follow-up was determined. Patients were stratified into several age groups (< 40, 40—49, 50—59, 60—69, 70—79, or > 80 years). The final study cohort included 3398 patients.

The incidence of new lung cancers at 90 days, 1 year, and 5 years were 1.1%, 1.7%, and 2.3%, respectively. Interestingly, no lung cancers were identified in patients aged under 40 years; only 3 patients younger than 50 years were diagnosed with a new lung cancer, and the incidence only rose in patients aged 50 to 60 years. The authors note that only 40% of patients had follow-up chest radiographs (despite recommendations for follow-up) and that the 90-day incidence of a new lung cancer was 2.5% in this subgroup.

The authors state that their study would suggest that restricting routine follow-up chest radiography to patients 50 years of age or older could triple current rates of lung cancer diagnosis within 90 days and miss only 1 of 57 lung cancers detected within a year. The authors estimate a cost of $1250 per lung cancer detected and state that this may seem inexpensive. However, they add that the 96% 1-year case fatality rate in the study suggests that the performance of routine radiography of asymptomatic patients does not reduce all cause or lung cancer—specific mortality. They state that whether this is a worthwhile expenditure should be debated.

Study limitations include the following:

- Histopathologic confirmation of lung cancer was not required.
- Patients diagnosed as having lung cancer after 90 days may have received an earlier diagnosis had a routine follow-up radiograph been performed.

- The baseline chest radiographs were not re-reviewed looking for underlying lung cancer.
- Although some patients received a follow-up chest radiograph, the exact reason for the radiograph was not determined.

The authors conclude that routine follow-up chest radiographs for patients with pneumonia are not warranted. They suggest restricting the use of such imaging for patients 50 years or older, particularly male smokers.

M. L. Rosado de Christenson, MD

Are Chest Radiographs Routinely Indicated After Chest Tube Removal Following Cardiac Surgery?
Eisenberg RL, Khabbaz KR (Beth Israel Deaconess Med Ctr, Boston, MA)
AJR Am J Roentgenol 197:122-124, 2011

Objective.—The purpose of this prospective study was to determine the incidence and clinical significance of pneumothoraces detected on routine radiography after chest tube removal following cardiac surgery and correlate those findings with an immediate postprocedure assessment of the likelihood of new pneumothorax.

Subjects and Methods.—Routine portable chest radiographs obtained after chest tube removal in 400 consecutive cardiac surgery patients were assessed by a radiologist to determine the incidence and grade of pneumothoraces and were correlated with the clinical estimation of the likelihood of this complication, and whether the radiographic finding changed medical management or led to surgical intervention.

Results.—Of 9.3% of cases (37/400) of new pneumothoraces after chest tube removal, 70.3% were tiny (barely perceptible), 27.0% were small (< 1 cm from the pleural line to the apex of the hemithorax), and 2.7% were medium (6–10 cm from the pleural line to the apex of the hemithorax). The incidences of small and medium pneumothoraces were substantially greater in patients with higher levels of clinical suspicion. All tiny pneumothoraces had no clinical importance. Not obtaining routine chest radiographs after chest tube removal in the 345 patients (86.3%) with the lowest level of clinical suspicion would have resulted in missing six small pneumothoraces (1.7%), none of which led to medical or surgical intervention or a delay in discharge.

Conclusion.—Chest radiography performed after chest tube removal following cardiac surgery is necessary only if the patient has respiratory or hemodynamic changes or if there are problems with the technical aspect of chest tube removal. Following this guideline in our patient population could have eliminated 86.3% of radiographs without missing any clinically significant pneumothoraces.

▶ The authors performed a prospective review to determine the prevalence of new pneumothorax or other abnormality on radiography obtained after chest tube removal following cardiac surgery and to determine how frequently such pneumothoraces required medical or surgical intervention. They also wanted to find out whether the incidence of these abnormalities could be correlated with an immediate postprocedure assessment by the cardiac surgeon as to the likelihood of pneumothorax or other complication.

The study population consisted of 400 consecutive patients who had routine radiography following chest tube removal after cardiac surgery procedures performed between May 2009 and March 2010. Before each chest tube removal, the cardiac surgeon filled out a form that indicated the likelihood of pneumothorax using a 5-point scale based on clinical parameters. In each case, a radiologist interpreted the images to confirm the presence of pneumothorax and categorized the pneumothoraces found as tiny, small, moderate (1–5 cm of pleural separation), medium (6–10 cm of pleural separation), or severe (substantial collapse of the lung). When pneumothorax was found, comparison images were reviewed to determine whether the pneumothorax had been previously present. When there was a new pneumothorax, chart reviews were performed to determine whether the finding led to a change in medical management.

Pneumothorax was detected in 12.8% of patients (51 of 400), and 74.5% were tiny, 23.5% were small, and 2.5% were medium; 17.5% were unchanged; 9.3% of patients had a new pneumothorax, of which, 70.3% were tiny, 27.0% were small, and 2.7% were medium. Two new pneumothoraces were symptomatic and led to placement of chest tube and discharge delay.

The authors found that not obtaining routine chest radiographs after chest tube removal in the 345 patients (86.3%) with the lowest level of clinical suspicion would have resulted in missing small pneumothoraces in 6 patients. In these specific cases, no pneumothorax led to medical or surgical intervention or discharge delay.

The authors state that the study results support performing chest radiography after chest tube removal only if the patient is symptomatic or if there are technical difficulties with the removal of the chest tube.

M. L. Rosado de Christenson, MD

Central Venous Line Placement in the Superior Vena Cava and the Azygos Vein: Differentiation on Posteroanterior Chest Radiographs
Haygood TM, Brennan PC, Ryan J, et al (Univ of Texas M D Anderson Cancer Ctr, Houston; Univ of Sydney, Australia; et al)
AJR Am J Roentgenol 196:783-787, 2011

Objective.—The purpose of this study was to determine, first, the accuracy with which radiologists reading posteroanterior chest radiographs differentiate whether a central venous line is in the superior vena cava or the azygos vein and, second, the circumstances in which radiologists may omit the lateral view to determine the position of a central venous line.

Materials and Methods.—Twenty-four radiologists evaluated 60 posteroanterior chest radiographs to determine the position of a central venous line in the superior vena cava or azygos vein. Investigators evaluated the appearance of the central venous lines to refine rules for determining central venous line position on a frontal radiograph and omitting the lateral view.

Results.—The accuracy of posteroanterior radiography for determining central venous line position was 90% at one study location and 85.5% at the other. No central venous line in the azygos vein extended more than 10.9 mm caudal to the cephalic edge of the right main bronchus. No central venous line in the superior vena cava had a down-the-barrel or curved appearance at the caudal edge.

Conclusion.—For central venous lines extending at least 15 mm caudal to the cephalic edge of the right main bronchus and having no down-the-barrel or curved caudal appearance, categorization was nearly 100% accurate. Therefore, if desired to save radiation exposure and cost, it may be feasible to omit lateral views in radiography of patients with central venous lines extending at least 15 mm caudal to the cephalic edge of the right main bronchus in whom the caudal edge does not have a down-the-barrel or curved appearance (Fig 5).

▶ The authors state that the placement of central venous catheters is characteristically documented with chest radiography, often including only frontal imaging. While lateral radiography can help distinguish superior vena cava (SVC) versus azygos vein location of the catheter tip, there may be specific catheter appearances on frontal radiographs that would increase confidence of likelihood of azygos vein catheter placement and necessity for repositioning. They state that approximately a quarter of azygos line placements are not recognized. They also state that azygos vein placement of central catheters carries higher complication rates than SVC or right atrium placement to include perforation, thrombosis, stenosis, and extravasation. Pain may also result from administration of fluids through a malpositioned catheter in the azygos vein.

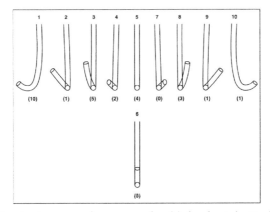

FIGURE 5.—Drawing shows range of appearances of caudal edge of central venous lines in azygos vein (*n* = 30). Values in parentheses indicate number of central venous lines with that appearance. Intention is not to create new classification system but to illustrate range of appearances. (Reprinted from Haygood TM, Brennan PC, Ryan J, et al. Central venous line placement in the superior vena cava and the azygos vein: differentiation on posteroanterior chest radiographs. *AJR Am J Roentgenol.* 2011;196:783-787, with permission from the American Journal of Roentgenology.)

The authors describe the following findings as consistent with azygos placement (Fig 5):

- End-on (or down-the-barrel) appearance of the catheter as it turns posteriorly into the azygos arch. This finding may not occur at the tip of the central venous line.
- With catheter tips that turn left or right, there may be a curved or hook-like morphology of the distal catheter.

The authors describe the following findings as consistent with SVC placement:

- Straight craniocaudal path of catheter on frontal radiography
- Central venous line tip 1.5 cm below the tracheobronchial angle or cephalic bronchial wall without round or down-the-barrel appearance
- Tip at or below the level of the carina on supine frontal radiograph

The authors set out to determine the accuracy with which radiologists viewing such images can distinguish SVC from azygos vein location of a central venous catheter. The study was performed at 2 different sites, and the readers were attending radiologists. These radiologists evaluated 60 chest radiographs selected by 2 other chest radiologists who did not serve as readers. The radiographs were allocated to 2 study groups of 40 radiographs each, half of them with a central line tip in the SVC and the other half in the azygos vein. The radiologists read the images in 2 sessions separated by 3 days and indicated the catheter position and the level of confidence of their interpretation. The catheter appearance was also evaluated to determine characteristics of azygos and SVC catheter placements. Average sensitivities were calculated for the 2 reading sessions and an average area under a receiver operating characteristic analysis was determined.

According to the authors, using a 15-mm distance caudal to the cephalic bronchial wall or the tracheobronchial angle and absence of the down-the-barrel morphology of the catheter would allow confident identification of 17 of 30 of the central lines in the study located in the SVC. However, they add that applying these criteria would leave all central venous lines placed in the azygos and 13 of the 30 placed in the SVC in a group that could not be confidently categorized as being in the SVC. In fact, the percentage of correct interpretations decreased from an average of 99% for the 17 central lines satisfying the criteria to 92.1% for the 13 lines in the SVC that did not satisfy the criteria and for 78% for the 30 central lines in the azygos vein. However, the authors suggest that when the criteria are met, the lateral chest radiograph can be avoided.

Limitations:

- Central line position varies with the preferences of individuals placing them.
- Differences in experience may have existed between the 2 groups of radiologists.
- Differences in equipment may have affected the results.
- The images tested were posteroanterior chest radiographs. It is not known whether the study results would be similar with anteroposterior radiographs in the supine or semiupright position.

M. L. Rosado de Christenson, MD

Computed Tomography

Adaptive Statistical Iterative Reconstruction Technique for Radiation Dose Reduction in Chest CT: A Pilot Study

Singh S, Kalra MK, Gilman MD, et al (Massachusetts General Hosp, Boston; et al)
Radiology 259:565-573, 2011

Purpose.—To compare lesion detection and image quality of chest computed tomographic (CT) images acquired at various tube current-time products (40−150 mAs) and reconstructed with adaptive statistical iterative reconstruction (ASIR) or filtered back projection (FBP).

Materials and Methods.—In this Institutional Review Board−approved HIPAA-compliant study, CT data from 23 patients (mean age, 63 years ± 7.3 [standard deviation]; 10 men, 13 women) were acquired at varying tube current−time products (40, 75, 110, and 150 mAs) on a 64-row multi-detector CT scanner with 10-cm scan length. All patients gave informed consent. Data sets were reconstructed at 30%, 50%, and 70% ASIR-FBP blending. Two thoracic radiologists assessed image noise, visibility of small structures, lesion conspicuity, and diagnostic confidence. Objective noise and CT number were measured in the thoracic aorta. CT dose index volume, dose-length product, weight, and transverse diameter were recorded. Data were analyzed by using analysis of variance and the Wilcoxon signed rank test.

Results.—FBP had unacceptable noise at 40 and 75 mAs in 17 and five patients, respectively, whereas ASIR had acceptable noise at 40−150 mAs. Objective noise with 30%, 50%, and 70% ASIR blending (11.8 ± 3.8, 9.6 ± 3.1, and 7.5 ± 2.6, respectively) was lower than that with FBP (15.8 ± 4.8) ($P < .0001$). No lesions were missed on FBP or ASIR images. Lesion conspicuity was graded as well seen on both FBP and ASIR images ($P < .05$). Mild pixilated blotchy texture was noticed with 70% blended ASIR images.

Conclusion.—Acceptable image quality can be obtained for chest CT images acquired at 40 mAs by using ASIR without any substantial artifacts affecting diagnostic confidence (Fig 1).

▶ The authors report that in 2006, there were 70 million CT examinations performed in the United States, which translates into a doubling of the estimated effective dose per person in the U.S. to 6.2 mSv in 2006 from 3.6 mSv in 1980. In fact, it is estimated that in 2006, medical imaging contributed approximately 48% of the total radiation dose to patients, a contribution for which CT imaging is predominantly responsible. As the use of CT in the United States continues to increase, concerns about deleterious and carcinogenic effects have been voiced. Reduction in CT dose typically results in an increase in image noise, which may affect the quality of the imaging study. The authors state that dose reduction can be accomplished while maintaining image quality by optimization of various scanner parameters, including tube current, peak kilovoltage, and pitch and by

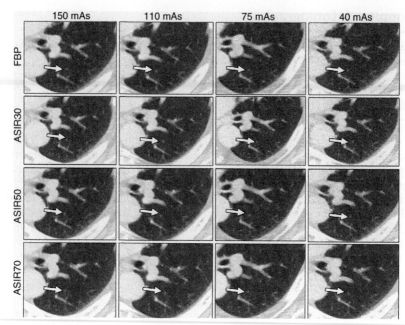

FIGURE 1.—Transverse chest CT images of a 61-year-old woman weighing 118 kg who had a history of left lower lobe pulmonary nodule (arrow). Images were reconstructed with FBP or ASIR at four tube current–time products. At 40 mAs, lesion conspicuity and diagnostic confidence was higher with ASIR images than with FBP images. (Reprinted from Singh S, Kalra MK, Gilman MD, et al. Adaptive statistical iterative reconstruction technique for radiation dose reduction in chest CT: a pilot study. *Radiology.* 2011;259:565-573. Copyright by the Radiological Society of North America.)

applying techniques that improve the quality of images obtained at a lower dose, including noise reduction filters (in filtered back projection) or use of iterative reconstruction techniques applied to the raw CT data.

The authors set out to compare images acquired at various tube current-time products (40–150 mAs) and reconstructed with filtered back projection (FBP) and adaptive iterative reconstruction (ASIR) techniques. This was a prospective study that included patients over age 50 who were scheduled to be imaged with chest CT, were able to give informed consent, and were hemodynamically stable. Pregnant patients were excluded. The study population was enrolled between February 9 and August 28, 2009. Study indications included evaluation of lung mass or lymphadenopathy, staging of lymphoma, evaluation of chest pain, hemoptysis, obstructive pulmonary disease, and abnormal chest radiographs.

After performance of the diagnostic chest CT, the patients underwent 4 additional sets of images with a scan length of 10 cm through the most subtle or smallest focal lung or mediastinal lesion within 1 minute of obtaining the diagnostic scan at 4 tube current-time products of 150, 110, 75, and 40 mAs. Automatic tube current modulation (ATCM) was not used for the additional images, and all other scanning parameters were held constant. The research images were reconstructed with FBP and ASIR (including 30%, 50%, and 70% ASIR).

All the data sets were randomized and assessed by 2 thoracic radiologists for image quality, grading noise on a 5-point scale and artifacts on a 4-point scale. Visualization of small structures was ranked on a 5-point scale. Lesion size was measured with a 4-point scale that addressed size and extent of involvement. In addition, the authors assessed subjective conspicuity of the lesions and diagnostic confidence on 5- and 4-point scales, respectively.

The authors noted the following:

ASIR

- Substantial reduction of subjective and objective image noise at a lower radiation dose (3.5 mGy) for chest CT
- Acceptable noise and diagnostic confidence at 40 mAs and 50% to 70% blending
- Objective noise measurements that were 52% lower for 70% ASIR than for FBP images
- Artifacts did not affect diagnostic information or interpretation
- Dose reduction of up to 75% achieved with ASIR

FBP

- Increase in subjective and objective noise on FBP images to suboptimal or unacceptable levels at 75 mAs (Fig 1)

The authors conclude that both ASIR and FBP allow substantial dose reduction with an unacceptable increase in image noise with FBP at 40 to 75 mAs. They allow that some small low-contrast lesions could be masked by unacceptably high noise on CT obtained at low doses and state that further studies are needed at the lower radiation dose levels. They also found that imaging at 40 mAs required higher proportions of ASIR blending (50% to 70%) compared with imaging at 75 mAs where 30% ASIR blending was sufficient for acceptable image quality and diagnostic confidence. This may also be affected by large patient size, which will contribute to increased noise. The authors state that, although not tested in this study, the addition of automatic tube current modulation may enable additional dose reduction with the ASIR technique and conclude that for patients under 90 kg, ASIR of 30% is optimal; for larger patients, scanned at 40 to 110 mAs ASIR of 50% is more appropriate.

Study limitations included a small sample size, failure of assessment of tube current-time products below 40 mAs, and failure to include ATCM.

M. L. Rosado de Christenson, MD

Incidental findings at chest CT: A needs assessment survey of radiologists' knowledge

Quint LE, Watcharotone K, Myles JD, et al (Univ of Michigan Health System, Ann Arbor; Univ of Michigan, Ann Arbor; et al)
Acad Radiol 18:1500-1506, 2011

Rationale and Objectives.—To assess practice patterns in evaluating incidental findings at chest computed tomography (CT) to determine the need for further education.

Materials and Methods.—A survey was given to 1600 radiologists, presenting four clinical case questions regarding the evaluation/significance of the following incidental findings at chest CT: thyroid lesion; enlarged mediastinal lymph nodes; asymptomatic, small pulmonary embolus; and small lung nodule. The respondents' answers were compared with "truth," as defined by the best evidence available in the medical literature. Additional questions elicited the respondents' demographics and comfort levels in addressing the findings. Analysis of variance models with a Tukey correction for post hoc comparisons and chi-square tests were used to determine if any demographic factors or comfort levels were predictive of higher correct response rates.

Results.—The overall survey response rate was 28% (445/1600). Correct case response rates ranged from 26% (115/442) to 79% (343/445). Only 6% (28/438) of respondents chose the correct answers for all cases. Up to 80% (353/440) of respondents felt comfortable in addressing findings, and only 57% (252/443) of respondents felt that they needed more training in this area. Fellowship training in cardiothoracic radiology, working in a teaching practice, and subspecialization in abdominal or cardiothoracic radiology were predictive of higher correct response rates. Except for one case question, the comfort level was not predictive of correct response rate.

Conclusions.—There was considerable variability among radiologists and substantial deviation from best medical practice with regard to the interpretation/evaluation of incidental findings at chest CT, signifying a significant need for further education.

▶ Incidental findings on cross-sectional imaging are common. The authors state that approximately 3% to 24% of chest computed tomography (CT) examinations show potentially significant incidental findings that may require further evaluation or follow-up. The purpose of their study was to learn about current practice patterns in management of incidental chest CT findings by surveying various groups of radiologists. In the survey, 4 clinical questions were posed to the participating radiologists regarding incidental findings, including a thyroid nodule, enlarged mediastinal lymph nodes, small peripheral pulmonary embolus, and small indeterminate lung nodule. The survey was presented as a series of multiple-choice questions that had a correct answer based on the best medical evidence currently available in the published literature.

The authors found considerable disagreement among radiologists in practice regarding the significance of the various incidental findings. Although a total of 94% of responders chose at least 1 option that was incorrect based on current published practice recommendations, 62% to 80% stated that they were comfortable or very comfortable in suggesting follow-up recommendations. In addition, 57% of participants stated that they required further training to make a determination for follow-up. Although there are well-defined evidence-based published guidelines (by the Fleischner Society) for the management of solid nodules found on CT, only 40% of responders had a correct answer with respect to the management of an incidental 4-mm nodule in a low-risk patient.

The authors list the low survey response rate (28%) as one of the limitations of the study and add that the responders may have represented a self-selected population that felt confident filling out the survey. The authors also admit that there may have been clues to the correct answers in the questions as presented and that the assumption of one of the answers as truth may also constitute a limitation.

However, they conclude that there may be a need for further education of radiologists in the area of incidental findings, given their prevalence, particularly in view of the increased utilization of thoracic CT.

M. L. Rosado de Christenson, MD

MDCT Bolus Tracking Data as an Adjunct for Predicting the Diagnosis of Pulmonary Hypertension and Concomitant Right-Heart Failure
Davarpanah AH, Hodnett PA, Farrelly CT, et al (Northwestern Univ, Chicago, IL)
AJR Am J Roentgenol 197:1064-1072, 2011

Objective.—The purpose of this study was to investigate the utility of bolus-triggering data from pulmonary CT angiography for predicting the diagnosis of pulmonary hypertension (PH) and right ventricular dysfunction (RVD) and to test its performance against previously established CT signs of PH.

Materials and Methods.—Automated bolus-triggering data from pulmonary CT angiograms of 101 patients were correlated with echocardiographic findings and a variety of CT-derived indexes of PH and RVD, including right and left ventricular minor axis diameter; pulmonary artery (PA), aortic, and superior vena caval diameters; right ventricular thickness; contrast reflux; and configuration of the interventricular septum. For bolus triggering, a region of interest was placed in the main PA. Time to threshold, defined as the time from the beginning of contrast injection to the time attenuation exceeded the threshold (100 HU), was measured. On the basis of results of two consecutive echocardiographic studies, subjects were divided into control and PH groups. The latter group was subdivided into PH without RVD and PH with RVD. Time to threshold values were compared between groups and correlated with standard CT-derived parameters.

Results.—Significant differences between groups were found in time to threshold, PA and right ventricular diameters, and PA-to-aorta and right ventricular—to—left ventricular ratios. Time to threshold had an incremental pattern from the control group (6.6 ± 1.0 seconds) to PH without RVD (9.2 ± 2.4 seconds) and PH with RVD (12.1 ± 3.4 seconds) ($p < 0.001$). The optimal diagnostic performance of time to threshold for revealing the presence of PH and RVD was at cutoff values of 7.75 and 8.75 seconds, respectively. Time to threshold had a strong direct correlation with PA diameter. In multivariable analyses, time to threshold was identified as a significant predictor of PH and RVD. The specificity of time to threshold and PA diameter together was higher than that of PA diameter alone.

Conclusion.—Measurement of time to threshold of contrast enhancement derived from bolus-timing data at MDCT may be a useful adjunctive tool for diagnosing PH and consequent RVD.

▶ The authors define pulmonary arterial hypertension or pulmonary hypertension as a disease of the pulmonary arteries that results in restriction of flow in the pulmonary circulation with a progressive increase in pulmonary vascular resistance and eventual right ventricular failure and death. Pulmonary hypertension is defined as mean pulmonary artery (PA) pressure of more than 25 mm Hg at rest or more than 30 mm Hg during exercise. Echocardiography is typically used to screen patients with possible pulmonary hypertension. CT pulmonary angiography (CTPA) has also been used in the assessment of affected patients and can be helpful in identifying causes of pulmonary hypertension, including chronic pulmonary thromboembolic disease. The authors set out to investigate the utility of bolus triggering data obtained during the performance of CTPA for predicting pulmonary hypertension and right ventricular dysfunction. They also wanted to compare the performance of bolus triggering data against previously established CT signs of pulmonary hypertension.

This was a retrospective study of 300 consecutive patients who underwent CTPA for suspected pulmonary thromboembolism at 1 institution between January and September 2008. Eligible patients underwent at least 2 echocardiograms within a month of the CTPA and had no evidence of pulmonary embolism. One hundred and twelve patients met the inclusion criteria. These patients were imaged on a variety of multidetector CT scanners, including 128-, 64-, and 16-channel scanners. They received 100 mL of low osmolar contrast material followed by a 50-ML saline chaser administered at a rate of 4 mL per second via an 18- or 20- antecubital venous access line. Five seconds after the beginning of the injection, CT images were obtained to trigger the CTPA when reaching a threshold of 100 HU over baseline in the pulmonary trunk.

The pulmonary trunk diameter and the inner lumen of the ascending aorta at the same level were measured, and the ratio between the pulmonary artery and aortic diameters was calculated. A ratio greater than 1 was considered indicative of pulmonary hypertension. The authors also measured the maximum minor axis diameters of the right and left ventricles at their widest, and the ratio between the right ventricular and left ventricular measurements was calculated. A ratio greater than 1 was considered an indication of right ventricular dysfunction. Other recorded findings included the appearance of the interventricular septum, the right ventricular thickness, the transverse diameter of the superior vena cava, and reflux of contrast into the inferior vena cava or hepatic veins. Interestingly, the authors found that using time/to/threshold together with pulmonary trunk diameter increases sensitivity to 94% and specificity to 94%.

The authors found that the time to threshold of contrast enhancement in the pulmonary trunk of patients with pulmonary hypertension may be prolonged and that this measurement correlated significantly with the diameter of the pulmonary trunk and with pressures measured at right heart catheterization in a subset of 31 patients with pulmonary hypertension who underwent this procedure. They found that the optimal cutoff value for detection of pulmonary hypertension was 7.75 seconds with 80% and 82% sensitivity and specificity, respectively. They also found that time to threshold of more than 8.75 seconds had 85% and 78% sensitivity and specificity, respectively, in the detection of right ventricular dysfunction.

The authors report several limitations of their study:

- Inclusion criteria required that patients have a series of imaging studies, which may have biased patient selection.
- Although echocardiography is frequently used in the evaluation of pulmonary hypertension, it may have several limitations for making this diagnosis.
- The study design was retrospective.

Because CTPA is often used in the evaluation of patients with suspected pulmonary hypertension and bolus timing data are routinely collected, the study results suggest that it may be worthwhile to collect such data during the performance of CTPA to help diagnose and monitor pulmonary hypertension and right heart failure.

M. L. Rosado de Christenson, MD

Interstitial Lung Disease

An Official ATS/ERS/JRS/ALAT Statement: Idiopathic Pulmonary Fibrosis: Evidence-based Guidelines for Diagnosis and Management
Raghu G, on behalf of the ATS/ERS/JRS/ALAT Committee on Idiopathic Pulmonary Fibrosis
Am J Respir Crit Care Med 183:788-824, 2011

This document is an international evidence-based guideline on the diagnosis and management of idiopathic pulmonary fibrosis, and is a collaborative effort of the American Thoracic Society, the European Respiratory Society, the Japanese Respiratory Society, and the Latin American Thoracic Association. It represents the current state of knowledge regarding idiopathic pulmonary fibrosis (IPF), and contains sections on definition and epidemiology, risk factors, diagnosis, natural history, staging and prognosis, treatment, and monitoring disease course. For the diagnosis and treatment sections, pragmatic GRADE evidence-based methodology was applied in a question-based format. For each diagnosis and treatment question, the committee graded the quality of the evidence available (high, moderate, low, or very low), and made a recommendation (yes or no, strong or weak). Recommendations were based on majority vote. It is emphasized that clinicians must spend adequate time with patients to discuss patients' values and preferences and decide on the appropriate course of action.

▶ Idiopathic pulmonary fibrosis (IPF) is an interstitial lung disease of unknown etiology that affects older adults who present with progressive dyspnea and increasingly worsening pulmonary function. It is a diagnosis that carries a poor prognosis.

This article outlines international evidence-based guidelines for the diagnosis and management of IPF. The work is a collaborative effort between the American Thoracic Society, the European Respiratory Society, the Japanese Respiratory Society, and the Latin American Thoracic Society. The GRADE system (Grades of Recommendation, Assessment, Development, and Evaluation) was used to formulate the recommendations. The multidisciplinary panel that participated in the formulation of the guidelines consisted of experts in the evaluation and management of IPF and included 24 pulmonologists, 4 thoracic radiologists, 4 pathologists, and 3 librarians. The guideline defines IPF as a "specific form of chronic, progressive fibrosing interstitial pneumonia of unknown cause, occurring primarily in older adults, limited to the lungs, and associated with the histopathologic and/or radiologic pattern of usual interstitial pneumonia (UIP)." It further highlights the importance of high-resolution CT (HRCT) in making the diagnosis of IPF.

The section of the article that defines the UIP pattern of IPF states that HRCT is an essential component of the diagnostic algorithm for IPF. The UIP pattern is characterized by parenchymal reticular opacities often associated with traction bronchiectasis and frequent honeycombing. Honeycombing is defined as clustered cystic air-containing spaces with well-defined walls that characteristically exhibit similar diameters (3–10 mm) but may be as large as 2.5 cm. Honeycombing typically affects the subpleural regions of the lung. Associated ground-glass opacity is common but is typically less extensive than the reticular opacities. Abnormalities forming part of the UIP pattern are usually basal and peripheral. The guideline states that HRCT findings of micronodules, air-trapping, non-honeycomb cysts, extensive ground-glass opacities, consolidation, and peribronchovascular distribution of lung disease should suggest an alternative diagnosis. Table 4 in the original article suggests that based on HRCT findings, the imaging pattern can be further characterized as "UIP pattern", "possible UIP pattern" or "inconsistent with UIP pattern."

Although the positive predictive value of an HRCT diagnosis of UIP is 90% to 100%, patients with HRCT studies that do not exhibit the UIP pattern may still have a histologic diagnosis of UIP on lung biopsy.

The authors remark that the accuracy of diagnosis of IPF increases with a multidisciplinary approach in which pulmonologists, radiologists, and pathologists with experience in the diagnosis of interstitial lung disease discuss the various features of each case to arrive at a diagnosis. Thus, radiologists must be familiar with the characteristic features of the UIP pattern to appropriately suggest the prospective diagnosis of IPF and to contribute to the multidisciplinary discussion and diagnosis of affected patients.

M. L. Rosado de Christenson, MD

Infection

CT of Viral Lower Respiratory Tract Infections in Adults: Comparison Among Viral Organisms and Between Viral and Bacterial Infections

Miller WT Jr, Mickus TJ, Barbosa E Jr, et al (Univ of Pennsylvania School of Medicine, Philadelphia; Allegheny General Hosp, Pittsburgh, PA; et al)
AJR Am J Roentgenol 197:1088-1095, 2011

Objective.—We retrospectively compared the CT findings of consecutive viral and bacterial lower respiratory tract infections (LRTIs) to determine their imaging appearance and any definable differences among the causative viruses and between the viral and bacterial infections.

Materials and Methods.—Imaging features of LRTI caused by influenza virus, respiratory syncytial virus (RSV), parainfluenza, adenovirus, and bacteria over a 33-month period were reviewed by three radiologists blinded to clinical and diagnostic information. Individual CT features and the dominant pattern of infection were recorded for each examination. Imaging characteristics were compared among the four respiratory viruses and between viral and bacterial infections.

Results.—One hundred fifteen chest CT scans were analyzed (60 influenza virus, 19 RSV, 10 adenovirus, four parainfluenza virus, and 22 bacterial pneumonia LRTIs). Individual imaging findings and imaging patterns were seen in similar frequencies when we compared viral and bacterial LRTIs, with the exception of the diffuse airspace pattern, which was seen more frequently in bacterial infections. Although there was overlap in the imaging appearance of individual viruses, RSV and adenovirus tended to have characteristic imaging appearances. RSV presented with an airway-centric pattern of disease (13/19 cases [68%]) characterized by varying

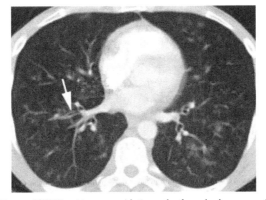

FIGURE 1.—41-year-old HIV-positive man with 1 month of cough, dyspnea, and night sweats. CT image shows multiple tree-in-bud opacities in lungs bilaterally, associated with mild bronchial wall thickening (*arrow*). Diagnosis was bronchiolitis as a result of respiratory syncytial virus infection. (Reprinted from Miller WT Jr, Mickus TJ, Barbosa E Jr, et al. CT of viral lower respiratory tract infections in adults: comparison among viral organisms and between viral and bacterial infections. *AJR Am J Roentgenol.* 2011;197:1088-1095, with permission from the American Journal of Roentgenology.)

mixtures of tree-in-bud opacities and bronchial wall thickening, with or without peribronchiolar consolidation. Adenovirus typically appeared as multifocal consolidation or ground-glass opacity without airway inflammatory findings (7/10 cases [70%]).

Conclusion.—There is considerable overlap in the imaging appearance of viral and bacterial respiratory infections. However, some characteristic differences can be seen, especially with RSV and adenovirus infections (Fig 1).

▶ With the objective of identifying and comparing CT features of viral and bacterial pulmonary infections, the authors retrospectively reviewed CT studies of patients with proved pulmonary infection by the 4 most common viruses responsible for community-acquired viral infection (influenza virus, respiratory syncytial virus (RSV), parainfluenza virus, and adenovirus) as well as patients with bacterial pulmonary infection. Patients with lower respiratory tract infection (LRTI) were defined on the basis of symptoms and laboratory evidence of bacterial or viral infection. Inclusion criteria included the following:

- Presentation with clinical symptoms of acute LRTI as an outpatient between November 1, 2005, and July 31, 2008
- Polymerase chain reaction (PCR) of respiratory secretions positive for the above-mentioned viruses
- Cultures positive for bacterial infection
- Chest CT within 72 hours of PCR

The study population included patients from 2 different affiliated medical centers who were divided into 4 different groups:

Group 1: evidence of viral infection without concurrent bacterial infection
Group 2: evidence of bacterial infection without concurrent viral infection
Group 3: evidence of concurrent viral and bacterial infection
Group 4: no evidence of viral or bacterial infection

Groups 3 and 4 were excluded. Ninety-three patients had evidence of viral infection, and 22 had evidence of bacterial infection.

The authors found that viral LRTI exhibited 1 of 4 imaging appearances: airway-centered abnormalities including tree-in-bud opacities, bronchial wall thickening and peribronchial consolidation, multifocal pneumonia (multifocal consolidation, ground-glass opacity, or both without airway findings), focal infection (focus of consolidation, ground-glass opacity, tree-in-bud opacities), or normal study. These findings had considerable overlap with the findings seen on patients with bacterial infection. The only pattern found to be significantly different between both types of infection was diffuse airspace disease, which was seen more frequently in patients with bacterial infection.

The authors confirmed that most patients with RSV infection (68%) exhibited a CT pattern of bronchiolitis (Fig 1). Most patients with adenovirus infection exhibited widespread multifocal pneumonia. They found that influenza pneumonia had the most variable imaging appearance and was most likely to exhibit normal CT imaging studies. Although patients with influenza virus had a low frequency of multifocal pneumonia, this virus was the most common viral cause for this pattern in the study.

The authors acknowledge several limitations to the study, including the facts that only a fraction of patients with viral LRTI had a chest CT that likely introduced selection bias and variable CT imaging techniques.

M. L. Rosado de Christenson, MD

Pulmonary Nocardiosis: Computed Tomography Features at Diagnosis
Blackmon KN, Ravenel JG, Gomez JM, et al (Med Univ of South Carolina, Charleston)
J Thorac Imaging 26:224-229, 2011

Purpose.—To review the computed tomography (CT) imaging features of pulmonary nocardiosis (PN) at the time of initial presentation.

Materials and Methods.—All patients from 1991 to 2008 with PN were identified (n=105). Patients without CT scan available at initial presentation were excluded (n=52). For the remaining 53 patients, standardized radiographic features were recorded. The patients were grouped by predisposing condition. Analysis includes descriptive summary statistics as well as associations among radiographic findings, associated findings, and host characteristics. Parametric and nonparametric statistical methods were used.

Results.—Median age of the patients was 52 years (range, 6 to 82 y). Some form of immunosuppression was present in 83% of the cases. Preexisting structural abnormalities of the lung were uncommon (bronchiectasis, 7; chronic obstructive pulmonary disease, 3). Twenty (38%) patients had interstitial opacities. Airspace disease was seen in 34 (64%) cases. Thirty (57%) cases revealed discrete nodules, 25 patients had 1 to 6 nodules (mean, 2), and 5 patients had fewer than 6 nodules, with the mean size of the largest nodule being 1.67 cm. Masses were seen in 11 patients (21%), 9 of whom had concomitant nodules. Cavitary lesions, including nodules, masses, or airspace disease, occurred in 40% of the cohort. Mediastinal lymphadenopathy was present in 8 (15%) patients. Fifteen patients (28%) had pleural effusions; the effusions were unilateral in 10 patients. Analysis of radiographic associations with patient groups found discrete nodules to be more often associated with immunosuppression compared with the nonimmunosuppressed group (66% vs. 11%; $P=0.0067$).

Conclusion.—The CT presentation of PN is heterogeneous. Airspace disease appeared most frequently (in 64% of the cases), and nodules were present in 57% of the cases. Nocardiosis should be considered in the differential diagnosis of immunosuppressed patients with new nodules or masses.

▶ The authors describe *Nocardia* sp. as an aerobic, gram-positive bacterium that exhibits partial acid-fast features, is soil-borne, and is not considered a typical laboratory contaminant or part of the normal human flora. Patients with nocardiosis are typically immunocompromised, although up to one-third of affected individuals have normal immunity. It is estimated that there are up to 1000 new *Nocardia* infections annually, but this may be an underestimation, as the organism often mimics other bacterial pulmonary infections. The route of infection is typically inhalation of the bacteria, and there is frequent hematogenous dissemination to the central nervous system and skin.

The authors undertook a retrospective review of all patients in their institution diagnosed with nocardiosis between January 1991 and May 2008 who also had computed tomography (CT), with the purpose of describing the CT manifestations of pulmonary infection. Fifty-three patients met inclusion criteria for the study.

The authors found that airspace consolidation was a common finding, seen in 64% of the patients. The most common abnormalities were airspace opacities and nodules (the latter found in 56% of cases). Nodules exhibited well-defined borders in 50% of cases. They found a significant association between immunosuppression and nodular disease on chest CT. Other findings included multiple or single pulmonary masses seen in 21% of cases. Of note, CT demonstrated cavitation in 60% of the nodules and 64% of the masses, which may relate to more confident identification of variations in attenuation of lesions on CT. Lymphadenopathy was seen in 15% of patients and pleural effusion in 28%. Interstitial lung disease was present in 15% of cases.

The authors acknowledge several limitations to the study, including the retrospective design and the variability of imaging technology during the study period. Nevertheless, this study emphasizes that nocardiosis should be considered in the differential diagnosis of patients with pulmonary infection, particularly those with immunosuppression.

M. L. Rosado de Christenson, MD

Screening of Asymptomatic Children for Tuberculosis: Is a Lateral Chest Radiograph Routinely Indicated?
Lee EY, Tracy DA, Eisenberg RL, et al (Children's Hosp Boston and Harvard Med School, Boston, MA; Beth Israel Deaconess Med Ctr, Boston, MA)
Acad Radiol 18:184-190, 2011

Rationale and Objectives.—The aim of this study was to determine whether a lateral chest radiograph provides additional diagnostic information to a posteroanterior (PA) radiograph in the screening of asymptomatic children with positive purified protein derivative (PPD) skin tests in a nonendemic area.

Materials and Methods.—This was an Institutional Review Board—approved, Health Insurance Portability and Accountability Act—compliant, retrospective study of 605 consecutive pediatric patients (294 males, 311 females; mean age, 10.8 ± 5.2 years) with positive PPD skin test results, who underwent PA and lateral chest radiographs between July 2003 and May 2009 at a tertiary care pediatric hospital in a nonendemic area for tuberculosis (TB). Two pediatric radiologists independently reviewed each chest radiograph for evidence of abnormalities that may be indicative of acute or chronic TB infection. The reviewers first analyzed the PA radiograph alone and subsequently evaluated the PA and the lateral radiograph together to determine whether any observed abnormality was identified only on the lateral radiograph. When an abnormality was detected on both PA and lateral radiographs, the reviewers determined whether the abnormality on the lateral radiograph changed the reviewer's decision based on the PA radiograph alone. Assessment of nonconcordance between PA and lateral chest radiographs for each reviewer was evaluated by the McNemar test of matched binary pairs. Agreement between reviewers for detecting abnormalities on radiographs was evaluated by using the kappa (κ) statistic.

Results.—The frequency of an abnormal chest radiograph related to TB was 1.8% (11/605). The PA radiograph showed abnormalities in all 11 (100%) children with radiographic abnormalities. Lateral radiographs showed abnormalities related to TB in 2 (18.2%) of 11 cases found to be abnormal on PA radiographs. Nine (81.8%) of 11 abnormalities on PA radiographs were not detected on the lateral chest radiographs. There was statistical evidence of nonconcordance between PA and lateral chest radiographs in detecting TB-related abnormalities for reviewer 1 ($P < .001$) and reviewer 2 ($P = .004$). In cases with abnormalities observed on both PA and lateral radiographs, there were no cases in which information obtained from the lateral chest radiograph resulted in a change in interpretation based on the PA radiograph alone. A high level of agreement was observed between the two independent reviewers in detecting TB-related abnormalities on PA radiographs ($\kappa = 0.84$, $P < .001$).

Conclusions.—A PA radiograph alone is sufficient for TB screening of asymptomatic pediatric patients with positive PPD skin test results in an area non-endemic for TB.

▶ Radiographic screening of tuberculosis is frequently used in the United States to further evaluate populations with positive tuberculin skin test results. The authors state that the Centers for Disease Control and the American Thoracic Society recommend that such radiographic screening should include posteroanterior (PA) and lateral chest radiographs for children less than 5 years of age and PA chest radiography alone for children over 5 years, with additional imaging at the discretion of the referring physician. In areas in which tuberculosis is endemic, it has been recommended that both PA and lateral chest radiographs should be obtained in children regardless of age.

The authors set out to determine whether the lateral chest radiograph provides additional information when added to the PA chest radiograph for imaging children being screened for tuberculosis. This was a retrospective review accomplished by identifying all pediatric patients (aged 18 years or less) who were screened with chest radiography for tuberculosis due to positive tuberculin skin test results between July 2003 and May 2009. The patients had a tuberculin skin test because they were considered at high risk for tuberculosis infection because of history of close contact with someone with tuberculosis or a positive skin test for tuberculosis, living with individuals who came to the United States from another country or living with or in contact with homeless adults, or adults with AIDS, HIV infection, or those using intravenous drugs or living in a congregate setting (including prison, nursing home, or mental institution). Two reviewers analyzed the PA chest radiographs first and then the PA and lateral chest radiographs. They determined whether observed abnormalities were only visible on the lateral chest radiograph and whether the findings on the lateral image changed the decision made based on the findings on PA chest radiography. In cases of discrepancies, the reviewers evaluated the cases together to reach a consensus decision, or a third reviewer served as the arbitrator and made the final decision. At least 1 reviewer noted an abnormal finding in 15 (2.5%) cases with a final 11 cases (1.8%) demonstrating abnormalities that included a calcified granuloma (6), noncalcified nodule (4), and apical pleural thickening (1). There were no findings of active tuberculosis. Incidental findings not related to tuberculosis were noted in 3 cases. Of interest, lateral radiographs did not show abnormalities in 9 of the 11 cases with abnormalities deemed abnormal on PA chest radiography. In the end, lateral chest radiographic findings did not result in the reviewers making a change in their diagnostic decisions. Thus, the authors conclude that the lateral chest radiograph did not provide diagnostic information that was not available on the PA chest radiograph. This would result in a reduction of radiation dose of 0.007 mSv and a cost savings of $87.00 per patient.

The authors point out several limitations to their study, including the fact that they studied a specific pediatric population in a specific clinical setting, the reviewers were aware that the patients had a positive tuberculin skin test, the reviewers were aware of the findings on PA chest radiography when interpreting the lateral chest radiographs, and the low yield of positive radiographic findings and absence of pathologic correlation.

M. L. Rosado de Christenson, MD

Pulmonary Thromboembolic Disease

Pulmonary CT Angiography Protocol Adapted to the Hemodynamic Effects of Pregnancy

Ridge CA, Mhuircheartaigh JN, Dodd JD, et al (St. Vincent's Univ Hosp, Elm Park, Dublin, Ireland; Univ College Hosp, Galway, Ireland)
AJR Am J Roentgenol 197:1058-1063, 2011

Objective.—The purpose of this study was to compare the image quality of a standard pulmonary CT angiography (CTA) protocol with a pulmonary CTA protocol optimized for use in pregnant patients with suspected pulmonary embolism (PE).

Materials and Methods.—Forty-five consecutive pregnant patients with suspected PE were retrospectively included in the study: 25 patients (group A) underwent standard-protocol pulmonary CTA and 20 patients (group B) were imaged using a protocol modified for pregnancy. The modified protocol used a shallow inspiration breath-hold and a high concentration, high rate of injection, and high volume of contrast material. Objective image quality and subjective image quality were evaluated by measuring pulmonary arterial enhancement, determining whether there was transient interruption of the contrast bolus by unopacified blood from the inferior vena cava (IVC), and assessing diagnostic adequacy.

Results.—Objective and subjective image quality were significantly better for group B—that is, for the group who underwent the CTA protocol optimized for pregnancy. Mean pulmonary arterial enhancement and the percentage of studies characterized as adequate for diagnosis were higher in group B than in group A: 321 ± 148 HU (SD) versus 178 ± 67 HU ($p = 0.0001$) and 90% versus 64% ($p = 0.05$), respectively. Transient interruption of contrast material by unopacified blood from the IVC was observed more frequently in group A (39%) than in group B (10%) ($p = 0.05$).

Conclusion.—A pulmonary CTA protocol optimized for pregnancy significantly improved image quality by increasing pulmonary arterial opacification, improving diagnostic adequacy, and decreasing transient interruption of the contrast bolus by unopacified blood from the IVC.

▶ It has been established that the hemodynamic effects of pregnancy affect the quality of CT pulmonary angiography (CTPA) and thus may contribute to indeterminate studies in this patient population. The authors state that dyspnea is a common complaint in the third trimester of pregnancy and that exclusion of pulmonary embolism (PE) is of importance, because it may account for 10% of pregnancy-related deaths in the United States.

The authors list the following hemodynamic effects of pregnancy: increased cardiac output (40%–50% increase predominantly in the second trimester), total vascular resistance, heart rate, and plasma volume (total blood volume increase by approximately 50% in early pregnancy). Inferior vena cava (IVC) pressure is also noted to increase because of the gravid uterus and may increase 6-fold in the third trimester in the supine position. The increased IVC pressure and the decreased pressure that results from deep inspiration results in a thoracoabdominal gradient of pressure with resultant increased venous return to the right heart (thoracoabdominal pump). These physiologic effects contribute to dilution of the contrast bolus and an increase in the pressure in the inferior vena cava, which may lead to the phenomenon of transient interruption of contrast by a bolus of unopacified blood.

The authors list several technical adjustments suggested in the literature to counteract the physiologic effects of pregnancy, including bolus tracking, short scan delay, high contrast medium flow rate, and high contrast medium concentration. In addition, it has been suggested that scans not be performed at deep inspiration, which has been shown to increase transient interruption of contrast due to increase of flow from the IVC into the right heart.

The study was a retrospective review of consecutive pregnant patients imaged with CTPA between July 1, 2006, and October 2010. The first 28 studies were performed on 25 pregnant patients using a standard protocol for CTPA characterized by injection of 75 mL of contrast via the antecubital vein with a flow rate of 4 mL per second followed by a 50-mL intravenous (IV) saline flush at deep inspiration. The next 20 pregnant patients in the study were imaged with antecubital injection of 95 mL of contrast with flow at

6 mL per second followed by a 50-mL intravenous saline flush obtained during shallow held inspiration and avoiding the Valsalva maneuver.

Images were analyzed by measuring attenuation in Hounsfield units at the pulmonary trunk, the right and left pulmonary arteries, and the right and left lower lobe pulmonary arteries proximal to the segmental divisions, with the area of interest measuring half the cross-sectional area of the vessel. The combined measurements were used to calculate the mean pulmonary opacification. Noise measurements and subjective image quality (including motion artifact) were also analyzed. The relative contribution of the IVC to the right heart was also evaluated.

The authors found that 90% of studies in group B were of diagnostic quality, compared with only 64% of studies in group A. In addition, 32.1% of studies in group A were categorized as of good quality as opposed to 80% of studies in group B. Study quality was categorized as poor in 39% of studies in group A versus 5% of studies in group B. Subjective image quality was also noted to be significantly better in group B with 90% of studies categorized as adequate as opposed to 64% of studies in group B. Finally, transient interruption of contrast was confirmed in 39% of studies in group A and in 10% of studies in group B.

Study limitations include the following:

- Retrospective study design
- Readers not blinded to protocol
- Consensus opinion used
- Left to right shunts not excluded echocardiographically
- The 2 groups varied in size and characteristics with fewer patients in group B

The authors conclude that optimized CTPA protocols in pregnancy increase the rate of diagnostically adequate studies and decrease the incidence of transient interruption of contrast.

M. L. Rosado de Christenson, MD

An Official American Thoracic Society/Society of Thoracic Radiology Clinical Practice Guideline: Evaluation of Suspected Pulmonary Embolism In Pregnancy
Leung AN, on behalf of the ATS/STR Committee on Pulmonary Embolism in Pregnancy
Am J Respir Crit Care Med 184:1200-1208, 2011

Background.—Pulmonary embolism (PE) is a leading cause of maternal mortality in the developed world. Along with appropriate prophylaxis and therapy, prevention of death from PE in pregnancy requires a high index of clinical suspicion followed by a timely and accurate diagnostic approach.

Methods.—To provide guidance on this important health issue, a multidisciplinary panel of major medical stakeholders was convened to develop evidence-based guidelines for evaluation of suspected pulmonary embolism in pregnancy using the Grades of Recommendation, Assessment, Development, and Evaluation (GRADE) system. In formulation of the recommended diagnostic algorithm, the important outcomes were defined to be diagnostic accuracy and diagnostic yield; the panel placed a high value on minimizing cumulative radiation dose when determining the recommended sequence of tests.

Results.—Overall, the quality of the underlying evidence for all recommendations was rated as very low or low, with some of the evidence considered for recommendations extrapolated from studies of the general population. Despite the low-quality evidence, strong recommendations were made for three specific scenarios: performance of chest radiography (CXR) as the first radiation-associated procedure; use of lung scintigraphy as the preferred test in the setting of a normal CXR; and performance of computed-tomographic pulmonary angiography (CTPA) rather than digital subtraction angiography (DSA) in a pregnant woman with a non-diagnostic ventilation—perfusion (V/Q) result.

Discussion.—The recommendations presented in this guideline are based upon the currently available evidence; availability of new clinical research data and development and dissemination of new technologies will necessitate a revision and update.

▶ The controversies regarding the diagnosis of pulmonary thromboembolic disease are highlighted by the relatively large proportion of articles that address this important topic within the literature. The authors state that pulmonary thromboembolism is a leading cause of mortality related to pregnancy in the developed world, accounting for 20% of maternal deaths in the United States. They add that the estimated incidence of pulmonary embolism (PE) in pregnant women is 10.6 per 100 000 with the highest risk during the postpartum period. The much-awaited guidelines outlined in this article resulted from a multidisciplinary effort and a project cosponsored by the American Thoracic Society and the Society of Thoracic Radiology. The guidelines were developed using the GRADE system (Grades of Recommendation, Assessment, Development, and Evaluation). The multidisciplinary panel that formulated the guidelines consisted of experts in the evaluation and management of pulmonary thromboembolic disease in pregnancy and included cardiothoracic radiologists, nuclear medicine physicians, pulmonary medicine specialists, obstetricians/gynecologists, medical physicists, and medical ethicists. The panel reviewed the relevant medical literature and formulated answers to a series of clinical questions using an evidence-based approach. The recommendations for or against a particular test required that at least 50% of participants be in favor with less than 20% preferring the alternative. Recommendations graded as strong had to be endorsed by at least 70% of the participants.

Seven recommendations are contained in the report. Strong recommendations include the following:

• Pregnant women with suspected PE should have a chest radiograph as the first radiation-associated procedure in the imaging workup.

- Pregnant women with suspected PE and a normal chest radiograph should have lung scintigraphy as the next imaging study (rather than CT pulmonary angiography [CTPA])
- Pregnant women with suspected PE and a nondiagnostic ventilation perfusion scan should undergo further diagnostic evaluation. In such cases, CT pulmonary angiography is recommended.

The authors acknowledge that the "low quality and limited amount of direct evidence pertaining to diagnostic test accuracy and patient-important outcomes in the pregnant population" are the main weaknesses of the study. They add that prospective studies are needed to validate the high negative predictive values of scintigraphy and CTPA reported in published retrospective reviews.

The authors state that combined use of chest radiography and scintigraphy allows definitive results in more than 90% of pregnant women with suspected pulmonary embolus and a normal chest radiograph. They also highlight the radiation-related risks associated with these imaging studies. They estimate that the fetal dose with either study is low and similar to the 0.5- to 1-mGy dose absorbed by the fetus from normal background radiation during the course of the pregnancy. They add that the maternal risk is higher and that it is related to radiation-induced cancer mortality related to breast and lung cancers. Given these issues, the authors advocate discussing the potential risks and benefits with the patient so that she can reach an informed decision.

The authors support minimizing radiation in the performance of the studies in the following manner:

- Use of technique adjusted to the size of the patient
- Use of collimation and other techniques to limit the fetal dose
- Using half the usual dose of technetium-99m (Tc-99m) macroaggregated albumin for the perfusion scan and increasing the scan time to achieve adequate counts
- Performing a Xenon-133 ventilation scan instead of a Tc-99m aerosol ventilation study to achieve a lower maternal dose
- Although some investigators recommend omitting the ventilation scan, the authors warn that this may decrease the diagnostic accuracy of the study
- Encouraging hydration and frequent voiding following scintigraphy to reduce the fetal dose
- Performing CTPA protocols that are optimized for the physiologic effects of pregnancy including automated bolus triggering, high iodinated contrast flow rate (4.5-6 mL/s), and/or high iodine concentration (350-400 mg I/mL) and clear instructions for breathing to minimize inadvertent Valsalva maneuver

M. L. Rosado de Christenson, MD

Does a Clinical Decision Rule Using D-Dimer Level Improve the Yield of Pulmonary CT Angiography?

Soo Hoo GW, Wu CC, Vazirani S, et al (West Los Angeles Med Ctr, CA)
AJR Am J Roentgenol 196:1059-1064, 2011

Objective.—The objective of our study was to evaluate the impact of incorporating a mandatory clinical decision rule and selective D-dimer use on the yield of pulmonary CT angiography (CTA).

Materials and Methods.—Guidelines incorporating a clinical decision rule (Wells score: range, 0—12.5) and a highly sensitive D-dimer assay as decision points were placed into a computerized order entry menu. From December 2006 through November 2008, 261 pulmonary CTA examinations of 238 men and 14 women (mean age ± SD, 65 ± 12 years; range, 31—92 years) were performed. Eight patients underwent more than one pulmonary CTA examination. Charts were reviewed. The results of pulmonary CTA, the clinical decision rule, and D-dimer level (if obtained) were analyzed with the Student t test, chi-square test, or other comparisons using statistical software (MedCalc, version 11.0).

Results.—Of the pulmonary CTA examinations, 16.5% (43/261) were positive for pulmonary embolism (PE) compared with 3.1% (6/196) during the previous 2 years. The mean clinical decision rule score and mean D-dimer level were 5.5 ± 2.4 (SD) and 4956 ± 2892 ng/mL, respectively, for those with PE compared with 4.5 ± 2.1 and 2398 ± 2100 ng/mL for those without PE (both, $p < 0.01$). The negative predictive value of a clinical decision rule score of 4 or less and D-dimer level of less than 1000 ng/mL was 1.0. A clinical decision rule of greater than 4 and a higher D-dimer level were better predictors for PE, especially a D-dimer level of greater than 3000 ng/mL (odds ratio – 6.69; 95% CI = 2.72—16.43).

Conclusion.—Guidelines combining a clinical decision rule with D-dimer level significantly improved the utilization of pulmonary CTA and positive yield for PE.

▶ The authors observed that computed tomography pulmonary angiogram (CTPA) requests increased by 56% in their institution between the years 2000 and 2005, without a significant change in the positivity rate for pulmonary embolism (PE) that was approximately 3.1% in the 2 years preceding the study. The authors describe the function of the Imaging Utilization Group that examined the institution's CTPA usage. This group (comprised of attending physicians from the medicine, surgery, radiology, and emergency medicine departments) determined that there were no protocol guidelines in place for the evaluation of suspected PE, specifically, no requirement of a clinical decision rule, a laboratory test, or a chest radiograph prior to placing an order for CTPA. In 2006, the group incorporated a clinical decision rule (Wells score), and the selective use of a highly sensitive D-dimer assay (the enzyme-linked immunosorbent assay [ELISA] D-dimer assay) into the computerized order entry menu. Physicians requesting CTPA were required to generate a composite Wells score. CTPA was automatically approved in patients with Wells scores greater than 4. For Wells scores equal to or less than 4, the physician was required to perform an ELISA D-dimer assay. If the level was 500 ng/mL or less, the study could be performed but only after consultation with the chest radiology attending physician. If the ELISA D-dimer level was greater than 500 ng/mL, the CTPA was automatically approved. The authors emphasized that no request was ever denied by the attending thoracic radiologist (Fig 1 in the original article). Referring physicians received continuing educational sessions to reinforce the need to adhere to the guidelines.

Imaging was performed after the administration of 100 mL of iodinated contrast, injected at a flow rate of 5 mL/s with bolus tracking, and scanning was triggered over the pulmonary trunk at 120 HU. Axial reconstructions of 1, 1.5, and 3 mm and 1.5-mm sagittal and coronal reconstructions were then obtained.

The study population included all CTPAs performed from December 1, 2006 to November 30, 2008. A total of 261 studies were performed on 252 patients (8 patients had more than 1 study). In addition, 57% of studies were obtained in hospitalized patients, and 43% were obtained from the emergency department.

The overall percentage of positive examinations increased to 13.4%, with 17.3% of positive studies in hospitalized patients and 15.3% of positive studies in outpatients in the emergency department. The authors note that 12.2% of patients with Wells scores of 4 or less had PE and that 20% of patients with Wells scores greater than 4 had PE. When patients had a Wells score of greater than 4 and a D-dimer greater than 3000 ng/mL, 72% of such patients had a positive study for PE.

The authors then conclude that CTPA utilization can be improved by incorporation of a clinical decision rule and ELISA D-dimer tests into the computerized order entry menu.

Limitations of the study:

- There are no data on patients that did not undergo CTPA.
- The study population was overwhelmingly male.
- Studies were read as positive or negative.
- There were no indeterminate scans.

M. L. Rosado de Christenson, MD

2 Breast Imaging

Introduction

It is a pleasure to present the selections of breast imaging articles for the 2012 YEAR BOOK OF DIAGNOSTIC RADIOLOGY. The articles selected are varied and interesting, and they reflect the broad range of issues we breast imagers encounter.

Pretty much all the bases are covered—mammography, breast ultrasound, and breast MRI. Whether you are a general radiologist, a breast imager, or a breast imager with a subspecialist interest, there is an article here for you.

Tanya W. Stephens, MD

Anatomy

The Nipple-Areolar Complex: A Pictorial Review of Common and Uncommon Conditions

An HY, Kim KS, Yu IK, et al (Eulji Univ Hosp, Daejeon, Korea; et al)
J Ultrasound Med 29:949-962, 2010

Objective.—The purpose of this presentation is to show the radiologic findings of normal variants and benign and malignant diseases that affect the nipple-areolar complex.

Methods.—We evaluated the imaging findings of nipple-areolar complex lesions, using multiple breast imaging modalities including mammography, sonography, galactography, contrast-enhanced magnetic resonance imaging (MRI), and positron emission tomography/computed tomography.

Results.—Radiologic features of nipple-areolar complex lesions, including Montgomery tubercles, nipple inversion, benign calcifications, inflammation, duct dilatations, intraductal papillomas, fibroadenomas, neurofibromatosis, dermatosis of the nipple, and breast malignancy, have been illustrated.

Conclusions.—A clinical examination is essential and an appropriate imaging evaluation with multiple modalities is often necessary to accurately diagnose an underlying abnormality of the nipple-areolar complex. Given the limitations of conventional mammography, supplemental mammographic views often are needed, and sonography may be performed to further characterize a mammographic or clinical finding. Also, contrast-enhanced MRI may be useful for additional evaluation.

▶ As a radiologist, I absolutely love images—pictures of things. Pictorial reviews tend to capture my attention. It is important for breast imagers to have a comprehensive understanding of the anatomic variants and benign and malignant processes, and the imaging features of these processes are key to accurate differentiation and diagnosis. The nipple-areolar complex may be affected by a large array of processes that can have similar imaging appearances. The authors of this pictorial review normal variants and benign and malignant diseases that involve the nipple-areolar complex. This review includes a spectrum of imaging modalities including mammograms, ultrasound, ductography, MRI, and CT/positron emission tomography. The authors include a comprehensive guide to deciding which imaging modality is appropriate for a variety of clinical histories.

T. W. Stephens, MD

The Augmented Breast

Challenges in Mammography: Part 2, Multimodality Review of Breast Augmentation—Imaging Findings and Complications
Venkataraman S, Hines N, Slanetz PJ (Beth Israel Deaconess Med Ctr and Harvard Med School, Boston, MA; Care Diagnostics for Women, Boca Raton, FL)
AJR Am J Roentgenol 197:W1031-W1045, 2011

Objective.—Breast augmentation is common throughout the world; however, there is variation in materials and surgical techniques. This review illustrates the mammographic, sonographic, and MRI characteristics of the different types of breast augmentation, including silicone, saline, polyacrylamide gel, and autologous fat augmentation.

Conclusion.—The imaging findings of complications such as implant rupture, free silicone, and fat necrosis in association with augmentation will be illustrated (Table 1).

▶ I have included 3 breast augmentation articles in this year's YEAR BOOK. These inclusions are secondary to an interesting 43-year-old woman whom I met last year. This lovely lady presented for a screening mammogram and told the technologist, "I have implants." When I reviewed her mammogram (she had no prior obtainable imaging), there were no visible implants, so I wondered if her implants were ruptured. Her mammograms were interesting. Although I saw no implants, I noted increased density throughout bilaterally, bilateral obscured masses, and dystrophic and ringlike calcifications associated with some of the obscured masses. I had her return for clinical examination with the possibility of additional imaging. With the help of an interpreter, we discovered that the patient did not have implants but had injections in her home country. The appearance of the breasts was most consistent with paraffin injections.

TABLE 1.—Appearance of Different Types of Breast Augmentation on Three Imaging Modalities

Type of Augmentation	Mammogram	Ultrasound	MRI
Silicone gel	Extremely dense oval masses	Anechoic with echogenic shell	T2, high signal; T1, low signal; silicone sensitive, high signal
Saline	Dense oval masses with visible folds and valve	Anechoic with echogenic shell	T2, high signal; T1, low signal; silicone sensitive, low signal
Free silicone liquid	Multiple extremely dense globular masses	Mixed hypoechoic, anechoic, and hyperechoic masses with dirty shadowing	T2, high signal; T1, low signal; silicone sensitive, high signal; no enhancement
Autologous fat	Multiple or single lucent masses with or without rim calcification	Variable: anechoic or complicated cyst; echogenic anterior margin and shadowing; solid hypoechoic mass	T2, high signal; T1, high signal; suppresses with fat suppression; with or without peripheral enhancement
Polyacrylamide gel	Single or multiple fluid density masses	Hypoechoic cysts with internal echoes	T2, high signal with foci of low signal; T1, low signal; silicone sensitive, low signal; with or without peripheral enhancement

This article provides a helpful review of the mammographic, sonographic, and MRI characteristics of different types of breast augmentation, including silicone, saline, polyacrylamide gel, and autologous fat augmentation.

T. W. Stephens, MD

Prosthetic Breast Implant Rupture: Imaging—Pictorial Essay

Colombo G, Ruvolo V, Stifanese R, et al (Koru Day Clinic Ctr, AL, Italy; Univ of Genoa, Italy; et al)
Aesthetic Plast Surg 35:891-900, 2011

In recent years, requests for breast implant surgery have occurred for several reasons. First, the number of diagnosed breast cancer cases has increased, and the number of reconstructive surgeries consequently has multiplied. Second, the number of patients who constantly try to achieve a better physical shape, corresponding in Western countries to the common image of prosperous and tonic breasts, has proliferated. These circumstances have led to an increasingly frequent need for more accurate and sophisticated imaging methods to study prosthetic breast implants and their integrity. Diagnostic imaging for the study of patients with suspected breast implant ruptures uses different techniques of radiologic investigation such as mammography and ultrasonography, even if the current gold standard is magnetic resonance imaging (MRI). This study aimed to draw attention to the main MRI signs capable of highlighting contractures or ruptures of the implants that are not always clinically detectable and thus to provide plastic surgeons with an adequate instrument for discerning any possible alterations in prosthetic implants. Furthermore, it was necessary to stress the importance of teamwork. In fact, proper cooperation and coordination between radiologists and dedicated plastic surgeons are fundamental for the proper management of patients and the complications they may experience.

▶ The increases in the number of breast cancer diagnoses and the increased number of women desiring breast cosmesis have increased the frequency of reconstructive breast plastic surgeries. The increases in surgeries have led to an increase in the amount of breast imaging studies for the evaluation of breast implants.

This article predominantly reviews the MRI features consistent with implant contractions or ruptures in single-lumen silicone implants and double-lumen saline (outer chamber)/silicone (inner chamber) implants. The authors also discuss the use of mammography and ultrasound in the evaluation of the integrity of implants.

It is important that we breast imagers are aware of the imaging features of intact and ruptured implants, so that we may assist our surgical colleagues in the proper management of our patients with breast implants.

T. W. Stephens, MD

The Augmented Breast: A Pictorial Review of the Abnormal and Unusual
Yang N, Muradali D (St Michael's Hosp, Toronto, Ontario, Canada)
AJR Am J Roentgenol 196:W451-W460, 2011

Objective.—This article reviews the multimodality imaging features of breast augmentation complications as well as appearances of unusual breast augmentation techniques.

Conclusion.—Cosmetic breast augmentation is an increasingly common procedure performed in our society. Although breast prosthesis implantation is the most common technique, other unusual techniques such as autologous fat implantation as well as direct liquid silicone and paraffin injections have also been used.

▶ Breast augmentation is the most common cosmetic surgical procedure performed in women. In 2010, there were about 300 000 procedures, which is an increase of 2% from 2009. Breast augmentations with silicone and saline implants are fairly straightforward for most breast imagers and for clinicians. Unusual and atypical techniques of breast augmentation, such as injections of foreign body substances, may limit the physical examination and may be difficult to interpret on breast imaging, both of which may lead to a delay in the diagnosis of breast cancer. It is important for radiologists to be aware of the abnormal and unusual features associated with breast augmentation.

T. W. Stephens, MD

Breast MRI

Background enhancement in breast MR: Correlation with breast density in mammography and background echotexture in ultrasound
Ko ES, Lee BH, Choi HY, et al (Korea Cancer Ctr Hosp, Nowon-Gu, Seoul, Republic of Korea; Gyeongsang Natl Univ Hosp, Jinju, Republic of Korea; et al)
Eur J Radiol 80:719-723, 2011

Objective.—This study aimed to determine whether background enhancement on MR was related to mammographic breast density or ultrasonographic background echotexture in premenopausal and postmenopausal women.

Materials and Methods.—We studied 142 patients (79 premenopausal, 63 postmenopausal) who underwent mammography, ultrasonography, and breast MR. We reviewed the mammography for overall breast density of the contralateral normal breast according to the four-point scale of the BI-RADS classification. Ultrasound findings were classified as homogeneous or heterogeneous background echotexture according to the BI-RADS lexicon. We rated background enhancement on a contralateral breast MR into four categories based on subtraction images: absent, mild, moderate, and marked. All imaging findings were interpreted independently by two readers without knowledge of menstrual status, imaging findings of other modalities.

Results.—There were significant differences between the premenopausal and postmenopausal group in distribution of mammographic breast density, ultrasonographic background echotexture, and degree of background enhancement. Regarding the relationship between mammographic density and background enhancement, there was no significant correlation. There was significant relationship between ultrasonographic background echotexture and background enhancement in both premenopausal and postmenopausal groups.

Conclusion.—There is a significant correlation between ultrasonographic background echotexture and background enhancement in MR regardless of menopausal status. Interpreting breast MR, or scheduling for breast MR of women showing heterogeneous background echotexture needs more caution.

▶ Breast magnetic resonance imaging (MRI) is an important tool for breast cancer detection. Current indications for breast MRI include extent of disease in patients with newly diagnosed breast cancer, screening of women at high risk, evaluation of patients with metastatic axillary adenocarcinoma and unknown primary site of malignancy, and assessment of silicone breast implant integrity.

Sure, breast MRI can find lesions that are clinically, mammographically, and sonographically occult, but what about the background enhancement? Can we use what we already know about breast density in mammography and background echotexture in ultrasound? That is what these authors asked.

First, breast tissue enhances on MRI. Sometimes it appears that everything is enhancing. Background enhancement is normal enhancement of breast tissue.

Usually background enhancement is symmetrical and bilateral. Background enhancement may decrease the sensitivity of MRI and may increase false-positive results. In fact, sometimes it is difficult to differentiate normal breast tissue enhancement from a true enhancing lesion. Background enhancement is usually categorized into 4 groups; absent or minimal, mild, moderate, and marked or severe.

You would think that the denser the breast tissue is on mammography, the more intense the enhancement would be on MRI. This was not confirmed by these authors or by Cubuk et al.[1] In fact, neither group found a relationship between background enhancement and breast density in either premenopausal or post-menopausal women. So if a woman has a mammographically dense breast (heterogeneously dense or extremely dense), there may be absent or minimal background enhancement on MRI and vice versa. The density of the breast on mammography does not predict the background enhancement on MRI.

The authors did find a statistically significant correlation between ultrasound background echotexture and background enhancement on MRI. Women with heterogeneous background echotexture displayed a higher degree of background enhancement. A higher degree of background enhancement can be associated with false-negative or false-positive results. So what does this mean? The authors recommend that interpreting or scheduling breast MRI of women showing heterogeneous background echotexture needs to be done with more caution. I would also recommend that when you encounter a higher degree of background enhancement on breast MRI, you review the breast ultrasound scan to determine if the background breast echotexture is heterogeneous. Please also review the prior mammograms carefully too, but if the background breast echotexture is heterogeneous, remember the authors' recommendation.

T. W. Stephens, MD

Reference

1. Cubuk R, Tasali N, Narin B, Keskiner F, Celik L, Guney S. Correlation between breast density in mammography and background enhancement in MR mammography. *Radiol Med.* 2010;115(3):434-441.

Nonmasslike Enhancement at Breast MR Imaging: The Added Value of Mammography and US for Lesion Categorization
Thomassin-Naggara I, Trop I, Chopier J, et al (Centre Hospitalo-Universitaire de Montréal, Canada; Université Pierre et Marie Curie, Paris, France)
Radiology 261:69-79, 2011

Purpose.—To determine the value of adding conventional imaging (mammography and ultrasonography [US]) to nonmasslike enhancement (NMLE) analysis with breast magnetic resonance (MR) imaging for predicting malignancy and for building an interpretation model incorporating all imaging modalities.

Materials and Methods.—The institutional ethics committees approved the study and granted a waiver of informed consent. In 115 women (mean age, 48.3 years; range, 21–76 years; 56 malignant, 12 high–risk, and 63 benign lesions), 131 NMLE lesions were analyzed. Two independent readers first classified MR images by using descriptive Breast Imaging Reporting and Data System (BI-RADS) criteria (BI-RADS classification with MR images alone [BI-RADS$_{MR}$]) and later repeated this classification, adding information from conventional imaging (BI-RADS classification with combination of MR images and conventional images [BI-RADS$_{MR+Con}$]). Lesion diagnosis was established with surgical histopathologic findings ($n = 68$), percutaneous biopsy results ($n = 25$), or 2 years of stability at MR imaging ($n = 38$). Receiver operating characteristic curves were built to compare BI-RADS$_{MR}$ with BI-RADS$_{MR+Con}$. A multivariate interpretation model was constructed and validated in a distinct cohort of 44 women.

Results.—Values for inter- and intraobserver agreement, respectively, were better for BI-RADS$_{MR+Con}$ ($\kappa = 0.847$ and 0.937) than for BI-RADS$_{MR}$ ($\kappa = 0.748$ and 0.861). For both readers, the areas under the receiver operating characteristic curve (AUCs) for diagnosis of malignancy were also superior when BI-RADS$_{MR+Con}$ (AUC $= 0.91$ [reader 1] and 0.93 [reader 2]) was compared with BI-RADS$_{MR}$ (AUC $= 0.84$ [reader 1] and 0.87 [reader 2]) ($P < .05$). An interpretation model combining conventional imaging with MR imaging criteria showed very good discrimination (AUC $= 0.89$ [training set] and 0.90 [validating set]).

Conclusion.—Adding conventional imaging to NMLE lesion characterization at breast MR imaging improved the diagnostic performance of radiologists, and the interpretation model used offers good accuracy with the potential to optimize the reproducibility of NMLE analysis at MR imaging.

▶ Breast MRI is an important tool for breast cancer detection. Current indications for breast MRI include extent of disease in patients with newly diagnosed breast cancer, screening of women at high risk, evaluation of patients with metastatic axillary adenocarcinoma and unknown primary site of malignancy, and assessment of silicone breast implant integrity.

I enjoy breast MRI...even the difficult cases...many of which involve non-masslike enhancement (NMLE). NMLE as defined by the American College of Radiology Breast Imaging Reporting and Data System (BI-RADS) lexicon is an area of enhancement without an associated mass. There is an overlap in the breast MRI features of benign and malignant NMLE. Segmental or clumped, linear, and ductal NMLE may be an imaging manifestation of ductal carcinoma in situ and benign lesions such as chronic mammary ductal ectasia and sclerosing adenosis.

The authors hypothesized that additional information gathered from clinical examination and from first-look and second-look conventional imaging (mammography and sonography) should improve MRI specificity in the analysis of NMLE. The additional information will lead to improved lesion characterization.

This study showed that for mammography, a positive correlate to an NMLE lesion was the identification of a mass, a distortion, an asymmetric density, or more than 3 not clearly benign calcifications in the territory of the NMLE. For ultrasonography (US), positive correlate to an NMLE lesion was the identification of a mass, an architectural distortion, or duct changes in the region of the NMLE.

The authors found that the most significant features predictive of malignancy at MRI were the presence of corresponding microcalcifications at mammography in the territory of NMLE (classified as BI-RADS category 4 or 5), segmental distribution, the presence of an ipsilateral suspicious mass, size greater than 31 mm, the presence of US abnormalities, and the presence of associated clinical symptoms.

The addition of conventional imaging findings to their interpretation model improved the analysis of NMLE. The detection of calcifications in the territory of NMLE becomes the most predictive feature of malignancy when the NMLE is greater than 20 mm. In the authors' experience, when not clearly benign calcifications are identified in the region of the NMLE, a biopsy must be performed even if the calcifications do not directly conform to the NMLE. The authors' model shows the added value of US in the analysis of NMLE. When there are no mammographically detected calcifications and when the NMLE displays a focal, linear, ductal, or regional distribution in women older than 45 years, a US correlate for the NMLE is associated with a greater risk of malignancy.

This article reminds us that the best interpretation of breast MRI occurs with review of prior mammograms and breast ultrasounds.

T. W. Stephens, MD

Follow-up Care

Use of BI-RADS 3—Probably Benign Category in the American College of Radiology Imaging Network Digital Mammographic Imaging Screening Trial

Baum JK, Hanna LG, Acharyya S, et al (Cambridge Health Alliance, MA; Brown Univ, Providence, RI; et al)
Radiology 260:61-67, 2011

Purpose.—To determine *(a)* how often the Breast Imaging Reporting and Data System (BI-RADS) category 3 was used in the American College of Radiology Imaging Network (ACRIN) Digital Mammographic Imaging Screening Trial (DMIST), either at the time of screening mammography or after work-up, *(b)* how often subjects actually returned for the recommended follow-up examination, and *(c)* the rate and stages of any malignancies subsequently found in subjects for whom short-term interval follow-up was recommended.

Materials and Methods.—This study was approved by the Institutional Review Board at all institutions where subjects were enrolled. All subjects participating in DMIST gave informed consent and the study was HIPAA-compliant. A total of 47 599 DMIST-eligible and evaluable subjects, all of whom consented to undergo both digital and screen-film mammography, were included in this analysis. Cases referred for short-term interval follow-up based on digital, screen-film, or both imaging examinations were determined. Compliance with the recommendations and the final outcome (malignancy diagnosis at biopsy or no malignancy confirmed through follow-up) of each evaluable case were determined.

Results.—A total of 1114 of the 47 599 (2.34%) subjects had tumors assigned a BI-RADS 3 category and were recommended to undergo short-interval follow-up. In this study, 791 of 1114 (71%) of the subjects were compliant with the recommendation and returned for short-interval follow-up. Of the women who did not return for short-interval follow-up, 70% (226 of 323) did return for their next annual mammography. Among all subjects whose tumors were assigned a BI-RADS 3 category either at screening mammography or after additional work-up, nine of 1114 (0.81%) were found to have cancer. Of the nine biopsy-proved cancers, six were invasive cancers and three were ductal carcinoma in situ stage Tis—T1c. The invasive cancers were all less than 2 cm in size.

Conclusion.—In DMIST, radiologists used the BI-RADS 3 classification infrequently (2.3% of patients). Tumors assigned a BI-RADS 3 category had a low rate of malignancy. The relatively high rate of noncompliance with short-interval follow-up recommendations (323 of 1114, or 29%) supports prior recommendations that radiologists thoroughly evaluate lesions before placing them in this category.

▶ In the article, Timeliness of Follow-up after Abnormal Screening Mammogram: Variability of Facilities, Rosenberg et al[1] found that when additional imaging (BI-RADS 0) or biopsies (BI-RADS 4 or 5) were recommended, patients returned in a timely fashion. One of the purposes of this study was to determine how often subjects actually returned for the recommended follow-up examination (BI-RADS 3). The authors found a relatively high rate of noncompliance with short-interval follow-up recommendations (323 of 1114 or 29%). So, bottom line, radiologists should thoroughly evaluate lesions carefully and should only place lesions with probability of malignancy less than 2% in category BI-RADS 3.

T. W. Stephens, MD

Reference

1. Rosenberg RD, Haneuse SJ, Geller BM; For Breast Cancer Surveillance Consortium. Timeliness of follow-up after abnormal screening mammogram: variability of facilities. *Radiology.* 2011;261:404-413.

Timeliness of Follow-up after Abnormal Screening Mammogram: Variability of Facilities
Rosenberg RD, For the Breast Cancer Surveillance Consortium (Univ of New Mexico-HSC, Albuquerque; et al)
Radiology 261:404-413, 2011

Purpose.—To describe the timeliness of follow-up care in community-based settings among women who receive a recommendation for immediate follow-up during the screening mammography process and how follow-up timeliness varies according to facility and facility-level characteristics.

Materials and Methods.—This was an institutional review board—approved and HIPAA-compliant study. Screening mammograms obtained from 1996 to 2007 in women 40–80 years old in the Breast Cancer Surveillance Consortium were examined. Inclusion criteria were a recommendation for immediate follow-up at screening, or subsequent imaging, and observed follow-up within 180 days of the recommendation. Recommendations for additional imaging (AI) and biopsy or surgical consultation (BSC) were analyzed separately. The distribution of time to follow-up care was estimated by using the Kaplan-Meier estimator.

Results.—Data were available on 214 897 AI recommendations from 118 facilities and 35 622 BSC recommendations from 101 facilities. The median time to subsequent follow-up care after recommendation was 14 days for AI and 16 days for BSC. Approximately 90% of AI follow-up and 81% of BSC follow-up occurred within 30 days. Facilities with higher recall rates tended to have longer AI follow-up times ($P < .001$). Over the study period, BSC follow-up rates at 15 and 30 days improved ($P < .001$). Follow-up times varied substantially across facilities. Timely follow-up was associated with larger volumes of the recommended procedures but not notably associated with facility type nor observed facility-level characteristics.

Conclusion.—Most patients with follow-up returned within 3 weeks of the recommendation.

▶ In the United States, of screened women who are recalled, about 1 in 5 will receive a recommendation for biopsy. How promptly recalled patients go on to further evaluation including biopsy is essential to the success of a screening program. Most recalled patients do not require a biopsy, so a prompt workup evaluation will greatly minimize patient anxiety. Prompt biopsy following a biopsy recommendation has even greater value.

The follow-up process involves several steps, and any of the steps may lead to delays. At screen-only facilities, further workup will need to be performed at another institution. At facilities providing screening and diagnostic mammograms, delays may occur between imaging and interpretation, between interpretation and contacting the patients, and between patient contact and the scheduling of follow-up imaging. The objective of this study was to describe the timeliness of follow-up care in community-based settings among women who received a recommendation for immediate follow-up based on screening mammography recommendation and how follow-up timeliness varies according to facility and facility-level characteristics.

Timeliness was not notably associated with facility type nor observed facility-level characteristics. One consistent characteristic associated with timely follow-up of additional imaging and biopsy or surgical consultation is larger mammography volumes. Time to follow-up varied widely between facilities, suggesting potential for improvement by many facilities. I would recommend that each breast screening mammography facility calculates its timeliness to ensure that most patients undergo follow-up with the minimum standard recommendations of the European guidelines, which is 95% of patients receiving a result within 15 working days and 90% offered the follow-up within 5 working days.

T. W. Stephens, MD

Image Quality

Mammography image quality: Model for predicting compliance with posterior nipple line criterion

Spuur K, Hung WT, Poulos A, et al (Univ of Sydney, New South Wales, Australia; Cancer Inst NSW, Sydney, Australia)

Eur J Radiol 80:713-718, 2011

Purpose.—To develop a model using measurements of pectoral muscle width and length together with the acceptability of the posterior nipple line criteria (PNL) to predict the acceptability of the presentation of the pectoral muscle in the mediolateral oblique view of the breast.

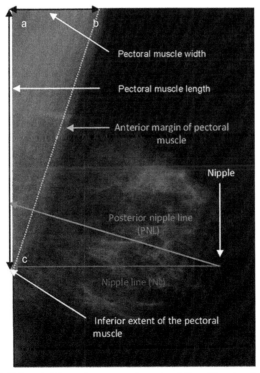

FIGURE 1.—Mediolateral oblique view—pectoral muscle width and length; relationship of pectoral muscle length to PNL and NL. The line b–c represents the anterior border of the pectoral muscle. *Source*: Private collection K. Spuur. (Reprinted from Spuur K, Hung WT, Poulos A, et al. Mammography image quality: model for predicting compliance with posterior nipple line criterion. *Eur J Radiol.* 2011;80:713-718, with permission from Elsevier Ireland.)

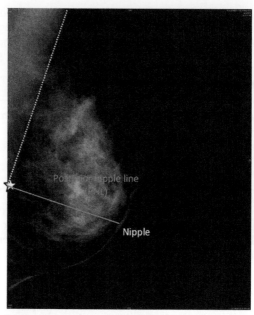

FIGURE 2.—Mediolateral oblique view—relationship of the inferior aspect of the pectoral muscle to the PNL in acceptable images. When the PNL is at the level of the inferior aspect of the pectoral muscle the image is acceptable. *Source*: Private collection K. Spuur. (Reprinted from European Journal of Radiology. Spuur K, Hung WT, Poulos A, et al. Mammography image quality: model for predicting compliance with posterior nipple line criterion. *Eur J Radiol.* 2011;80:713-718, with permission from Elsevier.)

Method.—A total of 400 mediolateral oblique mammogram images were randomly selected from BreastScreen NSW South West, Australia. Measurements of length and width of the pectoral muscle and the acceptability of the pectoral muscle position relative to the PNL were recorded. Data analysis involved logistic regression and ROC analysis to test the predictors of width and length and the performance of the model. The model was then used to predict the outcome of acceptable or unacceptable PNL criterion for each case.

Results.—The estimated odds ratio for an increase of 10 mm was 1.98 (CI = 1.68, 2.34) for the length predictor and 2.14 (CI = 1.56, 2.93) for the width predictor. A cut off point of 0.6083 was derived from the training set and applied with the developed model to the test set. The area under the ROC curve was 0.9339 demonstrating an accurate model.

Conclusion.—This paper describes a model to predict the acceptability of the PNL criterion using the width and length of the pectoral muscle. This model could be used in the automated assessment of image quality which has the potential to enhance the consistency in mammographic image quality evaluation. Optimising image quality contributes to increased accuracy in radiological interpretation, which maximises the early detection of breast cancer and potentially reduces mortality rates (Figs 1 and 2).

▶ During my oral boards I was asked about the posterior nipple line (PNL). The PNL may be defined as a reference line drawn from the nipple at right angles to the anterior aspect of the pectoralis muscle contour or to the back of the image, whichever comes first, or as a reference line 10 mm above or below the inferior aspect of the pectoralis muscle.

This study used measurements of width and length in conjunction with the acceptability of the PNL criteria to develop an automated model that predicts the acceptability of the imaging to the pectoralis muscle relative to the PNL. This model could be used as an automated assessment of mammographic image quality of the mediolateral oblique view. An automated assessment has the potential to reduce subjective evaluation of image quality.

This article is an excellent reminder of the importance of high-quality mammography. High-quality mammography is essential for the early detection of breast cancer.

T. W. Stephens, MD

Screening Mammography

Accuracy of Screening Mammography in Older Women

Sinclair N, Littenberg B, Geller B, et al (Brown Univ, Providence, RI; Univ of Vermont School of Medicine, Burlington; Univ of Vermont, Burlington; et al)
AJR Am J Roentgenol 197:1268-1273, 2011

Objective.—The objective of our study was to determine the accuracy and cancer detection rate of screening mammography in women as they age.

Materials and Methods.—Using data from the Vermont Breast Cancer Surveillance System (1996–2006), we calculated the sensitivity, specificity, positive predictive value, negative predictive value, and cancer detection rate by decade of age for 403,448 mammograms of 96,193 women 50–101 years old. Confounding variables were assessed using logistic regression analysis.

Results.—The sensitivity of screening mammography increased from 77.3% for the 50-to 59-year-old group to 93.8% for the 90- to 101-year-old group ($p = 0.015$). Specificity increased from 98.7% to 98.8% at age 50–59 compared with age 90–101 ($p < 0.001$), respectively. The cancer detection rate increased from 3.7 cases per 1000 mammograms at age 50–59 to 14.4 cases per 1000 mammograms at age 90–101 ($p < 0.001$). The prevalence of breast cancer increased from 4.8% to 15.4% across age groups ($p < 0.001$) as did the positive predictive value from 22.2% to 55.6% ($p < 0.001$). There was no evidence of confounding by body mass index, breast density, or other factors. Tumors were more likely to be small, hormone receptor—positive, and more invasive as women aged. Accuracy parameters were all associated with age without evidence of confounding by regression analysis.

Conclusion.—Screening mammography is more accurate in older women than in younger women, suggesting that it may be of value in assessing women in all age groups. These data do not address the impact of mammography screening on mortality or breast cancer outcomes.

▶ Just this week I read the mammogram of an active 71-year-old woman. I met her at the gym and never knew her age. She is vivacious and full of love for life that some 20-year-old people don't have. Then there is the 82-year-old woman whose needle localization I did. She informed me that the key secret to long life is having children after age 40 years. Smile. So it is for these 2 ladies that I read this article with much interest.

The data from this study showed that mammography for breast cancer screening among women older than 70 years seems to detect smaller, earlier-stage, invasive rather than noninvasive, receptor-positive tumors.

The authors found that screening mammography is more accurate in older women than in younger women. This finding suggests that mammography may be valuable in assessing women of all ages. The authors recommend discussing the potential benefits of mammography screening with women older than 65 years with reasonable life expectancy.

So I guess I can look forward to an annual mammogram when I'm 100 years old.

T. W. Stephens, MD

Mammography in 40-Year-Old Women: What Difference Does It Make? The Potential Impact of the U.S. Preventative Services Task Force (USPSTF) Mammography Guidelines
Shen N, Hammonds LS, Madsen D, et al (Univ of Missouri School of Medicine, Columbia)
Ann Surg Oncol 18:3066-3071, 2011

Background.—This 10-year retrospective chart review evaluates the potential impact the most recent U.S. Preventative Services Task Force (USPSTF) report recommending against annual mammographic screening of women aged 40–49 years.

Methods.—The medical record database was systematically searched to discover all women aged 40–49 years treated for breast cancer over a 10-year period. These women were separated into 2 cohorts—mammographically detected cancer (MDC) and nonmammographically detected cancer (NMDC). Statistical analysis of the cohorts was performed for family history (FH), sentinel lymph node (SLN) status, tumor size at presentation, and disease-free and overall survival.

Results.—A total of 1581 women were treated for breast cancer; of these, 311 were between the ages of 40 and 49 years with complete diagnostic information, 145 were MDC, and 166 were NMDC. The average tumor diameter of the MDC group was 20.68 mm, which was significantly smaller than that of the NMDC group at 30.38 mm (*P* < .0001). Women with MDC had a significantly lower incidence of SLN positive cancer than the NMDC group, 28 of 113 (24.78%) vs. 85 of 152 (55.92%; *P* < .0001), respectively. The 5-year disease-free survival for both groups was MDC 94% (95% confidence interval [95% CI], 87–97%) and NMDC 71% (95% CI 62–78%). The overall 5-year survival estimates were MDC 97% (95% CI 92–99%) and NMDC 78% (95% CI 69–85%), respectively.

Conclusion.—This review demonstrates the significance of mammographic screening for early detection and treatment of breast cancer. Mammographic screening in women aged 40–49 detected smaller tumors with less nodal metastasis, resulting in improved survival, which supports annual mammographic screening in this age group.

▶ A 40-year-old women's lifetime risk for breast cancer development is 1 in 8 (12.5%), and her risk of breast cancer development over the next 10 years is 1 in 69 (1.44%). The mortality rates of breast cancer have decreased since 1990, and this mortality rate decrease has been attributed to screening mammography.

The U.S. Preventative Services Task Force (USPSTF) gave screening mammography in women 40 to 49 a grade B recommendation in 2002. In 2009, the task force felt that the harms of screening in women in this age group outweighed the benefits of early detection and early intervention, so the USPSTF recommended against screening mammography in women 40 to 49, which is a grade C recommendation.

The authors compared cancers detected by mammography and nonmammographically detected cancers. This study's results found that mammographic screening in women age 40 to 49 detected smaller tumors with less nodal metastasis, which results in improved survival (Table 1 in original article). These findings support annual mammography and challenges publications suggesting that better treatment and breast cancer awareness, not screening mammography, are responsible for the declines in breast cancer mortality.

T. W. Stephens, MD

Screen-detected breast cancer: Does presence of minimal signs on prior mammograms predict staging or grading of cancer?
Bansal GJ, Thomas KG (Univ Hosp of Wales, Cardiff, UK; Breast Test Wales, Cardiff, UK)
Clin Radiol 66:605-608, 2011

Aim.—To investigate whether the presence of minimal signs on prior mammograms predict staging or grading of cancer.

Materials and Methods.—The previous mammograms of 148 consecutive patients with screen-detected breast cancer were examined. Women with an abnormality visible (minimal signs) on both current and prior mammograms formed the study group; the remaining patients formed the control group. Age, average size of tumour, tumour characteristic, histopathology, grade, and lymph node status were compared between the two groups, using Fisher's exact test. Cases in which earlier diagnosis would have made a significant prognostic difference were also evaluated.

Results.—Eighteen percent of patients showed an abnormality at the site of the tumour on previous mammograms. There was no statistically significant difference between the two groups with respect to age, average size of tumour, histopathology, grade or lymph node status with p-values being 0.609, 0.781, 0.938, and 0.444, respectively. The only statistically significant difference between the two groups was tumour characteristics with more microcalcifications associated with either mass or asymmetrical density seen in the study group ($p = 0.003$). Five patients in the study group showed lymph node positivity and were grade 3, and therefore, may have had possible gain from earlier diagnosis.

Conclusion.—The present study did not demonstrate a statistical difference in grading or staging between the group that showed "minimal signs" on prior mammograms versus normal prior mammograms. Microcalcification seems to be the most common characteristic seen in the missed cancer and a more aggressive management approach is suggested for breast microcalcifications.

▶ Learning about minimal signs can enhance our performance in reading screening mammograms and can improve the sensitivity of screening mammography for breast malignancy. For the purpose of this study, the following criteria were used for minimal signs on prior mammograms: vague densities, subtle architectural distortion or asymmetric density, subtle clustered microcalcifications, or a combination of these findings.

False-negative mammograms can lead to a delay in the detection of breast cancer, so it is of the utmost importance that we decrease our number of false-negative mammograms by reducing our errors of perception and interpretation.

In the present study, about 18% of the screen-detected cancers showed minimal signs on prior mammograms. Although, in general, cancer with prior minimal signs did not show favorable staging or grading (the study did not show a statistical difference in grading or staging between the group that showed minimal signs on prior mammograms and the group that showed normal prior mammograms), microcalcifications associated with masses or asymmetric densities seem to be the most significant characteristic on prior mammograms. The authors recommend a more aggressive management approach for breast microcalcifications.

Familiarity with minimal signs and an appropriate management approach are recommended for the diagnosis of these lesions to avoid subsequent diagnosis of high-grade advanced cancer.

T. W. Stephens, MD

Breast surgical specimen radiographs: How reliable are they?
Britton PD, Sonoda LI, Yamamoto AK, et al (Cambridge Univ Hosps NHS Foundation Trust, Cambridge, UK)
Eur J Radiol 79:245-249, 2011

Radiography of the excised surgical specimen following wire guided localisation of impalpable breast lesions is standard surgical practice. The aims of the study were to establish the reliability of the breast specimen radiograph (SR) in determining lesion excision and to determine whether the radiographic margin correlated with the histological margin.

The clinical, imaging, SR and pathological details of 106 patients with a pre-operative diagnosis of breast cancer were retrospectively reviewed. The reliability of orientation was estimated and the appearance and distance from the mammographic abnormality to each radial margin were measured and correlated with surgical histological findings.

The overall accuracy of the specimen radiograph in determining whether the mammographic lesion was present was 99%. The SR could be orientated "very reliably" or "reliably" in 80% of patients, however in only 48% of patients did the closest margin on the SR correspond with the same nearest margin at final histology. A maximum measurement of 11 mm or more from the lesion to the specimen edge was associated with a 77% likelihood of having a clear final histological margin (taken as 5 mm or more) and if <11 mm a 58% chance of having involved final histological margins. There was however a wide overlap in the results with patients having an apparently wide SR margin but histologically involved margins and vice versa.

The SR is reliable at determining whether the target lesion has been removed. The correlation of SR margin orientation and measurement with final histological measurement is however far less reliable.

▶ The aims of this study were to examine whether breast specimen radiographs may reliably determine lesion excision and to evaluate radiologic/histopathological correlation of specimen margins.

If a lesion is mammographically visible, it stands to reason that it will be visible on the specimen radiograph. The authors' findings confirmed this. At our institution, we also perform specimen radiographs of mammographically occult lesions, some of which will be visible on specimen radiograph after excision. The now mammographically visible lesions are believed to be visible because of the removal of overlapping breast parenchyma.

Radiologic/histopathological correlation is essential to achieving tumor-free margins. At our institution, the surgeons orient the specimen for the specimen radiograph. Once the specimen margins are labeled, we radiologists review the radiographs with our pathology and surgical colleagues. If we are concerned about close radiologic margins, our surgical colleagues will obtain more breast tissue from the surgical cavity.

Interestingly, these authors' data showed that although the vast majority of specimen radiographs were believed to be reliably orientated, in only slightly less than half of cases did the close margin on the specimen radiograph correspond with the same nearest margin on final histology.

The authors found that when the edge of a lesion on a specimen radiograph is ill defined, the most reliable results are obtained by taking the maximum distance from the edge of the specimen to the closest, unequivocal site of a lesion.

The authors concluded that the maximum measurement to the specimen edge of 11 mm or more corresponded to a greater likelihood of a clear histological margin.

Obtaining tumor-free margins is a collaborative effort among pathologists, surgeons, and radiologists. The closer we work together, the better the final results for our patients.

T. W. Stephens, MD

Patient Perceptions

Attitudes of women in their forties toward the 2009 USPSTF mammogram guidelines: a randomized trial on the effects of media exposure
Davidson AS, Liao X, Magee BD (Univ of Massachusetts Med School, Worcester)
Am J Obstet Gynecol 205:30.e1-30.e7, 2011

Objective.—The objective of the study was to assess women's attitudes toward 2009 US Preventive Services Task Force mammography screening guideline changes and evaluate the role of media in shaping opinions.

Study Design.—Two hundred forty-nine women, aged 39-49 years, presenting for annual examinations randomized to read 1 of 2 articles, and survey completion comprised the design of the study.

Results.—Eighty-eight percent overestimated the lifetime breast cancer (BrCa) risk. Eighty-nine percent want yearly mammograms in their 40s. Eighty-six percent felt the changes were unsafe, and even if the changes were doctor recommended, 84% would not delay screening until age 50 years. Those with a friend/relative with BrCa were more likely to want annual mammography in their forties (92% vs 77%, $P = .001$), and feel changes unsafe (91% vs 69%, $P \leq .0001$). Participants with previous false-positive mammograms were less likely to accept doctor-recommended screening delay until age 50 years (8% vs 21%, $P = .01$).

Conclusion.—Women overestimate BrCa risk. Skepticism of new mammogram guidelines exists, and is increased by exposure to negative media. Those with prior false-positive mammograms are less likely to accept changes.

▶ It has been about a year since the US Preventive Services Task Force (USPSTF) published its updated mammogram screening guideline recommendations. The recommendations generated much controversy and many questions. The authors of this article ask 3 questions: Are women's attitudes influenced by the popular media? What personal factors may affect their attitudes? How are the new recommendations being received?

So what did the authors conclude? Most women in the study overestimated their risk of getting breast cancer. The majority of the participants did not feel that the new guidelines were safe, and the majority did not intend to follow the guidelines, even with their doctor's recommendation. Of the patients who felt that the new guidelines were safe, nearly half did not intend to delay the onset of regular mammograms. Seventy-six percent of patients in their 40s had friends or family members with breast cancer, and the majority of these women felt that they should personally continue to have yearly mammograms. These findings show that the public interprets health policy in relation to their personal experiences. The USPSTF concluded that psychological harm from false-positives is a major risk of screening mammography. The present study showed that patients were more likely to see the additional imaging and resultant biopsy(ies) associated with a false-positive mammogram as a near miss rather than a false alarm.

So, bottom line, patients do not plan to delay the onset of regular mammograms, and if they are recalled for additional imaging with a resultant biopsy with benign result, they will view the event as a near miss rather than a false alarm.

T. W. Stephens, MD

Postneoadjuvant Pathologic Tumor Response

Accuracy of Clinical Examination, Digital Mammogram, Ultrasound, and MRI in Determining Postneoadjuvant Pathologic Tumor Response in Operable Breast Cancer Patients
Croshaw R, Shapiro-Wright H, Svensson E, et al (Allegheny General Hosp, Pittsburgh, PA; St Clare Hosp, Fenton, MO)
Ann Surg Oncol 18:3160-3163, 2011

Background.—To determine the accuracy, positive predictive value (PPV), and negative predictive value (NPV) of clinical examination and breast imaging techniques in determining pathologic complete response in patients with locally advanced breast cancer after neoadjuvant therapy.

Methods.—A retrospective review was performed of data collected from patients treated with either neoadjuvant hormonal or chemotherapy between January 2005 and September 2010. Patients were evaluated by one of three surgical breast oncologists before neoadjuvant therapy and within 1 month before surgery by clinical breast examination (CBE), digital mammogram, breast ultrasound, and/or magnetic resonance imaging (MRI). The accuracy, NPV, and PPV of each modality was calculated on the basis of the final pathologic report. Available data from the literature was synthesized.

Results.—Sixty-two tumors in 61 patients with a mean age of 56 (range 34—87) years were evaluated. Overall accuracy ranged from 54% (CBE) to 80% (breast ultrasound). All modalities had a PPV greater than 75% for identifying the presence of residual disease. The PPV of each modality was generally higher in the younger patients. The NPV of all methods was less than 50%. The accuracy and NPV were compromised even further in younger patients. The combination of our own data with data available from the literature revealed MRI to be superior with regard to accuracy and PPV, but the NPV of MRIs remained poor at 65%.

Conclusions.—All measured tests are good at predicting the presence of disease on final pathology, but none are able to reliably predict a pathologic complete response.

▶ Will imaging ever replace breast surgery in the evaluation of patients with locally advanced breast cancer after neoadjuvant chemotherapy? Is surgery always necessary?

This study evaluated the accuracy, positive predictive value (PPV), and negative predictive value (NPV) of clinical examination and breast imaging (mammography, ultrasound [US], MRI) in determining pathologic complete response (pCR) in patients with locally advanced breast cancer after neoadjuvant chemotherapy.

The authors found that mammography, US, and MRI all have the ability to reliably predict the presence of disease on final pathology in patients younger and older than 50 years. Therefore, a positive result by any modality does not likely need to be confirmed before surgical intervention. Although MRI is the most accurate imaging modality in determining the presence or absence of disease on final pathology, it is still not reliable in predicting a pCR because its NPV is 65%. No other imaging modality had an NPV greater than 50%.

Although at this time imaging is not reliable enough to confirm a pCR, breast imagers and breast imaging play an important role in the evaluation of breast tumor response to neoadjuvant chemotherapy.

T. W. Stephens, MD

Post-Surgical Breast

Lower sensitivity of screening mammography after previous benign breast surgery

van Breest Smallenburg V, Duijm LEM, Voogd AC, et al (Catharina Hosp, Eindhoven, The Netherlands; Comprehensive Cancer Centre South (IKZ)/ Eindhoven Cancer Registry, The Netherlands; et al)
Int J Cancer 130:122-128, 2012

Few data are available on the effect of previous benign breast surgery on screening mammography accuracy. We determined whether sensitivity of screening mammography and tumor characteristics are different for women with and without previous benign breast surgery. We included a consecutive series of 317,398 screening mammograms of women screened between 1997 and 2008. During 2-year follow-up, clinical data, breast imaging, biopsy and surgery reports were collected from women with screen-detected or interval breast cancers. Screening sensitivity, tumor biology and tumor stages were compared between 168 women with breast cancer and prior ipsilateral benign breast surgery and 2,039 women with breast cancer but without previous ipsilateral, benign breast surgery. The sensitivity of screening mammography was significantly lower for women with prior surgery [64.3% (108/168) *versus* 73.4% (1,496/2,039), $p = 0.01$]. The concomitant increased interval cancer risk remained significant after logistic regression adjustment for age and breast density (OR = 1.5, 95% CI: 1.1–2.1). Comparing screen-detected cancers in women with and without prior breast surgery, no significant differences in estrogen receptor status ($p = 0.56$), mitotic activity ($p = 0.17$), proportions of large (T2+) tumors ($p = 0.6$) or lymph node positive tumors ($p = 0.4$) were found. Also for interval cancers, no differences were found in estrogen receptor status ($p = 0.41$), mitotic activity ($p = 0.39$), proportions of large tumors ($p = 0.9$) and lymph node positive tumors ($p = 0.5$) between women with and without prior breast surgery. We conclude that sensitivity of screening mammography is significantly lower in women with previous benign breast surgery than without, but tumor characteristics are comparable both for screen detected cancers and interval cancers.

▶ This interesting study from the Netherlands determined whether the sensitivity of screening mammography and tumor characteristics are different for women who have had previous benign breast surgery and for women who have not.

The authors did not find significant differences in estrogen receptor status, mitotic activity, proportions of large tumors, or lymph node status between screen-detected and intervals cancer in women with and without prior benign breast surgery. The authors did find in women with prior benign breast surgery that sensitivity of screening mammography is significantly lower.

Two other articles have addressed the effect of previous benign breast surgery on screening mammography.[1,2] Banks et al[1] found a borderline significantly lower sensitivity after breast surgery for a condition other than breast cancer. Taplin et al[2] found a significantly lower specificity after previous benign breast surgery but no difference in sensitivity.

The screening intervals are different among the studies. I think the difference is reflective in the differing results of the 3 studies. The Banks et al study[1] from the United Kingdom used a 3-year screening interval, the Taplin et al article[2] from the United States used annual screening mammography, and these authors from the Netherlands used a biennial screening interval.

The authors acknowledge that the difference in the screening interval among all 3 studies limits comparison with this study. I would like to see additional studies that study the effect of previous benign breast surgery on screening mammograms. But in the meantime I would recommend that, given the results of this study, breast imagers more carefully evaluate screening mammograms in patients with previous benign breast surgeries.

T. W. Stephens, MD

References

1. Banks E, Reeves G, Beral V, et al. Influence of personal characteristics of individual women on sensitivity and specificity of mammography in the Million Women Study: cohort study. *BMJ.* 2004;329:477.

2. Taplin SH, Abraham L, Geller BM, et al. Effect of previous benign breast biopsy on the interpretive performance of subsequent screening mammography. *J Natl Cancer Inst.* 2010;102:1040-1051.

Pregnant and Lactating Women

Accuracy of Diagnostic Mammography and Breast Ultrasound During Pregnancy and Lactation

Robbins J, Jeffries D, Roubidoux M, et al (Univ of Wisconsin Hosps and Clinics, Madison; Univ of Michigan Health System, Ann Arbor)
AJR Am J Roentgenol 196:716-722, 2011

Objective.—The purpose of this article is to determine the accuracy of mammography and sonography in evaluating pregnant, lactating, and postpartum women.

Materials and Methods.—We retrospectively reviewed diagnostic breast imaging examinations of 155 pregnant, lactating, and postpartum women with 164 lesions presenting to our breast imaging department from 2004 to 2005. Records were reviewed for clinical presentation, reported sonographic or mammographic findings with BI-RADS assessment, histologic results, and clinical outcomes. Examinations rated as BI-RADS categories 4 and 5 were considered positive. One hundred thirty-four (82%) of 164 lesions had pathology results available or longer than 12 months follow-up in our study group. Of these lesions, 12 (9%) were evaluated by mammography alone, 49 (37%) were evaluated by ultrasound alone, and 73 (54%) were evaluated by both techniques.

Results.—Of 134 lesions, 87 (65%) were in patients who presented during lactation, 34 (25%) who presented during pregnancy, and 13 (10%) who presented postpartum. The presenting symptom for 86 lesions (64%) was a palpable mass. Biopsies were performed for 40 lesions. Of these lesions, four were malignant and 36 were benign. Mammograms were dense or heterogeneously dense in 88% of patients. All four malignancies were BI-RADS category 4 or 5 according to both mammography and ultrasound. For the 85 lesions evaluated with mammography, there was 100% sensitivity, 93% specificity, 40% positive predictive value, and 100% negative predictive value. For the 122 lesions evaluated with sonography, there was 100% sensitivity, 86% specificity, 19% positive predictive value, and 100% negative predictive value.

Conclusion.—Among lactating and pregnant women, both mammography and sonography had a negative predictive value of 100% and accurately revealed the few cancers that were present in our study group.

▶ The majority of the patients in this study were lactating (65%); however, a quarter of the patients were pregnant and it is upon this subset of pregnant patients that I will focus my attention.

There is a bit of consternation with both patients and breast radiologists when it comes to imaging pregnant patients with mammography. Pregnancy-associated breast cancer (PABC) is rare and seen in 1 in 3000 to 10 000 pregnancies. The incidence of PABC is expected to increase as more and more women delay childbearing into and beyond the fourth decade.

The authors found that both mammography and sonography had a negative predictive value of 100% and accurately revealed the few cancers present in this study. While it is well known and widely accepted that sonography may be performed in pregnant patients, there is controversy surrounding the use of mammography in pregnant patients. The National Comprehensive Cancer Network guidelines state that mammography of the breast with shielding can be done safely.[1]

The majority of the pregnant patients in the study were symptomatic; however, a few were undergoing follow-up or routine breast imaging. The most common symptom was a palpable mass. Of the 4 malignancies in this study, 1 was identified in a pregnant patient. All the malignancies showed calcifications on mammography. One of the malignancies was also associated with a mass, another with architectural distortion. Three of the malignancies were seen on ultrasound as a solid mass and 1 was seen as dilated ducts with a solid intraductal component.

A standard formal breast imaging protocol for the evaluation of pregnant and lactating women has not been established. Previous studies[2-4] have shown that ultrasound was more sensitive than mammography in the detection of breast cancer. These authors did not see a difference in the sensitivity of mammography and sonography; however, the study sample size was very small.

More research is necessary to develop a formal breast imaging protocol for the evaluation of pregnant and lactating women. Until a protocol is developed, mammography of the breast with shielding can be done safely in pregnant patients.

T. W. Stephens, MD

References

1. National Comprehensive Cancer Network. *Clinical practice guidelines in oncology: breast cancer.* 2008;Vol 2. Fort Washington, PA: National Comprehensive Cancer Network.
2. Yang WT, Dryden MJ, Gwyn K, Whitman GJ, Theriault R. Imaging of breast cancer diagnosed and treated with chemotherapy during pregnancy. *Radiology.* 2006;239:52-60.
3. Ahn BY, Kim HH, Moon WK, et al. Pregnancy- and lactation-associated breast cancer: mammographic and sonographic findings. *J Ultrasound Med.* 2003;22: 491-497.
4. Liberman L, Giess CS, Dershaw DD, Deutch BM, Petrek JA. Imaging of pregnancy-associated breast cancer. *Radiology.* 1994;191:245-248.

Ultrasound

Complex cystic lesions of the breast on ultrasonography: Feature analysis and BI-RADS assessment

Hsu H-H, Yu J-C, Lee H-S, et al (Tri-Service General Hosp, Taipei, Taiwan, ROC)
Eur J Radiol 79:73-79, 2011

Purpose.—To analyze the features of breast complex cystic lesions at ultrasonography (US) and to determine appropriate Breast Imaging

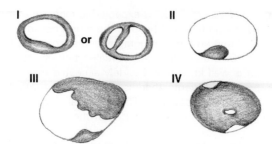

FIGURE 1.—Schema of the four US types of the complex cystic lesion is shown. (Reprinted from European Journal of Radiology. Hsu H-H, Yu J-C, Lee H-S, et al. Complex cystic lesions of the breast on ultrasonography: feature analysis and BI-RADS assessment. *Eur J Radiol.* 2011;79:73-79, Copyright 2011, with permission from Elsevier.)

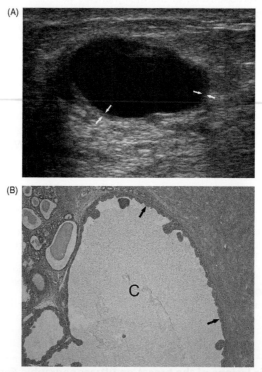

FIGURE 2.—Type I complex cystic lesion; fibrocystic change. (A) US image shows a circumscribed thick-walled complex cystic mass (arrows) with posterior acoustic enhancement. (B) Photomicrograph of the subsequent excised specimen shows apocrine metaplasia with cyst formation (C) and reactive stromal changes, findings consistent with cyst wall (arrows). Haematoxylin-eosin (H & E) stain, 100×. (Reprinted from European Journal of Radiology. Hsu H-H, Yu J-C, Lee H-S, et al. Complex cystic lesions of the breast on ultrasonography: feature analysis and BI-RADS assessment. *Eur J Radiol.* 2011;79:73-79, Copyright 2011, with permission from Elsevier.)

Reporting and Data System (BI-RADS) categories and management recommendations for these lesions based on US findings with pathologic correlation.

Materials and Methods.—From July 2001 to June 2007, 152 consecutive pathologically proven complex cystic lesions on US were retrospectively reviewed. All lesions at US were evaluated for size, lesion characteristics, margins, and presence of abnormal axillary nodes. US features of lesions were classified into four types, and positive predictive values (PPVs) were calculated for each type. Clinical, imaging, and histopathological findings were reviewed.

Results.—Of the 152 lesions based on US appearance, 36 (24%) were classified as type I, 49 (32%) as type II, 28 (18%) as type III, and 39 (26%) as type IV. The PPVs for malignancy in each type were 14% for type I, 16% for type II, 14% for type III, and 41% for type IV. There was a significantly higher frequency of malignancy among lesions of type IV compared with the other three types ($16/39 = 41\%$ vs $5/36 = 14\%$, $p = 0.0089$; $16/39 = 41\%$

(A)

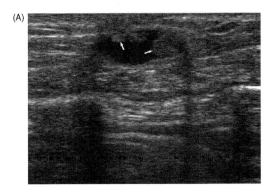

(B)

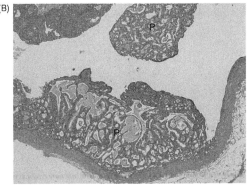

FIGURE 3.—Type II complex cystic lesion; intracystic papillomas. (A) US image reveals a cystic mass with internal mural nodules (arrows) and anechoic portion. (B) Corresponding to the US finding, papillary projections emanated from fibrovascular cores of papillomas (P) and attached to the cystic wall. H & E stain, 100×. (Reprinted from European Journal of Radiology. Hsu H-H, Yu J-C, Lee H-S, et al. Complex cystic lesions of the breast on ultrasonography: feature analysis and BI-RADS assessment. *Eur J Radiol.* 2011;79:73-79, Copyright 2011, with permission from Elsevier.)

vs $8/49 = 16\%$, $p = 0.0098$; and $16/39 = 41\%$ vs $4/28 = 14\%$, $p = 0.018$ [Chi-squared test]). Lesions with maximum diameter equal to or larger than 20 mm, not circumscribed margins, or a mammographic finding of suspected malignancy had a high probability of malignancy ($p < 0.05$ for each).

Conclusion.—US is useful in evaluating the complex cystic lesions and in clarifying the indication for biopsy of these lesions. The four types of US classifications used in our study establish accepted benchmarks for these breast abnormalities when stratified according to BI-RADS categories (Figs 1-5).

▶ Cystic breast lesions may be categorized as simple, complicated, or complex. Simple cysts are anechoic with imperceptible walls. Complicated cysts contain homogeneous low-level internal echoes and include cystic lesions with a layered fluid-debris level or brightly echogenic foci. Complex cystic lesions have thick walls, thick septa, and intracystic masses or may present as a complex mass containing both anechoic (cystic) and echogenic (solid) components.

The ultrasonography features characterizing complex cystic masses may be classified into 4 types: (1) in type I, the masses have a thick outer wall, thick

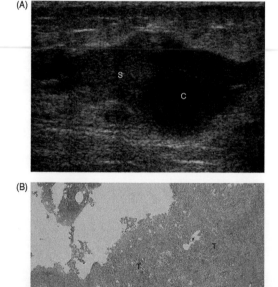

FIGURE 4.—Type III complex cystic mass; infiltrating ductal carcinoma. (A) US image shows a complex cystic (C) and solid (S) mass with at least 50% cystic portion. (B) Corresponding to the US finding, an infiltrating ductal carcinoma (T) with central haemorrhage and necrosis is demonstrated. H & E stain, 40×. (Reprinted from European Journal of Radiology. Hsu H-H, Yu J-C, Lee H-S, et al. Complex cystic lesions of the breast on ultrasonography: feature analysis and BI-RADS assessment. *Eur J Radiol.* 2011;79:73-79, Copyright 2011, with permission from Elsevier.)

(A)

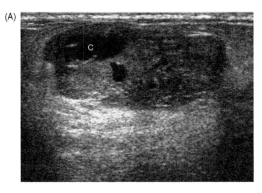

(B)

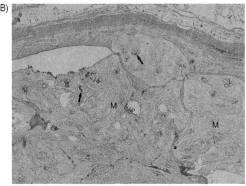

FIGURE 5.—Type IV complex cystic mass; mucinous carcinoma. (A) US image shows a heterogeneous (hypoechoic) mass with eccentric cystic components (C). (B) Photomicrograph of an excised specimen demonstrates nests of tumour cells (arrows) floating within extracellular mucin (M) lakes, corresponding to cystic areas of a complex cystic mass on US. H & E stain, 100×. (Reprinted from European Journal of Radiology. Hsu H-H, Yu J-C, Lee H-S, et al. Complex cystic lesions of the breast on ultrasonography: feature analysis and BI-RADS assessment. *Eur J Radiol*. 2011;79:73-79, Copyright 2011, with permission from Elsevier.)

internal septa, or both; (2) in type II, the masses are an intracystic type with 1 or more discrete solid mural lesions within a cyst; (3) in type III, the masses contain mixed cystic and solid components and have at least a 50% cystic portion in a mass; (4) in type IV, there are predominantly (at least 50%) solid masses with eccentric or central cystic foci.

Complex cystic lesions of the breast encompass a heterogeneous group of lesions, including intraductal or intracystic papillomas, fibrocystic changes, fibroadenomas, atypical ductal hyperplasia, and ductal carcinoma in situ, intracystic carcinoma, and invasive ductal carcinoma.

Although malignancy was noted with all 4 types of complex cystic lesions, the authors found a significantly higher frequency of malignancy among the type IV complex cystic lesions. This reminds us to carefully examine and characterize cystic lesions.

T. W. Stephens, MD

Hyperechoic Lesions of the Breast: Not Always Benign

Linda A. Zuiani C, Lorenzon M, et al (Univ of Udine, Italy; et al)
AJR Am J Roentgenol 196:1219-1224, 2011

Objective.—The purposes of our study were, first, to evaluate the frequency, clinical presentation, and associated imaging findings of malignant breast lesions presenting as hyperechoic nodules in a large series of consecutive sonographically guided core needle biopsies (CNBs) and, second, to investigate sonographic features that are able to predict malignancy in hyperechoic breast lesions.

Materials and Methods.—The radiologic and pathologic records for 4511 consecutive sonographically guided CNBs were retrospectively reviewed. Hyperechoic lesions were identified, and clinical notes and related mammography or MRI reports were reviewed. The sonographic images were evaluated according to the BI-RADS lexicon by two experienced breast radiologists. Surgical pathology results and follow-up served as the reference standard for lesions diagnosed as malignant or high-risk and benign at CNB, respectively. The frequency of hyperechoic carcinomas among all carcinomas was calculated. Differences in sonographic appearance between hyperechoic benign and malignant lesions were evaluated using the chi-square test or the Fisher exact test.

Results.—Of all biopsied lesions, 25 (0.6%) were hyperechoic. Among the 1849 malignant lesions, nine (0.4%) were hyperechoic. The remaining 16 were benign. None of the hyperechoic malignancies was a "purely" sonographic lesion, because all were palpable, mammographically visible, or detectable on breast MRI. Malignant lesions were more likely than benign lesions to have noncircumscribed margins (9/9 vs 7/16; $p = 0.008$) and nonparallel orientation (6/9 vs 1/16; $p = 0.003$).

Conclusion.—When encountering a hyperechoic nodule, malignant nature cannot be excluded. Suspicious sonographic signs and correlation with other imaging techniques may help avoid misdiagnosis (Table 2).

▶ The authors of this article retrospectively reviewed the radiology and pathology for 4511 consecutive ultrasound-guided core needle biopsies. A total of 1849 malignancies were found, and 9 of the malignancies were hyperechoic. The authors report that 5 of the 9 hyperechoic lesions were palpable, 5 of 8 evaluated with mammography had a mammographic correlate seen on mammography, and 3 of 5 evaluated with breast magnetic resonance imaging (MRI) had a MRI correlate seen on breast MRI.

Although hyperechogenicity in itself may suggest benignity, to deem a mass a BI-RADS category 2 lesion, radiologists cannot depend solely on one criterion, such as hyperechogenicity or parallel orientation, but must take all the sonographic features into account.[1] One suspicious feature prevents a lesion from having a benign designation.

It is interesting to note that all 9 hyperechoic malignancies in this study had noncircumscribed margins. Six of 9 of the hyperechoic lesions had nonparallel

TABLE 2.—Sonographic Features of 25 Hyperechoic Lesions of the Breast

Feature, Findings	No. (%) of Malignant Lesions ($n = 9$)	No. (%) of Benign Lesions ($n = 16$)	p^a
Shape			NS
Oval or round	0 (0)	2 (12)	
Lobular or irregular	9 (100)	14 (88)	
Orientation			0.003
Parallel	3 (33)	15 (94)	
Nonparallel	6 (67)	1 (6)	
Margin			0.008
Circumscribed	0 (0)	9 (56)	
Noncircumscribed	9 (100)	7 (44)	
Hypoechoic areas			NS
Present	7 (78)	7 (44)	
Absent	2 (22)	9 (56)	
Posterior acoustic features			NS
Absent	3 (33)	11 (69)	
Shadowing	6 (67)	5 (31)	
Enhancement	0 (0)	0 (0)	
Vascularity			NS
Present	6 (67)	7 (44)	
Absent	3 (33)	9 (56)	

Note—NS = not significant.
^{a}Chi-square or Fisher exact test; $p < 0.05$ is considered as statistically significant.

orientation. Any one suspicious feature precludes benignity and a BI-RADS category 2 designation.

Bottom line: Hyperechoic breast lesions are not always benign. The same sonographic features used to characterize breast masses by ultrasound scan should be applied to all lesions whether hyperechoic, hypoechoic, or isoechoic. Any suspicious sonographic features that correlate with other imaging and clinical information must be taken into account.

T. W. Stephens, MD

Reference

1. Stavros AT, Thickman D, Rapp CL, Dennis MA, Parker SH, Sisney GA. Solid breast nodules: use of sonography to distinguish between benign and malignant lesions. *Radiology.* 1995;196:123-134.

Miscellaneous

Full-Field Digital Mammographic Interpretation With Prior Analog Versus Prior Digitized Analog Mammography: Time for Interpretation

Garg AS, Rapelyea JA, Rechtman LR, et al (The George Washington Univ Med Ctr, DC)
AJR Am J Roentgenol 196:1436-1438, 2011

Objective.—The purpose of our study was to quantitatively compare the time for interpretation of screening full-field digital mammography

(FFDM) images using prior analog film mammograms for comparison versus digitized prior analog mammograms.

Materials and Methods.—Images from 100 FFDM studies were interpreted by four radiologists. All FFDM images had comparison analog mammograms obtained a minimum of 1 year earlier that were digitized using a 43-μm film digitizer. Initially, the FFDM images were interpreted using the digitized prior mammogram on two, 5-megapixel monitors and PACS. All available PACS tools could be used. Four weeks later, the same 100 screening FFDMs were interpreted using the original analog mammograms on an alternator at 90° to the monitors used to interpret the screening FFDMs. The interpretation times were recorded and compared. The results were compared and evaluated for statistical significance using statistical software, with statistical significance set at $p < 0.05$.

Results.—For each radiologist, the mean reading time for FFDM with digitized priors was significantly shorter in length in comparison with the mean reading time calculated for interpreting FFDM using analog film priors. The differences in times recorded between digitized analog versus analog ranged from 11.31 to 74.18 seconds. The reading times for the four readers ranged from 17.32 to 185.94 seconds, with a mean of 58.56 seconds when using analog film prior mammograms. When using digitized analog prior mammograms, the reading times for the four readers ranged from 11.32 to 109.11 seconds with a mean of 39.76 seconds. The average difference in reading time was calculated to be 18.80 seconds, showing that there is a 32% increase in interpretation speed when using a digitized prior analog for comparison studies as opposed to an analog prior.

Conclusion.—There is a statistically significant 32.1% average improvement in interpretation time when FFDM screening mammograms use digitized analog comparison mammograms than if FFDM is interpreted with the original analog film mammograms. This should allow more FFDMs to be interpreted in the same amount of time if digitized prior analog mammograms are used.

▶ With the increase in our daily workload and the shortage of breast imagers, workflow is a critical issue.

Whether digital or analog, comparison with prior mammograms is key to the early diagnosis of malignancy. In fact, comparison mammograms are essential in the detection and diagnosis of smaller, earlier-stage breast cancers.

Comparison of full-field digital mammography (FFDM) with digitized analog films and analog films is not without difficulties. With contrast differences, it may be difficult to determine if a finding is new or not. Taking the time to distinguish differences may add to the interpretation time. With nondigitized analog films, interpretation times may be increased from repeatedly looking away from the monitor to review the priors. The need to manually hang and remove the analog nondigitized films is also time consuming.

The purpose of this study was to compare the time of mammographic interpretation of FFDM with prior analog mammograms versus prior digitized analog mammograms, thus quantifying the assumed increased efficiency of using digitized prior mammograms. The authors concluded that interpretation times were shorter when comparison was made with digitized analog mammograms. Decreased time was seen for all readers regardless of the level of experience. This leads to greater efficiency, which is believed to be secondary to an increase in workflow. Digitization of mammograms leads to optimization of the image, which gives radiologists the ability to manipulate the contrast and to utilize the magnification feature. A decrease in the time for interpretation should allow for the interpretation of more mammograms in the same amount of time.

T. W. Stephens, MD

3 Musculoskeletal

Introduction

It is my pleasure to present the following selections from the musculo-skeletal imaging literature for review. Included are original scientific articles that seek to expand our understanding, reviews that serve to improve our imaging, and interventional techniques and offerings from related publications in fields such as rheumatology that lend an important clinical perspective to the practicing radiologist.

Included are musculoskeletal tumor imaging articles that detail factors contributing to success in imaging-guided biopsy and articles that are important in the evaluation of liposarcoma. A review of clavicle and acromioclavicular joint injuries is included as it details the change in the clinical and surgical approach to injuries of these structures. As the orthopedic community adopts a more aggressive surgical approach, it is important for the imager to be aware of surgical techniques and possible complications.

Two recent contributions to the literature improve our understanding of bisphosphonate-related atypical subtrochanteric fractures. This topic has attracted much attention recently and it is important for the musculoskeletal radiologist to be aware of recent developments as well as clinical perspectives. We have encountered several cases at our institution and discussions with our colleagues in endocrinology demonstrate the interest they have in the topic as well.

New surgical approaches and devices continue to be developed in the field of spine surgery. A helpful imaging review of fixation devices is included that serves to keep the imager up to date with new hardware that may be encountered. Also included is a study evaluating the role of early radiographic surveillance following spine surgery. A review of imaging findings and complications in the resurfaced hip is particularly timely given the recent attention paid to the issue in both the medical literature and lay press.

Several articles are included that relate to joint and sports injury. Two articles update the reader on imaging of the anterior cruciate ligament and one describes an oblique imaging technique designed to evaluate the ligament bundles. The potential morbidity of direct arthrography is also explored in a particularly interesting and informative scientific article. The relative frequency of symptoms that patients may experience in the days following this procedure reminds us to have a detailed discussion with our patients before they undergo arthrography. In our section, we have begun calling patients the day after procedures to check in on them and to monitor for possible discomfort or complication. Several articles dealing with imaging in the hip are included and reflect recent interest in hip imaging and arthroscopic intervention. A discussion of the postoperative acetabular labrum is particularly helpful given the increasing number of patients who have undergone debridement or repair.

I hope that these selections are informative and that the reader finds them useful in daily practice.

Colin Strickland, MD

Tumors

Revisiting CT-Guided Percutaneous Core Needle Biopsy of Musculoskeletal Lesions: Contributors to Biopsy Success

Omura MC, Motamedi K, UyBico S, et al (David Geffen School of Medicine at UCLA; et al)
AJR Am J Roentgenol 197:457-461, 2011

Objective.—The purpose of this article is to investigate potential technical, imaging, and histopathologic contributors to the success of CT biopsy.

Materials and Methods.—Four hundred forty-four consecutive CT biopsies of musculoskeletal lesions performed from 2005 to 2008 were retrospectively classified as diagnostic or nondiagnostic and as accurate or inaccurate. A biopsy was considered as diagnostic if it provided a definitive pathologic diagnosis or was clinically useful; as accurate if it was concordant with the ultimate diagnosis with respect to identification of malignancy, grade, and histopathologic features; and as successful if it was both diagnostic and accurate. Biopsy success rate, diagnostic yield, and accuracy were assessed according to lesion location, use of sedation, biopsy equipment type, bone lesion matrix type, and lesion histologic type (i.e., bone or soft-tissue origin, malignant or benign neoplasm, and low- or intermediate-to-high-grade neoplasm).

Results.—Of 444 biopsies, 71% were diagnostic, 86% were accurate, and 70% were successful. Biopsy success and diagnostic yield were greater in bone lesions, malignant neoplasms, and intermediate-to-high-grade neoplasms compared with soft-tissue lesions ($p < 0.01$), benign neoplasms ($p < 0.0001$), and low-grade neoplasms ($p < 0.0001$). Success and diagnostic yield were not significantly associated with technical or imaging factors. Biopsy accuracy was not associated with any of the tested variables. Of the 128 nondiagnostic biopsy results, 53% were accurate with respect to subsequent surgical pathologic findings. Most of these biopsy results were of benign soft-tissue lesions.

Conclusion.—CT biopsy of musculoskeletal lesions is accurate and effective. It may be limited in the evaluation of benign and low-grade soft-tissue neoplasms.

▶ Omura et al examine the practice of CT-guided core needle biopsy in this retrospective review. The authors examine the results of CT-guided biopsy at their institution with regard to how frequently a biopsy is diagnostic and/or accurate. A successful result was declared for biopsies deemed both diagnostic and accurate, and the reported rate was 70% for this study. This result is similar to that reported in earlier literature. Some limitations of CT-guided biopsy that have been reported in the past were not shown to be statistically significant in this sample; however, distribution of the included cases into subtypes such as sclerotic bone lesions yielded small groups of cases, and thus the statistical analysis was limited.

The authors raise the possibility that lower biopsy success rates with soft-tissue lesions in their sample may reflect the limited characterization of soft-tissue lesions typically allowed by radiologic imaging studies. An integrated approach to evaluation and characterization of bone and soft tissue lesions using both biopsy specimens and radiologic features is critical to arrive at a successful result. Our trainees are frequently surprised to see pathologists questioning radiologists during multidisciplinary conferences about the imaging characteristics of lesions and using this information to inform their final diagnoses.

Another point made by the authors is the importance of appropriate sampling of complex lesions. Necrotic or hemorrhagic regions of a lesion often look particularly strange on imaging, and, when planning a procedure, it is critical to sample living tissue rather than hemorrhage or debris. Obtaining samples in different regions of a lesion is also mentioned as a useful approach and may prove necessary for a successful result. For each biopsy being considered, it is important to review all available imaging studies, clinical information, and potential complications before proceeding. It is also important to recognize that features well seen by MRI may be invisible by CT and the use of bony or soft tissue landmarks may be necessary. Planning goes a long way toward securing a successful result.

C. Strickland, MD

Imaging of Liposarcoma: Classification, Patterns of Tumor Recurrence, and Response to Treatment

O'Regan KN, Jagannathan J, Krajewski K, et al (Dana Farber Cancer Inst, Boston, MA)
AJR Am J Roentgenol 197:W37-W43, 2011

Objective.—The purpose of this study was to illustrate the subtypes of liposarcoma (LPS) and the significance of the nonlipomatous tumor components using multiple imaging modalities.

Conclusion.—The subtypes of LPS with greater nonlipomatous soft-tissue components on imaging studies tend to show less differentiation and are usually more aggressive both histologically and clinically. Imaging plays an important role in the diagnosis, surveillance, and response assessment of LPS.

▶ O'Regan et al provide a useful overview of the variability of liposarcoma in this pictorial review. Awareness of the myriad possible appearances is important to radiologists in any subspecialty given the relatively high prevalence of the tumor. Particularly important to note is the variable fat content seen in liposarcoma. Trainees are often surprised to learn that fat may not be seen at all in such lesions. Early in training, they may leave the appropriate diagnosis out of the differential diagnosis for a soft-tissue mass when such a poorly differentiated lesion is encountered.

The categories of atypical lipomatous tumors are discussed and examples provided. The need for surgical resection is important to note for such lesions. Of particular value is the discussion of retroperitoneal lipomatous tumors. Such lesions may be inconspicuous and tempting to dismiss given their well-differentiated appearance. The extremely high recurrence rate of well-differentiated liposarcoma in the retroperitoneum also deserves specific attention and is highlighted in the review.

The authors make the important point that when following patients for site recurrence, particular attention must be paid to portions of a lipoma that demonstrate the most aggressive features. The absence of a new fatty mass at a site of prior resection does not ensure that no recurrence has occurred. Rather, a small enhancing soft-tissue nodule may indicate local recurrence.

Discussion of the imaging appearance of myxoid liposarcomas is also of value. Such masses can appear "cystic" on fluid-sensitive sequences. I have frequently used a case of one such tumor at our institution to stress the role of enhancement characteristics on MRI in evaluation of a soft-tissue mass.

C. Strickland, MD

Trauma

Clavicle and acromioclavicular joint injuries: a review of imaging, treatment, and complications
Melenevsky Y, Yablon CM, Ramappa A, et al (Beth Israel Deaconess Med Ctr, Boston, MA)
Skeletal Radiol 40:831-842, 2011

Fractures of the clavicle account for 2.6–5% of all fractures. Clavicular fractures have traditionally been treated conservatively, however, there has recently been increased interest in surgical repair of displaced clavicular fractures, with resultant lower rates of nonunion and malunion. Treatment of acromioclavicular (AC) separation has traditionally been conservative, with surgery reserved for patients with chronic pain or significant dislocation and acute soft tissue injury. It is important for the radiologist to become familiar with the surgical techniques used to fixate these fractures as well as the post-operative appearance and potential complications.

▶ With this review, Melenevsky et al provide a helpful update on the important imaging features of clavicle and acromioclavicular joint injuries. Although treatment of such injuries has been largely conservative in past years, increasing numbers of patients are undergoing surgical repair. This trend becomes clear to anyone interpreting radiographs for a busy orthopedic surgery department.

This article describes the classification systems used to describe clavicle fractures. Although several exist, it is less important to know the specifics of each one than it is to know what goes into the grading systems and thus what is important to the treating surgeon. Describing the fracture site and the degree of comminution and displacement is important, as is the case with all fractures. The probable status of the acromioclavicular and coracoclavicular ligaments may also be assessed by the degree of displacement of adjacent fragments. The importance of these features is discussed in the review because they form the basis for determining whether conservative or surgical management will be applied.

The discussion of currently favored fixation hardware and potential complications is useful, as are images illustrating each one. The authors also draw attention to repair methods that are subtle on radiographic follow-up studies. Coracoclavicular ligament reconstruction with tendon graft or suture may leave only subtle lucent tunnels in the distal clavicle as evidence of a prior intervention. Awareness of such surgical approaches is necessary for accurate interpretation. Another important point is that of MRI assessment. The authors describe helpful imaging planes that demonstrate pathology. It is also important to consider the site of injury and type of repair when designing an appropriate MRI protocol. Expanding the field of view may be necessary in cases in which patients report shoulder pain that may be related to an intra-articular derangement or complication related to a clavicle or AC joint intervention.

Although interest in more aggressive management of these injuries grows, it will be important for all imagers to have a working knowledge of repair techniques and factors that dictate the appropriate clinical approach.

C. Strickland, MD

Systemic

Bisphosphonate-Related Complete Atypical Subtrochanteric Femoral Fractures: Diagnostic Utility of Radiography

Rosenberg ZS, Vieira RLR, Chan SS, et al (New York Univ Hosp for Joint Diseases; et al)
AJR Am J Roentgenol 197:954-960, 2011

Objective.—The objective of our study was to evaluate the diagnostic utility of conventional radiography for diagnosing bisphosphonate-related atypical subtrochanteric femoral fractures.

Materials and Methods.—Retrospective interpretation of 38 radiographs of complete subtrochanteric and diaphyseal femoral fractures in two patient groups—one group being treated with bisphosphonates (19 fractures in 17 patients) and a second group not being treated with bisphosphonates (19 fractures in 19 patients)—was performed by three radiologists. The readers assessed four imaging criteria: focal lateral cortical thickening, transverse fracture, medial femoral spike, and fracture comminution. The odds ratios and the sensitivity, specificity, and accuracy of each imaging criterion as a predictor of bisphosphonate-related fractures were calculated. Similarly, the interobserver agreement and the sensitivity, specificity, and accuracy of diagnosing bisphosphonate-related fractures (i.e., atypical femoral fractures) were determined for the three readers.

Results.—Among the candidate predictors of bisphosphonate-related fractures, focal lateral cortical thickening and transverse fracture had the highest odds ratios (76.4 and 10.1, respectively). Medial spike and comminution had odd ratios of 3.8 and 0.63, respectively. Focal lateral cortical thickening and transverse fracture were also the most accurate factors for detecting bisphosphonate-related fractures for all readers. The sensitivity, specificity, and overall accuracy for diagnosing bisphosphonate-related fractures were 94.7%, 100%, and 97.4% for reader 1; 94.7%, 68.4%, and 81.6% for reader 2; and 89.5%, 89.5%, and 89.5% for reader 3, respectively. The interobserver agreement was substantial ($\kappa > 0.61$).

Conclusion.—Radiographs are reliable for distinguishing between complete femoral fractures related to bisphosphonate use and those not related to bisphosphonate use. Focal lateral cortical thickening and transverse fracture are the most dependable signs, showing high odds ratios and the highest accuracy for diagnosing these fractures.

▶ Rosenberg et al provide a timely and instructive investigation of bisphosphonate-related femur fractures. The topic has generated much interest in recent years as increasing numbers of radiologists, surgeons, and providers from multiple specialties have recognized a pattern of femur fractures previously described as quite rare occurring with some frequency. The study describes the attempt to distinguish between bisphosphonate-related fractures and those related to a traumatic mechanism. Not surprisingly, the investigators demonstrated a statistically significant difference in 4 important radiographic features between the 2 groups. Focal lateral cortical thickening stands out particularly as an important distinguishing feature with an associated high odds ratio of associated bisphosphonate therapy. Although the results of the study are not surprising, they serve to reinforce the fact that the imaging features of bisphosphonate-related fractures (focal lateral cortical thickening, transverse fracture orientation, medial spike, and lack of comminution) are well described and accurate in clinical practice.

The mechanism of fractures included in the study could also be determined by the clinical history. In fact, all patients with bisphosphonate-related fractures reported "minimal or no trauma," whereas patients in the other group all had a history of major trauma. This underscores the importance of going beyond the commonly unhelpful study indication of "pain" to seek an accurate clinical history from the medical record or ordering provider when necessary.

Other important points made by the authors are recommendations to image the opposite femur because a developing fracture may be found there as well. The description of prodromal mild or vague pain is also worth noting, and patients imaged at our institution with bisphosphonate-related fractures have reported these symptoms. The appropriateness of treatment options (surgery, hiatus from medication) is under debate, but it will remain important for radiologists to have knowledge of these fractures and to communicate to clinicians the importance of the imaging findings described in this study.

C. Strickland, MD

Bisphosphonates in the treatment of osteoporosis: a review of their contribution and controversies

Reid IR (Univ of Auckland, New Zealand)

Skeletal Radiol 40:1191-1196, 2011

The bisphosphonates have revolutionized the therapy of osteoporosis, particularly the prevention of vertebral and hip fractures. The development of tools for defining absolute fracture risk facilitates their targeting to appropriate, at-risk individuals. Prescribers need to be aware of their common side effects (gastrointestinal intolerance with oral dosing and flu-like illness following intravenous use). Whether these agents carry a real risk of other problems such as osteonecrosis of the jaw and subtrochanteric fractures remains uncertain at the present time. If the association of these problems with bisphosphonates is real, it is important that the major therapeutic benefits that can accrue from bisphosphonates' appropriate targeted use are not lost as a result of the anxiety concerning these extremely rare adverse events.

▶ In his review of bisphosphonate usage for osteoporosis, Reid offers clinical perspectives regarding a class of medications that have attracted recent attention from the musculoskeletal radiology community. The brief history provided reveals the relatively recent expansion of clinical use of bisphosphonates. He also details the biochemical nature and effects of the class of medications on living bone.

Osteonecrosis of the jaw and atypical femoral stress fractures have captured recent attention and forced reevaluation of the safety profile of bisphosphonates. It is important to consider the efficacy of these medications and the reduction in fracture incidence borne out in earlier literature. Atypical stress fractures may occur, although this risk needs to be weighed against the proven benefits of treatment. What remains largely unknown is the frequency of stress fractures related to bisphosphonate therapy. Given more recent widespread recognition, future studies should improve our understanding of this question. Certainly these atypical fractures have been encountered at our institution, and one could imagine that attention paid in recent literature will lead to more expansive studies aimed at nailing down the true prevalence.

The fact that the biologic effect of some agents lasts for years is important to consider and should be discussed with patients who present with problems potentially related to bisphosphonate therapy. Well-described adverse effects such as gastrointestinal intolerance are common and should be discussed and recognized when they occur.

Still needed is a clearer understanding of how to address treatment-related complications when they occur. Radiologists and others involved in the diagnosis and treatment of fractures continue to struggle with the management of patients who suffer complications from medications that have been shown to help so many.

C. Strickland, MD

Bone marrow MR imaging findings in disuse osteoporosis

de Abreu MR, Wesselly M, Chung CB, et al (Hospital Mãe de Deus, Porto Alegre, Brazil; Univ of California, San Diego)
Skeletal Radiol 40:571-575, 2011

Objective.—To demonstrate MR imaging findings in the cortical and trabecular bone as well as marrow changes in patients with disuse osteoporosis (DO).

Materials and Methods. Sixteen patients (14 men, 2 women, aged 27–86 years) with clinical and radiographic evidence of DO of a lower limb joint (10 knees, 6 ankles) with MR examination of the same joint performed within a 1-month period were selected, as well as 16 healthy volunteers (7 men, 9 women, aged 25–75 years, 10 knees and 6 ankles). MR imaging findings of the bone marrow were analyzed by 2 musculoskeletal radiologists in consensus regarding: diffuse or focal signal alteration, reinforcement of vertical or longitudinal trabecular lines, and presence of abnormal vascularization.

Results.—All patients (100%,16/16) with DO presented MR imaging abnormalities of the bone marrow, such as: accentuation of vertical trabecular lines (50%, 8/16), presence of subchondral lobules of fat (37.5%, 6/16), presence of horizontal trabecular lines (31%, 5/16), prominence of bone vessels (25%, 4/16), and presence of dotted areas of high signal intensity on T2-weighted fat-suppressed sequences (12.5%, 2/16). Such MR findings did not appear in the control individuals.

Conclusion.—There are several MR imaging findings in bones with DO that range from accentuation of vertical and horizontal marrow lines, presence of subchondral lobules of fat, prominent bone vascularization and the presence of dotted foci of high signal intensity on T2-weighted fat-suppressed sequences. Recognition of these signs may prove helpful in the identification of DO as well as distinguishing these findings from other entities.

▶ This article provides an insightful look at bone marrow signal in patients with disuse osteoporosis (DO). The radiographic findings associated with this condition have long been recognized and include bandlike or spotty regions of osteoporosis, cortical lamellation, or scalloping and trabecular coarsening. A diffuse pattern of demineralization may also be seen. Disuse osteoporosis is commonly encountered on MR studies in routine clinical practice, and some understanding and recognition of imaging findings is important.

MR imaging features of DO determined by consensus opinion of the authors include accentuation of vertical and horizontal marrow lines, the presence of subchondral fat lobules, and prominent vessels in the medullary space. The described features correspond well with those long described on radiographs and underscore the importance of interpretation of MR studies with corresponding radiographs when possible.

The number of patients with DO included in the study is small, so the relative frequency or importance of each imaging finding is difficult to determine.

Similarly, the imaging findings on accompanying radiographs were used as the gold standard. Perhaps MR findings may predate radiographic findings in the development of DO, but more studies will be needed to clarify this point. What is important to recognize is the probable relation between the described MR findings and those that are observed commonly on radiographs. Differentiation of marrow signal abnormalities from DO from those related to other conditions such as complex regional pain syndrome (CRPS) presents a challenge for future research. The authors hypothesize that the use of contrast with associated soft-tissue enhancement in CRPS may be helpful. Indeed, comparison with patients with other global marrow abnormalities may also be useful to further define the specific imaging features of DO.

C. Strickland, MD

Sclerosing Bone Dysplasias: Review and Differentiation from Other Causes of Osteosclerosis
Ihde LL, Forrester DM, Gottsegen CJ, et al (Univ of Southern California, Los Angeles; et al)
Radiographics 31:1865-1882, 2011

Sclerosing bone dysplasias are skeletal abnormalities of varying severity with a wide range of radiologic, clinical, and genetic features. Hereditary sclerosing bone dysplasias result from some disturbance in the pathways involved in osteoblast or osteoclast regulation, leading to abnormal accumulation of bone. Several genes have been discovered that, when disrupted, result in specific types of hereditary sclerosing bone dysplasia (osteopetrosis, pyknodysostosis, osteopoikilosis, osteopathia striata, progressive diaphyseal dysplasia, hereditary multiple diaphyseal sclerosis, hyperostosis corticalis generalisata), many of which exhibit similar pathologic mechanisms involving endochondral or intramembranous ossification and some of which share similar underlying genetic defects. Nonhereditary dysplasias include intramedullary osteosclerosis, melorheostosis, and overlap syndromes, whereas acquired syndromes with increased bone density, which may simulate sclerosing bone dysplasias, include osteoblastic metastases, Paget disease of bone, Erdheim-Chester disease, myelofibrosis, and sickle cell disease. Knowledge of the radiologic appearances, distribution, and associated clinical findings of hereditary and nonhereditary sclerosing bone dysplasias and acquired syndromes with increased bone density is crucial for accurate diagnosis.

▶ Ihde et al provide in this pictorial review an approach to sclerosing bone dysplasias that serves as a useful exercise for the experienced musculoskeletal radiologist and trainee alike. The article is richly filled with imaging examples, and a chart summarizes genetic, clinical, and imaging features of each disease. Particularly useful is the categorization of diseases into hereditary and nonhereditary groups. The inclusion of more commonly encountered mimics such as Paget disease and osteoblastic metastatic disease is also helpful in recognizing features that should lead the interpreter to the correct diagnosis or at least to recognize when the differential diagnosis should include a sclerosing dysplasia.

The authors go beyond the "aunt-minnie" descriptions for diseases and provide additional commentary and demographic information. Melorheostosis lesions may progress, and knowledge of this evolving appearance is useful, as lesions seen in any given patient will likely be encountered again and again over the years during imaging performed for other reasons, such as osteoarthrosis of the knee.

The authors also stress the importance of correlation with clinical history. This concept always bears repeating when interpreting imaging studies of any kind. Distinguishing features, such as the reported sparing of the skull in hereditary multiple diaphyseal sclerosis, are also described. These features are helpful when entertaining the diagnosis of a sclerosing bone dysplasia.

The review appropriately concentrates on the radiographic appearance of each disease. Future discussion of magnetic resonance imaging correlation would be helpful as well as several diseases described that may be detected incidentally. The fact that characteristic features are seen best with radiographs does stress their continued importance relative to more advanced imaging techniques when confronting a rare or unexpected disease of bone.

C. Strickland, MD

Effect of Spinal Segment Variants on Numbering Vertebral Levels at Lumbar MR Imaging

Carrino JA, Campbell PD Jr, Lin DC, et al (Johns Hopkins Univ School of Medicine, Baltimore, MD; Booth Radiology, Woodbury, NJ; et al)
Radiology 259:196-202, 2011

Purpose.—To verify iliolumbar ligament (ILL) location, to evaluate magnetic resonance (MR) imaging morphologic features for detecting lumbosacral transitional vertebrae (TVs) (LSTVs), and to determine whether transitional situations are associated with anomalous vertebral numbering.

Materials and Methods.—Investigational review board approval was obtained for this HIPAA-compliant retrospective study. A review of 147 subjects was performed by using spine radiography as the reference standard to determine total and segmental vertebral count and transitional anatomy. Thoracolumbar TVs (TLTVs) and LSTVs were identified. The lumbosacral intervertebral disk angle (LSIVDA), defined as the angle between the endplates, was measured, S1-2 disk morphology was rated according to the classification by O'Driscoll et al, and the ILL level was determined from MR images. Statistical analysis was performed by using χ^2 tests for dichotomous and ordinal variables and the *t* test for continuous variables.

Results.—An anomalous total number of vertebrae were present in 12 (8.2%) of 147 subjects. The ILL was identified in 126 (85.7%) of 147 subjects and was present at L5 in 122 (96.8%) subjects; the remaining four (3.2%) subjects had an anomalous total number of vertebrae.

A complete S1-2 intervertebral disk was associated with LSTVs ($P = .004$); however, LSIVDA was not ($P = .2$). TLTVs were present in six (4.1%) and LSTVs were present in 22 (15.0%) of 147 subjects. Both were present in four (2.7%) subjects. The presence of a TLTV was associated with a higher incidence of a concomitant LSTV and vice versa ($P < .001$; odds ratio [OR], 13.7; 95% confidence interval [CI]: 2.7, 68.4]). A TLTV was not associated with an anomalous total number of vertebrae ($P = .46$), but an LSTV was ($P < .001$; OR, 7.4; 95% CI: 2.2, 24.8).

Conclusion.—The ILL denotes the lowest lumbar vertebra, which does not always represent L5. A well-formed, complete S1-2 intervertebral disk is associated with LSTVs, but alteration in LSIVDA is not. LSTVs are associated with anomalous vertebral numbering.

▶ Carrino et al address an important issue that comes up almost daily in the clinical interpretation of spine imaging studies. Transitional thoracolumbar and lumbosacral vertebrae are frequently encountered and need to be recognized and acknowledged in reports for radiographic, computed tomography (CT) and magnetic resonance imaging (MRI) studies. First-year residents often are surprised to learn the frequency with which transitional levels occur and the issues that they create with accurately assigning numbers to the spinal segments under evaluation. Multiple landmarks (both bony and soft tissue) have been proposed over the years as ways of determining how to number spinal levels. Several are discussed and problems with each identified. While the iliolumbar ligament has been described as a reproducible way of identifying L5, even this method is flawed. The important point is made in this series that the iliolumbar ligament identifies the lowest lumbar level, although this is not always L5. This simple point is crucial to recognize and to avoid mislabeling lumbar spinal segments. It is interesting to note that the lumbosacral intervertebral disc angle was not associated with a lumbosacral transitional vertebra.

As with any potentially confusing issue, the presence of ambiguous segmentation requires diligent communication between radiologists and surgeons participating in the patient's care. At our institution, the first statement in the body of any lumbar spine radiograph is an assessment of the number of lumbar vertebrae present. Similarly, when interpreting lumbar spine CT and MRI studies, the radiographs are consulted to make sure there is agreement in the numbering system described in each report. The medical record is also consulted to ensure that our surgical colleagues are describing the same levels we are reporting in their clinical and preoperative notes. As the authors of this series recommend, explicit statements are made declaring the numbering system used. This is important to ensure that everyone is on the same page, particularly when an intervention is being considered.

C. Strickland, MD

Can Necrotizing Infectious Fasciitis Be Differentiated from Nonnecrotizing Infectious Fasciitis with MR Imaging?

Kim KT, Kim YJ, Won Lee J, et al (Inha Univ Hosp, Incheon, South Korea)
Radiology 259:816-824, 2011

Purpose.—To retrospectively evaluate whether magnetic resonance (MR) imaging findings can be used to differentiate necrotizing infectious fasciitis (NIF) from nonnecrotizing infectious fasciitis (non-NIF).

Materials and Methods.—Institutional review board approval was obtained, but patient consent was not required for this retrospective review of records and images because patient anonymity was preserved. Thirty patients (seven with NIF, 23 with non-NIF) were included in the study. The following imaging findings were analyzed on fat-suppressed T2-weighted MR images: *(a)* signal intensity in the deep fascia (low, high, or mixed high and low), *(b)* thickness of abnormal signal intensity in the deep fascia (≥ 3 mm or <3 mm), *(c)* pattern of abnormal signal intensity in muscle (no abnormality, peripheral bandlike signal intensity, or patchy high signal intensity), *(d)* degree of deep fascia involvement (partial or extensive), and *(e)* degree of compartment involvement (fewer than three compartments or three or more compartments). On contrast material–enhanced fat-suppressed T1-weighted images, the contrast enhancement patterns of the abnormal deep fascia (no enhancement, enhancement, or enhancement with nonenhancing portion) and the muscle (no abnormality, peripheral bandlike signal intensity, or patchy high signal intensity) were evaluated. The presence of abscesses in the subcutaneous fat layer was evaluated with all sequences.

Results.—The patients with NIF had a significantly greater frequency of *(a)* thick (≥ 3 mm) abnormal signal intensity on fat-suppressed T2-weighted images, *(b)* low signal intensity in the deep fascia on fat-suppressed T2-weighted images, *(c)* a focal or diffuse nonenhancing portion in the area of abnormal signal intensity in the deep fascia, *(d)* extensive involvement of the deep fascia, and *(e)* involvement of three or more compartments in one extremity ($P < .05$).

Conclusion.—MR imaging is potentially helpful for differentiating NIF from non-NIF.

▶ Necrotizing infectious fasciitis continues to present a challenging diagnosis. The disease can be rapidly fatal and may be confused clinically with cellulitis and other less-aggressive entities. Imaging features (particularly early in the disease process) overlap with cellulitis, adding further complexity to medical management. It is with this in mind that this retrospective case-control study seeks to shed light on features that may help specifically identify cases of necrotizing fasciitis by magnetic resonance imaging (MRI). The important features are discussed in the study and include thick abnormal fascial signal, areas of decreased T2 signal, nonenhancement, deep fascial involvement, and extensive disease involving 3 or more fascial compartments. Awareness of these features is important and may prompt recognition of a potential severe disease process at work.

This analysis, however, also brings up some important points. While certain features are helpful in making a specific diagnosis, overlap exists, making the task of "ruling out" necrotizing fasciitis a difficult one. Given the severity of the disease, it is often prudent to proceed to surgical biopsy or exploration, depending on clinical factors regardless of imaging findings. With the increasing use of MRI in the emergent setting, we have seen large numbers of cases of soft-tissue infection. In some cases, a diagnosis can be made, but in others, a discussion with the clinicians is necessary to convey the meaning of a test result that may or may not answer the question at hand definitively. It is important that we communicate to clinicians the need to continue their assessment of patients if suspicion is high, despite potentially reassuring imaging findings. It is also important to note that in cases that need emergent surgical biopsy, it is necessary not to delay treatment for the sake of imaging.

C. Strickland, MD

Preoperative Diagnosis of Periprosthetic Joint Infection: Role of Aspiration
Squire MW, Della Valle CJ, Parvizi J (Univ of Wisconsin Hosps and Clinics, Madison; Rush Univ Med Ctr, Chicago, IL; Rothman Inst at Jefferson, Philadelphia, PA)
AJR Am J Roentgenol 196:875-879, 2011

Objective.—The purpose of this article is to illustrate how total knee arthroplasty (TKA) and total hip arthroplasty (THA) aspiration by the radiologist can assist the health care team in determining the presence or absence of periprosthetic joint infection.

Conclusion.—The increasing incidence of periprosthetic TKA and THA infection, as well as the changing role of aspiration for diagnosing periprosthetic joint infection, will likely increase demand for this important procedure in the future.

▶ Squire et al provide a useful clinical perspective on the role of aspiration in detection and characterization of periprosthetic infection in hip and knee prostheses. Fluoroscopic- or ultrasound-guided aspiration of the knee and hip is an important procedure with which every radiologist should be familiar. The fact that infection is the leading cause of knee arthroplasty revision and the third most frequent cause of hip arthroplasty revision in the United States underscores the importance of the procedure. An ordered approach to the patient with possible infection is necessary to arrive at the appropriate diagnosis or to at least decide which (if any) intervention is indicated.

The authors review the imaging literature as well as clinical and laboratory factors that aid in diagnosis. Results from studies indicating that false-positive results are encountered in 3% to 16% of cases are helpful and should be communicated to clinicians asking for an aspiration. These findings also serve to remind the operator of the importance of strict aseptic technique. This is particularly true when an intervention may lead to the infection of a prosthesis that is currently sterile.

The powerful negative predictive value of C-reactive protein and erythrocyte sedimentation rate in excluding infection is helpful to bear in mind, and requesting these tests may help to avoid an unnecessary intervention.

Synovial fluid white blood cell counts encountered in infected joints are commonly much lower than those seen in native joints. This point is described along with implications for treatment decisions, and it is important to recognize when helping clinicians to interpret imaging and aspiration results.

A general discussion of surgical technique, including the need for a 2-stage surgical approach when treating an infected prosthesis, lends important clinical perspective to the radiologist who does not work closely with orthopedic colleagues on a daily basis. Finally, the authors discuss the utility of withholding antibiotics when planning an aspiration. Although this can be achieved with planning and communication, in practice this may be difficult to coordinate, particularly when patients present through the emergency department.

C. Strickland, MD

Arthritis

New Techniques in Lumbar Spinal Instrumentation: What the Radiologist Needs to Know
Murtagh RD, Quencer RM, Castellvi AE, et al (Univ Diagnostic Inst, Tampa, FL; Univ of Miami, FL; Florida Orthopedic Inst, Tampa; et al)
Radiology 260:317-330, 2011

Lumbar spinal fusion is a commonly performed procedure, and, despite changes in cage types and fixation hardware, radiologists have, over the years, become familiar with the imaging features of typical spinal fusion and many of the complications seen in patients after surgery, including pseudoarthrosis, hardware loosening, and recurrent or residual disk herniation. Recently, however, novel approaches and devices have been developed, including advances in minimally invasive surgery, the increasing use of osteoinductive materials, and a wide variety of motion-preserving devices. These new approaches and devices manifest with characteristic imaging features and the potential for unusual and unexpected complications. Several of these devices and approaches are experimental, but many, including those devices used in lateral approaches to fusion, as well as the use of bone morphogenic protein, disk arthroplasty, and interspinous spacers, are seen with increasing frequency in daily clinical practice. Given the recent advances in spinal fusion surgery, it is important that radiologists have a basic understanding of the rationale behind these procedures, the common imaging features of the devices, and the complications associated with their use.

▶ Murtagh et al provide a valuable review of current lumbar spinal instrumentation techniques in this timely article. Any radiologist who interprets spine studies will appreciate the comprehensive approach and brief discussions of surgical technique. New devices frequently enter the market, and it is always helpful to have knowledge of what one may encounter.

In addition to describing hardware, the review also discusses the current role of osteoinductive bone graft substitutes including bone morphogenic protein (BMP). The inflammatory response that may be seen following its use is important to recognize, as it may masquerade as infection. At our institution, BMP is not used in the cervical spine because of reported complications.

The discussion of motion preservation devices is also helpful, given their proliferation. Results have been variable, and it is not uncommon at our institution to see a disk replacement device inserted at a diseased level and then months or years later fusion hardware placed at the same level because of ongoing or new symptoms.

Interspinous transplant devices are frequently used at our institution and require scrutiny during radiographic evaluation, as complications, including spinous process fracture, may be very subtle. Surgeons at our institution also pay particular attention to the size and shape of spinous processes at levels where placement of an X-Stop device is being considered.

As is always true in musculoskeletal radiology, it is important to understand the surgical hardware utilized by referring physicians if we are to have a helpful and meaningful clinical impact. A weekly spine conference at our institution helps to introduce us to new techniques and hardware employed by our spine surgeons.

C. Strickland, MD

The Utility of Repeated Postoperative Radiographs After Lumbar Instrumented Fusion for Degenerative Lumbar Spine
Yamashita T, Steinmetz MP, Lieberman IH, et al (Cleveland Clinic, OH; Metro Health Med Ctr, Cleveland, OH; Texas Back Inst, Plano)
Spine 36:1955-1960, 2011

Study Design.—Retrospective chart review.

Objective.—To assess the impact that routine postoperative radiographs have in clinical outcome and clinical decision-making.

Summary of Background Data.—No standard exists that outlines how often and when radiographs should be taken after lumbar fusion. Routine postoperative radiographs can be a source of inconvenience and cost to patients, radiation exposure, and possibly, confounding information.

Methods.—The patients who underwent a single or multilevel lumbar instrumented fusion were investigated. At each time-point after surgery, it was noted if they demonstrated new symptoms or clinical deterioration. The Fisher exact test was used to analyze the categorical data.

Results.—Sixty-three patients (25 males and 38 females) were identified with a mean age of 52 years (range, 20–87). Plain radiographs were taken at 269 visits including all time-points. In 17 (6.3%) visits, abnormal findings were found in 13 patients, including suspected pseudoarthrosis on radiographs (n = 10) and adjacent segment disease on radiographs (n = 3).

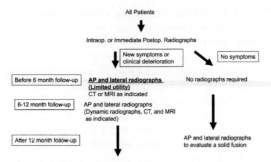

FIGURE 1.—Algorithm describing a proposed method for choosing an appropriate postoperative imaging modality after lumbar instrumented fusion. (Reprinted from Yamashita T, Steinmetz MP, Lieberman IH, et al. The utility of repeated postoperative radiographs after lumbar instrumented fusion for degenerative lumbar spine. *Spine*. 2011;36:1955-1960, with permission from North American Spine Society.)

They were found during 11 of 50 visits (22%) in the patients with new symptoms or clinical deterioration and during 6 of 219 visits (2.7%) in the asymptomatic patients. The probability of an abnormal finding was significantly lower in the asymptomatic patients ($P < 0.001$). Before the 6-month follow-up, abnormal findings were found in 1 of 111 visits (0.9%) and in 16 of 158 visits (10%) at the 6-month follow-up or later. The probability of an abnormal finding was significantly lower before the 6-month follow-up ($P < 0.001$). In six of the seven symptomatic patients (86%) with suspected pseudoarthrosis on radiographs, pseudoarthrosis was initially suspected between 6 and 12 months after surgery.

Conclusion.—This study suggests that plain radiographs should be performed as indicated clinically rather than routinely after instrumented lumbar fusion. The vast majority of asymptomatic patients do not require routine postoperative radiographs (Fig 1).

▶ Yamashita et al investigate the use of routine postoperative lumbar spine radiographs in this retrospective review. While the practice of obtaining early postoperative studies intuitively makes sense, the authors make several important points regarding the outcomes in their study group. Few patients proved to have complications, and most were accompanied by symptoms that could have directed appropriate imaging. In addition, those who did exhibit complications demonstrated symptoms that would prompt additional workup in the 6 months following surgery. Based on these findings, routine postoperative studies in the weeks to months following surgery were discouraged. This conclusion does, however, leave the reader with some questions. In our practice, postoperative studies establish a new baseline that is helpful in the evaluation of future studies. It would be interesting to compare the accuracy and sensitivity of radiographs obtained at 12 months both with and without earlier studies available for comparison. In addition, early complications such as discitis that may complicate fusion would require rapid diagnosis. Certainly we would expect such a scenario to be clinically apparent, although comparison radiographs obtained in the first 6 months after surgery would likely be necessary to detect subtle new findings such as endplate erosion or disc space narrowing. It is unclear how the absence of such postoperative imaging would affect such a scenario. It is also important to consider the use of imaging techniques such as computed tomography and magnetic resonance imaging (MRI) in cases of clinical deterioration. Clearly, radiographs play a role in the evaluation of new symptoms, but an MRI may be necessary to identify a new disc herniation or evidence of infection. Future study will be necessary to more fully evaluate the use of the new algorithm proposed for postoperative imaging (Fig 1).

C. Strickland, MD

Identification of Intraarticular and Periarticular Uric Acid Crystals with Dual-Energy CT: Initial Evaluation
Glazebrook KN, Guimarães LS, Murthy NS, et al (Mayo Clinic, Rochester, MN)
Radiology 261:516-524, 2011

Purpose.—To estimate the accuracy, sensitivity, specificity, and interobserver agreement of dual-energy computed tomography (CT) in detection of uric acid crystals in joints or periarticular structures in patients with arthralgia and patients suspected of having gout, with joint aspiration results as reference standard.

Materials and Methods.—With institutional review board approval, patient consent, and HIPAA compliance, 94 patients (age range, 29–89 years) underwent dual-source, dual-energy (80 and 140 kVp) CT of a painful joint. A material decomposition algorithm was used to identify uric acid. Two blinded musculoskeletal radiologists evaluated the dual-energy CT images and classified the examination findings as positive or negative for the presence of uric acid crystals. Reference standard was the result of joint aspiration.

Results.—Forty-three of 94 patients (46%) underwent attempted joint aspiration within 1 month of dual-energy CT. Aspiration was successful in 31 of 43 patients (72%). In 12 of 31 patients (39%), uric acid crystals were identified at joint aspiration; in 19 patients, they were not. Readers 1 and 2 had no false-negative findings for uric acid at dual-energy CT. Sensitivity was 100% (12 of 12; 95% confidence interval (CI): 74%, 100%) for both readers. Specificity was 89% (17 of 19; 95% CI: 67%, 99%) for reader 1 and 79% (15 of 19; 95% CI: 54%, 94%) for reader 2, with near-perfect agreement between the readers($\kappa = 0.87$; range, 0.70–1.00) in the 31 patients who underwent aspiration.

Conclusion.—Initial retrospective assessment suggests that dual-energy CT is a sensitive, noninvasive, and reproducible method for identifying uric acid deposits in joints and periarticular soft tissues in patients suspected of having gout.

▶ Diagnosis and characterization of arthritis is one of the major duties of the musculoskeletal radiologist. Technical advances in dual-energy computed tomography (CT) scanning have allowed for characterization of specific materials, including uric acid crystals. The use of CT in identification of uric acid crystal deposits around joint spaces is described in this study by Glazebrook et al.

This exciting technique appears to be useful, and the agreement between dual-energy CT and aspiration is impressive, although the number of cases tested in this study is small. Discussion of cases in the study that were regarded as false-positives is informative. Two cases are described in which dual-energy CT identified deposits in patients later believed to have gout despite initially negative aspirations. These examples illustrate the potential utility of CT evaluation and may help guide aspiration to appropriate sites if it needs to be performed.

Given that the diagnosis of gout often relies on secondary criteria, inclusion of dual-energy CT results with criteria such as serum uric acid levels may improve diagnostic accuracy in the future.

An important limitation of the study to consider is the use of Siemens software in the analysis that may not be available at all centers. Similarly, the technical parameters used may also prevent adoption of the technique described in the article until similar imaging scanners are in widespread clinical use.

The small sample size and selection bias limit the external validity of the study. Aspiration was only performed in 31 of 94 patients, so this too limits the statistical significance. On the other hand, given the complexity and number of secondary signs used in the diagnosis, dual-energy CT may provide much needed additional diagnostic information. The performance of the technique in other inflammatory and degenerative forms of arthritis will need to be considered when assessing the role of CT in the clinical setting.

C. Strickland, MD

Rheumatoid Arthritis: Ultrasound Versus MRI
Rowbotham EL, Grainger AJ (Chapel Allerton Hosp, Leeds, UK)
AJR Am J Roentgenol 197:541-546, 2011

Objective.—Rheumatoid arthritis is a predominantly joint-based disease affecting approximately 1% of the world's population. This article will address the increasing use of both ultrasound and MRI in the diagnosis and monitoring of rheumatoid arthritis and will highlight both the strengths and weaknesses of these two imaging modalities, with particular reference to bone erosions and synovitis.

Conclusion.—Because they can detect early disease, both ultrasound and MRI will become increasingly important in the diagnosis and management of rheumatoid arthritis. Future studies with increased patient numbers will be necessary if one of these two modalities is to emerge as a clear winner as the imaging modality of choice (Table 1).

▶ This review provides valuable insight into the evaluation of early rheumatoid arthritis with ultrasound and MRI. As is the case with many diagnostic techniques, neither is clearly superior, and each offers strengths. See Table 1 for a comparison of the modalities. The ease, low cost, safety, and high spacial resolution of ultrasound compare well with MRI. On the other hand, the ability

TABLE 1.—Comparison of Modalities

Ultrasound		MRI	
Strengths	Weaknesses	Strengths	Weaknesses
Real-time and dynamic imaging	Unable to image within bone	Ability to image deep within the joint and bone (e.g., marrow edema)	Contraindications (e.g., pacemaker)
Immediately accessible	Difficulties with temporal comparison	More complete assessment of whole joint including all articular surfaces	Time and patient tolerance
Allows operator to undertake clinical assessment	Poor depth penetration for larger joints and difficulty accessing parts of some joints	Proven correlation of synovitis and histopathology	Limited to one body region
Power Doppler imaging correlates well with disease activity	Specialist training not always available	Quantitative measurement of synovium	Ideally IV contrast administration needed for synovitis assessment
Relatively easy to examine multiple body regions	Operator dependent	Readily reproducible	Potential for motion artifact

to evaluate deep structures and bone edema and to offer a global assessment make MRI an attractive technique. Comparison over time is also easier with MRI studies. Indeed, MRI commonly serves as the gold standard when comparing the sensitivity of other modalities in the detection and characterization of bony erosions. In a sense, the debate of ultrasound versus MRI for early RA is similar to that surrounding the use of these modalities in the shoulder. Each has its own strengths and weaknesses, and it is important to communicate to our referring clinicians these unique characteristics. What is certain is that an appropriate skill level is necessary with both for appropriate clinical care.

The authors make additional points that are worth noting. It is interesting from a historical perspective that radiographic features were added in 1987 and removed in 2010 as criteria for the diagnosis of rheumatoid arthritis. This recent change is in recognition of the fact that erosions are a late manifestation of disease. The improving clinical utility of current therapies (and rising cost) mandate that we diagnose and treat the disease appropriately in early clinical stages.

As noted in the conclusion, more studies will be needed to clearly define the role of each modality.

C. Strickland, MD

Radiology of the resurfaced hip

Rahman L, Hall-Craggs M, Muirhead-Allwood SK (The London Hip Unit, UK; Univ College London Hosp, UK)
Skeletal Radiol 40:819-830, 2011

Hip resurfacing arthroplasty is an increasingly common procedure for osteoarthritis. Conventional radiographs are used routinely for follow-up assessment, however they only provide limited information on the radiological outcome. Various complications have been reported in the scientific literature although not all are fully understood. In an effort to investigate problematic or failing hip resurfacings, various radiological methods have been utilized. These methods can be used to help make a diagnosis and guide management. This paper aims to review and illustrate the radiographic findings in the form of radiography, computerized tomography (CT), magnetic resonance imaging (MRI), and ultrasound of both normal and abnormal findings in hip resurfacing arthroplasty. However, imaging around a metal prosthesis with CT and MRI is particularly challenging and therefore the potential techniques used to overcome this are discussed.

▶ As surgical approaches to diseases change, so too does the skill set of the radiologist need to evolve. In this review by Rahman et al, the reader is brought up to date on interpretation of radiographs and advanced imaging techniques used to evaluate the metal-on-metal resurfaced hip prosthesis. At our institution, we have observed a similar increase in the number of resurfacing procedures reported by the authors. Briefly reviewed in the article are the manufacturers and types of prostheses that may be encountered, which serves to highlight subtle differences between implants. Ultimately, it is critical to be aware of what types of prosthesis are used at one's own institution, as each may have specific imaging features.

Particularly useful to the practicing radiologist is the review of radiographic assessment of prosthesis placement and common complications including specific patterns of loosening, subsidence, impingement, and femoral neck narrowing. Metal hypersensitivity reactions associated with metal-on-metal prostheses are of particular concern and require extensive laboratory and imaging evaluation.

Evaluation of metal-on-metal hip prostheses with CT and MRI is complicated by artifact, and this review also includes a discussion of strategies that may be used to improve image quality around the joint. The same methods are useful when applied to total or hemiarthroplasties and should be techniques with which the musculoskeletal radiologist is familiar.

C. Strickland, MD

Joints/Sports Injuries

Three tesla magnetic resonance imaging of the anterior cruciate ligament of the knee: can we differentiate complete from partial tears?
Van Dyck P, Vanhoenacker FM, Gielen JL, et al (Univ of Antwerp, Belgium; et al)
Skeletal Radiol 40:701-707, 2011

Purpose.—To determine the ability of 3.0T magnetic resonance (MR) imaging to identify partial tears of the anterior cruciate ligament (ACL) and to allow distinction of complete from partial ACL tears.

Materials and Methods.—One hundred seventy-two patients were prospectively studied by 3.0T MR imaging and arthroscopy in our institution.

MR images were interpreted in consensus by two experienced reviewers, and the ACL was diagnosed as being normal, partially torn, or completely torn. Diagnostic accuracy of 3.0T MR for the detection of both complete and partial tears of the ACL was calculated using arthroscopy as the standard of reference.

Results.—There were 132 patients with an intact ACL, 17 had a partial, and 23 had a complete tear of the ACL seen at arthroscopy. Sensitivity, specificity, and accuracy of 3.0T MR for complete ACL tears were 83, 99, and 97%, respectively, and, for partial ACL tears, 77, 97, and 95%, respectively. Five of 40 ACL lesions (13%) could not correctly be identified as complete or partial ACL tears.

Conclusion.—MR imaging at 3.0T represents a highly accurate method for identifying tears of the ACL. However, differentiation between complete and partial ACL tears and identification of partial tears of this ligament remains difficult, even at 3.0T.

▶ Imaging at high field strength has resulted in increased imaging performance in a wide number of musculoskeletal applications; however, some tasks remain stubbornly difficult. Such is the case with the characterization of partial anterior cruciate ligament (ACL) tears as described in this study in a comparison between 3.0-T MRI and arthroscopy. The experience described here again demonstrates the importance of both clinical and imaging findings in deciding which treatment is appropriate for any given patient. Particularly interesting here are the example cases that illustrate how imaging and arthroscopic findings may differ. Several illuminating examples are included. The authors postulate that the injury pattern of the ACL may change between imaging and arthroscopy. Although surgical correlation is critical, this confounding factor likely comes into play in countless studies with surgical findings as the gold standard. This limitation is important to keep in mind when considering the reported performance of imaging studies. The authors also discuss the selection bias inherent in this study, which may skew reported accuracy of diagnostic tests.

C. Strickland, MD

Oblique axial MR imaging of the normal anterior cruciate ligament bundles
Ng AWH, Griffith JF, Law KY, et al (Chinese Univ of Hong Kong, Hong Kong SAR)
Skeletal Radiol 40:1587-1594, 2011

Background.—Most anterior cruciate ligament (ACL) tears extend across both the anteromedial and the posterolateral bundles. Although complete tears cannot heal, partial tears, which may involve predominantly one or both bundles, may be able to heal because of a blood supply via the medial geniculate artery. Correctly assessing partial tears with early in the process may avoid their progression into complete tears. If one bundle is involved predominantly, the surgeon can perform single bundle reconstruction rather than full ACL graft reconstruction. The two bundles are comparable in size and consistency, and both attach to the medial aspect of the lateral femoral condyle proximally and the anteromedial aspect of the tibial intercondylar area distally. Magnetic resonance (MR) imaging is used to delineate the bundles, but orthogonal planes can identify normal ACL bundle structure in only 42% of knees. The usefulness of an oblique axial plane for the MR imaging of normal ACL bundles was compared to that of standard sagittal, coronal, and axial planes. Normal MR appearance was also described.

Methods.—Sixty knees in 34 male and 26 female patients (mean age 37.1 years) were evaluated. Twenty subjects were healthy volunteers with no knee symptoms or injury; 40 subjects had no history of knee injury but were being evaluated for knee pain. None had clinical symptoms of knee laxity. All underwent MR examinations using a 3T imaging system with a phased array knee coil of eight elements. The components of the knee examination included turbo-spin-echo sagittal intermediate-weighted imaging in a plane parallel to the outer cortex of the lateral femoral condyle, coronal T2-weighted fat suppression imaging, and axial intermediate-weighted fat-suppressed imaging, followed by oblique axial imaging of the ACL, which included intermediate-weighted images obtained in a plane aligned perpendicularly to the course of the ACL, with sagittal and coronal images used for positioning and alignment. The extra sequence took about 4 minutes. Ability to delineate the two bundles near the tibial insertion, at the mid-portion, and near the femoral origin was classified as good, adequate, or poor. The ACL's typical appearance was defined as the appearance of both bundles commonly found in most oblique axial images at the three levels. Additional structures were also reported.

Results.—It was possible to delineate the two bundles in all cases. Ninety-nine percent of the combined assessments yielded good or adequate delineation of both bundles using oblique axial imaging. Only 43% of the standard sagittal, 47% of the standard coronal, and 39% of the standard axial images could delineate the bundles as clearly. Delineation was especially poor close to the femoral attachment using the sagittal, coronal, and axial images.

Eighty-two percent of the ACLs demonstrated typical appearances, with the anteromedial bundle at the anteromedial aspect of the ACL and the posterolateral bundle more posterolaterally. Near the tibial insertion, 95% of the anteromedial bundles had a thick C-shaped hypointense rim with a central hyperintense zone. Posterolateral bundles appeared as a more loosely arranged group of ligament fibers separated by fatty-type tissues. At the mid-point, both bundles were more compact and rounded, whereas near the femoral attachment, both were more oblong. The anteromedial bundle was typically uniformly hypointense, with the posterolateral bundle slightly less so. Atypical appearances were noted in 18% of the knees and included a larger central hyperintense zone at the tibial and mid-points of the anteromedial bundle (5% of cases), an intermediate bundle (5%), a ligamentum mucosum (2%), a moderately attenuated posterolateral bundle throughout the ACL's length (2%), and small ganglion cysts (5%).

TABLE 1.—Delineation of Anteromedial and Posterolateral ACL Bundles on Oblique Axial and Standard Sagittal and Coronal Imaging. Comparisons were Made at the Tibial Insertion, at the Mid-Portion, and at the Femoral Origin of the ACL. The Delineation of the Two Bundles was Graded as Good, Adequate, or Poor. Differences in Delineation of Both Bundles Between the Oblique Axial and Standard Sagittal, Coronal, and Axial Planes were Highly Significant ($P<0.0001$) at All Levels

		Good Delineation	Adequate Delineation	Poor Delineation
Tibial insertion	Oblique axial	40 (60%)	20 (40%)	0
	Standard sagittal	18 (30%)	25 (41.7%)	17 (28.3%)
	Standard coronal	17 (28.3%)	37 (61.7%)	6 (10%)
	Standard axial	16 (26.7%)	18 (30%)	26 (43.3%)
Mid-portion	Oblique axial	32 (53.3%)	28 (46.7%)	0
	Standard sagittal	7 (11.7%)	24 (40%)	29 (48.3%)
	Standard coronal	4 (6.7%)	12 (20%)	44 (73.3%)
	Standard axial	6 (10%)	10 (16.7%)	44 (73.3%)
Femoral origin	Oblique axial	31 (51.7%)	27 (45%)	2 (3.3%)
	Standard sagittal	1 (1.7%)	3 (5%)	56 (93.3%)
	Standard coronal	2 (3.3%)	12 (20%)	46 (76.7%)
	Standard axial	5 (8.3%)	15 (25%)	40 (66.7%)

Conclusions.—Oblique axial plane imaging of the ACL was significantly more effectively in delineating both ACL bundles than the standard sagittal, coronal, and axial imaging. Clearer delineation may improve the recognition of partial tears and clinical management (Table 1).

▶ This study describes the use of an oblique axial imaging sequence for evaluation of the anterior cruciate ligament (ACL) and differentiation of anteromedial and posterolateral bundles. The sequence studied does allow for improved visualization of structures and demonstrates well the 2 discreet bundles. Other oblique planes such as an oblique coronal plane have been studied, and it would be interesting to see how each compares with standard planes and with each other. Also important to consider is that the ACL is evaluated in all 3 standard planes. Although any given sequence may not perform particularly well (see Table 1), taken together, confident assessment seems more likely. Certainly in the clinical setting, all sequences are scrutinized for signs of injury and findings are corroborated.

Although the data presented demonstrate the improved visualization of structures in the study, one wonders how much of an improvement this would yield in the clinical setting. In normal volunteers, the sequence may perform well, but the injured ligament may be demonstrated by standard sequences as well. Clearly, additional study will be necessary to answer the question. The appearance of the ACL bundles is certainly striking on the oblique axial image.

The use of such an oblique axial sequence for evaluation of double-bundle repairs is also an interesting issue. That particular surgical repair is not commonly performed at our institution but may be common elsewhere.

Investigation of global assessment of the knee using three-dimensional sequences with multiplanar reconstruction capabilities is ongoing, and, although not clinically ready, such techniques in the future may allow for inclusion of such an oblique axial image without penalty in scan time.

C. Strickland, MD

Shoulder US: Anatomy, Technique, and Scanning Pitfalls
Jacobson JA (Univ of Michigan Med Ctr, Ann Arbor)
Radiology 260:6-16, 2011

The accuracy of shoulder ultrasonography (US) is largely dependent on the US examination technique. It is essential that the individual performing the US examination has an understanding of pertinent anatomy, such as bone surface anatomy and tendon orientation. It is also important to be familiar with imaging pitfalls related to US technique, such as anisotropy. In this article, shoulder US scanning technique, as well as related anatomy and scanning pitfalls, will be reviewed. The use of a protocol-driven shoulder US examination is important to ensure a comprehensive and efficient evaluation. An on-line video tutorial demonstrating a shoulder US also accompanies this article.

▶ Dr Jacobson once again provides us with an excellent review and demonstration of ultrasound technique in the evaluation of the shoulder. With increasing interest in musculoskeletal ultrasound, it is critical that all those performing and interpreting these examinations have a solid foundation of knowledge when it comes to sonographic anatomy, imaging technique, and pitfalls. This review expertly discusses each and leaves the reader with a greater understanding, a useful reference, and a valuable educational tool.

Important anatomic landmarks are discussed, including the relative coverage of the superior and middle facets of the greater tuberosity of the humerus by the supraspinatus and infraspinatus tendons. Differentiation of fibers from each of the rotator cuff tendons is also discussed.

Perhaps most useful is the detailed description of an imaging protocol and the structures that should be evaluated at each location of the shoulder. A 5-step approach is illustrated with photographs of correct transducer placement and corresponding sonographic images. Operators new to the technique of shoulder ultrasound scan will find the approach useful and reproducible. In addition, the supplemental video reinforces the points discussed in the article, particularly with regard to transducer placement, which can prove challenging. Ultimately, those involved in shoulder ultrasound scan interpretation will need to scan many patients themselves to attain adequate facility with the technique. This article serves as a useful guide during that training period.

Pitfalls of the examination are discussed, including anisotropy, which is an important consideration in all musculoskeletal ultrasound examinations. Complete evaluation of anterior supraspinatus fibers and use of the biceps tendon in the rotator interval as an important landmark are appropriately emphasized.

C. Strickland, MD

Morbidity of Direct MR Arthrography

Giaconi JC, Link TM, Vail TP, et al (Univ of California, San Francisco)
AJR Am J Roentgenol 196:868-874, 2011

Objective.—The purpose of this study was to determine the incidence and severity of arthrographic pain after intraarticular injection of a gadolinium mixture diluted in normal saline for direct MR arthrography.

Subjects and Methods.—From March 2009 until January 2010, 155 consecutive patients underwent direct MR arthrography; 20 patients were lost to follow-up. Patients were contacted by telephone between 3 and 7 days after joint injection. Using an 11-point numeric pain rating scale, patients were asked to report if they had experienced joint pain that was different or more intense than their preinjection baseline, the severity of pain, the duration of pain, time to onset of pain, and eventual resolution of pain.

Results.—The incidence of postarthrographic pain was 66% (89/135), with an average intensity of pain of 4.8 ± 2.4 (range, 1–10). Postarthrographic pain lasted an average of 44.4 ± 30.5 hours (range, 6–168 hours). The time to onset of pain after joint injection was on average 16.6 ± 13.1 hours (range, 4–72 hours). There was no significant difference regarding the severity or incidence of postarthrographic pain between groups on the basis of patient age ($p = 0.20$ and 0.26), patient sex ($p = 0.20$ and 0.86), contrast mixture contents ($p - 0.83$ and 0.49), or joint injected ($p = 0.51$ and 0.47). No patients experienced any other serious side effects.

Conclusion.—Sixty-six percent of patients who undergo direct MR arthrography will experience a fairly severe delayed onset of pain that completely resolves over the course of several days.

▶ Direct MR arthrography is a commonly performed procedure with well-documented utility and safety. The recent study by Giaconi et al sheds important light on the experience of patients undergoing this routine minimally invasive procedure. Sixty-six percent of patients in their study went on to have significant pain following direct arthrography.

Interestingly, no significant differences among postprocedure pain levels at different joints could be detected, although the authors point out that the small sample size of some injection sites may hide any true difference. Similarly, the inclusion or exclusion of epinephrine in the arthrographic cocktail did not alter the degree of pain reported. While the exact mixtures used at different institutions vary, the results presented here are likely applicable to most practices, given the relative required concentrations of gadolinium and iodinated contrast that allow for optimized MR imaging.

The mechanisms proposed for the cause of pain and delayed onset are also useful and raise interesting questions that may lead to further study. Whether extravasation from the injected joint plays an important role remains an interesting question. Perhaps the experience of the operator performing the procedure may play a role by affecting the number of needle repositionings or time of needle in the joint? The direct arthrography in this study was performed by musculoskeletal radiology fellows with supervision, and one might wonder how patient symptoms may differ following procedures by those without subspecialty training or extensive experience.

This study helps reinforce the need to understand the effects that our interventions have on patients. It is interesting to note that the authors describe their practice of routine clinical follow-up by way of a phone call with patients 3 to 7 days after arthrography. This practice was prompted by reports from referring physicians that the patients they had sent for MR arthrograms had experienced pain after the procedure.

Discussion of this postprocedure pain phenomenon by the radiologist performing the arthrogram with the patient should serve to make patients less anxious and help identify the radiologist as a physician involved and interested in their care. For these reasons, pain following the procedure is a routine point of discussion when obtaining consent for such procedures in our department.

C. Strickland, MD

MR Arthrographic Appearance of the Postoperative Acetabular Labrum in Patients With Suspected Recurrent Labral Tears
Blankenbaker DG, De Smet AA, Keene JS (Univ of Wisconsin School of Medicine and Public Health, Madison)
AJR Am J Roentgenol 197:W1118-W1122, 2011

Objective.—The objective of our study was to evaluate the MR arthrographic appearance of the acetabular labrum in patients with a suspected recurrent acetabular labral tear after previous arthroscopic resection of a labral tear.

Conclusion.—The labrum after excision will appear shortened on MR arthrography. A recurrent labral tear can be diagnosed by the identification on MR arthrography of a new line to the labral surface, an enlarged and distorted labrum, or a new paralabral cyst.

▶ The acetabular labrum has attracted much attention of late as the use of hip arthroscopy in clinical practice has expanded. This study provides helpful insight to all who interpret hip magnetic resonance (MR) images. As the authors point out, enough patients have undergone labral debridement or repair that some of them are starting to show up again with recurrent hip pain. For many such patients, the next stop is the radiology department for MR arthrography. By review of imaging findings both without and later with correlative surgical information, the authors describe the features that are expected in a recurrent labral tear. Namely, the presence of a new high-signal intensity line extending to the labral surface, enlargement and distortion of the labrum, and the presence of a new paralabral cyst allow for the diagnosis to be made. As is pointed out in the article, further study will be necessary to test the accuracy of such criteria.

Surgical correlation in such studies is critical when defining the imaging features of pathology. The need for anatomic correlation also presents an obstacle in the study of the labrum. One wonders how commonly similar imaging features described in the study could be found in patients years after a repair or debridement but who don't have any new or recurrent symptoms and thus no arthroscopic data. Perhaps some of these patients would be proven to have tears as well at arthroscopy. It seems likely that the challenge of accurate diagnosis of acetabular labral pathology will follow us to postoperative evaluation.

In addition, the nonarthrographic appearance of recurrent labral tearing warrants investigation. Comparison of accuracy between arthrographic and nonarthrographic studies is eagerly awaited.

C. Strickland, MD

Indirect MR Arthrographic Findings of Adhesive Capsulitis
Song KD, Kwon JW, Yoon YC, et al (Sungkyunkwan Univ School of Medicine, Seoul, Korea)
AJR Am J Roentgenol 197:W1105-W1109, 2011

Objective.—The objective of our study was to compare the indirect MR arthrographic findings of patients with adhesive capsulitis and patients without adhesive capsulitis.

Materials and Methods.—Indirect MR arthrograms of 35 patients (21 women, 14 men; mean age, 50.1 years) diagnosed with adhesive capsulitis clinically were compared with indirect MR arthrograms of 45 patients (23 women, 22 men; mean age, 48.9 years) without adhesive capsulitis. Joint capsule thickness in the axillary recess and the thicknesses of the enhancing portion of the axillary recess and the rotator interval were, respectively, evaluated on coronal T2-weighted images and coronal and sagittal fat-suppressed enhanced T1-weighted images by two radiologists independently. Reliability was studied using the intraclass correlation coefficient (ICC). Receiver operating characteristic (ROC) curves were compared.

Results.—Patients with adhesive capsulitis had significantly thickened joint capsules in the axillary recess and a thickened enhancing portion in the axillary recess and in the rotator interval. The difference in the thicknesses of the enhancing portion in the axillary recess and in the rotator interval were significantly greater than the difference in joint capsule thicknesses in the axillary recess between the adhesive capsulitis group and the control group ($p < 0.001$). Interobserver reliability was good for all three indexes (ICC ≥ 0.80). The area under the ROC curve for the thickness of the joint capsule in the axillary recess and the thicknesses of the enhancing portion of the axillary recess and the rotator interval were 0.797, 0.861, and 0.847, respectively.

Conclusion.—An abundance of enhancing tissue in the rotator interval and thickening and enhancement of the axillary recess are signs suggestive of adhesive capsulitis on indirect MR arthrography.

▶ Adhesive capsulitis, or frozen shoulder, is a relatively common clinical diagnosis with which radiologists come into contact. While the diagnosis is commonly made without imaging, knowledge of characteristic imaging features is important to the musculoskeletal radiologist. Song et al discuss the findings on indirect arthrography and show the relative differences in enhancing tissue seen at the rotator interval and axillary recess. Differences between patients with and without the condition are shown, although the differences are small, particularly in the case of the axillary recess.

The use of magnetic resonance imaging (MRI) in the evaluation of adhesive capsulitis is aimed largely at the exclusion of other possible diagnoses. It would be interesting to study the relative sensitivity of indirect (or even direct) arthrography and nonenhanced MRI in the diagnosis in a single study. Whether indirect arthrography offers sufficient additional diagnostic accuracy to advocate its use routinely in the setting of adhesive capsulitis remains unanswered.

At our institution, we are frequently asked to perform therapeutic injections in patients with adhesive capsulitis with the purpose of speeding recovery and allowing the patient to make greater progress with physical therapy. The typical arthrographic approach we use brings the needle through the rotator interval, which often complicates evaluation of that region if MRI imaging is also performed after the intervention. Typically, this does not present a problem given that the diagnosis has already been established. Another perplexing question is how well imaging findings correlate with the clinical course of the disease. Findings that suggest a rapid return to normal activity or a long complicated course would require a large group for study but would also provide helpful information to our referring providers.

C. Strickland, MD

Displaceability of SLAP lesion on shoulder MR arthrography with external rotation position
Jung JY, Ha DH, Lee SM, et al (CHA Univ, Gyeonggi-do, Korea; et al)
Skelet Radiol 40:1047-1055, 2011

Objective.—To investigate the usefulness of the external rotation (ER) position on magnetic resonance (MR) arthrography for the diagnosis of superior labral anterior to posterior (SLAP) lesion.

Materials and Methods.—Approval of institutional review board was obtained, and informed consent was waived. The MR arthrograms of 210 shoulders that were arthroscopically confirmed as SLAP lesion in 163 shoulders and intact superior labrum in 47 shoulders were retrospectively reviewed in each neutral and ER position for the diagnosis of SLAP lesion, the extent of distraction of the torn labrum, and the external rotation angle. The sensitivity, specificity, and diagnostic accuracy of MR arthrograms for determining SLAP lesion were assessed in each position. For the arthroscopically confirmed group, the diagnosis of SLAP lesion and the extent of distraction about the tear were compared between neutral and ER positions by Fisher's exact test and the paired *t*-test. The correlation between the external rotation angle and the diagnosis of SLAP lesion, and between the external rotation angle and the differences in the extent of distraction were evaluated in the ER position using the ANOVA test.

Results.—Sensitivity and diagnostic accuracy of MR arthrography for SLAP lesion increased from 64.4% and 71.0% in the neutral position to 78.5% and 81.9% in the ER position, respectively, without change of specificity, which was 93.6% in both positions. The diagnosis of SLAP lesion was changed from negative to SLAP lesion in 16.0% of the arthroscopically confirmed group. Mean difference in the extent of distraction about the tear was 0.69 mm (range −1.40 ~ 6.67 mm), which was statistically significant. There was no relationship between the external rotation angle and the diagnosis of SLAP lesion, and between the external rotation angle and the differences in the extent of distraction.

Conclusion.—Shoulder MR arthrography with additional ER positioning helps in the diagnosis of SLAP lesion and provides information about the displaceability of the torn labrum.

▶ Kwak et al[1] published in 1998 that positioning the arm in external rotation (ER) optimizes visualization of the labral biceps anchor compared with neutral or abduction external rotation (ABER) arthrography. Yet over the last decade, imaging in external rotation imaging has not been significantly analyzed, whereas articles on ABER positioning abound. The article by Jung et al addresses this expertly in a study of 210 subjects. The authors report an increase in sensitivity from 64% to 79% in comparing the neutral thumbs-up position with external rotation for MR arthrography of superior labral (SLAP) tears at the biceps anchor. Additionally, proven SLAP tears demonstrated an average displacement of 0.7 mm between the 2 positions, simulating the clinical significance of unstable tears as seen by the arthroscopist. While the mean patient achieved 34° of arc in rotating the shoulder, as little as 5° of added external rotation is shown to be adequate for increasing accuracy and demonstrating displaceability. External rotation for arthrography is also presented as an obtainable position for this patient population, with only a relatively small number of patients (15) excluded from the study because of inadequate rotation. The various accepted mechanisms of superior labral tearing, including forced shoulder adduction, biceps tension, and posterior peel-back, suggest external rotation as a helpful method to demonstrate SLAP tears. Jung et al have nicely quantitated the added value of external rotation in evaluating superior labral tears at the biceps anchor.

R. Chapin, MD

Reference

1. Kwak SM, Brown RR, Trudell D, Resnick D. Glenohumeral joint: comparison of shoulder positions at MR arthrography. *Radiology.* 1998;208:375-380.

Evaluation of the Glenoid Labrum With 3-T MRI: Is Intraarticular Contrast Necessary?

Major NM, Browne J, Domzalski T, et al (Hosp of the Univ of Pennsylvania, Philadelphia; Duke Univ Med Ctr, Durham, NC)
AJR Am J Roentgenol 196:1139-1144, 2011

Objective.—The purpose of this study was to evaluate the diagnostic accuracy of 3-T MRI versus 3-T MR arthrography for assessing labral abnormalities in the shoulder using arthroscopy as the gold standard.

Subjects and Methods.—Forty-two patients (28 men, 14 women; mean age, 33 years) underwent MR arthrography and conventional MRI of the same shoulder. Two patients underwent bilateral shoulder examinations, for a total of 44 shoulder examinations. Twenty-two shoulders underwent arthroscopy. The results of arthroscopy were used as the reference standard. Three musculoskeletal radiologists prospectively and independently interpreted MRI and MR arthrography examinations. Differences in performance of conventional MRI and MR arthrography were analyzed for statistical significance by the two-tailed McNemar test.

Results.—Of the 22 arthroscopies performed, 26 labral tears were found in 18 shoulders and four shoulders were normal with respect to the labrum. There were 12 superior, nine posterior, and five anterior labral tears identified at arthroscopy. By consensus review, conventional MRI identified nine of 12 superior (sensitivity, 75%; specificity, 100%), seven of nine posterior (sensitivity, 78%; specificity, 92%), and three of five anterior (sensitivity, 60%; specificity, 94%) labral tears. MR arthrography identified nine of 12 superior (sensitivity, 75%; specificity, 100%), eight of nine posterior (sensitivity, 89%; specificity, 100%), and five of five anterior (sensitivity, 100%; specificity, 100%) labral tears.

Conclusion.—Although the power of our preliminary study is small, the results suggest that intraarticular contrast material is helpful in diagnosing labral tears in the shoulder, particularly tears of the anterior labrum. Our preliminary results suggest that MR arthrography adds value for diagnosing labral tears in the shoulder compared with conventional MRI even at 3 T.

▶ The necessity of direct arthrography remains a topic of continued debate. Widespread clinical introduction of 3-T imaging systems has added to the debate by providing interpreting radiologists with images demonstrating improved signal-to-noise characteristics and higher quality. Major et al. provide additional important insight into the question with a series of 44 shoulders imaged with both MRI and MR arthrography. A particular strength of the study is the fact that the MRI and MR arthrogram studies were performed on the same day and on the same scanner, which dispenses with several potential confounding factors. Twenty-two shoulders in the series ultimately underwent arthroscopy, and the results are of interest to all involved in imaging and treatment of the glenoid labrum. A trend toward increased sensitivity with arthrography was detected, although a significant difference could not be shown. The relatively small sample size likely contributes significantly to this finding, and clearly larger series are necessary to compare the techniques more completely. A few interesting points do emerge, however. All of the labral tears detected by MRI were also visible by MR arthrography, and all of the tears called on arthrographic studies turned out to be real in those patients who underwent arthroscopy. Interestingly, not all patients with positive MR arthrogram studies had surgical correlation, so it is possible that MR arthrography could have been shown to perform even more favorably if such data were available. This study also highlights the challenge in detecting and defining potentially small statistically significant differences in the performance of imaging techniques. The large sample sizes necessary to prove statistical significance are often difficult to recruit in a clinical setting.

Despite these limitations, however, this series suggests a continued important role for direct arthrography in the evaluation of the glenoid labrum. A larger series is needed to demonstrate whether significant superiority over conventional MRI exists.

C. Strickland, MD

Avascular necrosis (AVN) of the proximal fragment in scaphoid nonunion: Is intravenous contrast agent necessary in MRI?
Schmitt R, Christopoulos G, Wagner M, et al (Cardiovascular Ctr, Bad Neustadt an der Saale, Germany)
Eur J Radiol 77:222-227, 2011

Purpose.—The purpose of this prospective study is to assess the diagnostic value of intravenously applied contrast agent for diagnosing osteonecrosis of the proximal fragment in scaphoid nonunion, and to compare the imaging results with intraoperative findings.

Materials and Methods.—In 88 patients (7 women, 81 men) suffering from symptomatic scaphoid nonunion, preoperative MRI was performed (coronal PD-w FSE fs, sagittal-oblique T1-w SE nonenhanced and T1-w SE fs contrast-enhanced, sagittal T2*-w GRE). MRI interpretation was based on the intensity of contrast enhancement: $0 = $ none, $1 = $ focal, $2 = $ diffuse. Intraoperatively, the osseous viability was scored by means of bleeding points on the osteotomy site of the proximal scaphoid fragment: $0 = $ absent, $1 = $ moderate, $2 = $ good.

Results.—Intraoperatively, 17 necrotic, 29 compromised, and 42 normal proximal fragments were found. In nonenhanced MRI, bone viability was judged necrotic in 1 patient, compromised in 20 patients, and unaffected in 67 patients. Contrast-enhanced MRI revealed 14 necrotic, 21 compromised, and 53 normal proximal fragments. Judging surgical findings as the standard of reference, statistical analysis for nonenhanced MRI was: sensitivity 6.3%, specificity 100%, positive PV 100%, negative PV 82.6%, and accuracy 82.9%; statistics for contrast-enhanced MRI were: sensitivity 76.5%, specificity 98.6%, positive PV 92.9%, negative PV 94.6%, and accuracy 94.3%. Sensitivity for detecting avascular proximal fragments was significantly better ($p < 0.001$) in contrast-enhanced MRI in comparison to nonenhanced MRI.

Conclusion.—Viability of the proximal fragment in scaphoid nonunion can be significantly better assessed with the use of contrast-enhanced MRI as compared to nonenhanced MRI. Bone marrow edema is an inferior indicator of osteonecrosis. Application of intravenous gadolinium is recommended for imaging scaphoid nonunion.

▶ This study provides additional insight into the evaluation of the proximal scaphoid fracture fragment for osteonecrosis. Although various imaging strategies have been described by different groups, the experience described here with 88 patients provides additional evidence that contrast-enhanced studies improve sensitivity and potentially guide management. Surgical correlation in such a large number of patients lends important weight to the study, as does the follow-up period. Particularly useful is the discussion in the article of surgical assessment of bone viability (which involves directly visualizing sites of bleeding from the debrided bone surface) and differing treatments based on findings at the time of surgery. This background helps to illustrate the importance of MRI in this clinical scenario and how the clinical report will directly affect the patient management.

Important to consider, however, is that the surgical approach was the same for cases in the study and may not reflect those of referring surgeons everywhere. As with all musculoskeletal radiology interpretations, it is important to communicate with surgeons about the findings on studies we interpret and what they are likely to mean at time of surgery.

C. Strickland, MD

MR Arthrography of the Hip: Comparison of IDEAL-SPGR Volume Sequence to Standard MR Sequences in the Detection and Grading of Cartilage Lesions
Blankenbaker DG, Ullrick SR, Kijowski R, et al (Univ of Wisconsin School of Medicine and Public Health, Madison; et al)
Radiology 261:863-871, 2011

Purpose.—To compare the diagnostic performance of iterative decomposition of water and fat with echo asymmetry and least-squares estimation (IDEAL)–spoiled gradient-recalled echo (SPGR) with that of standard magnetic resonance (MR) arthrography sequences for detecting and grading cartilage lesions within the hip joint during MR arthrography.

Materials and Methods.—Following institutional review board approval, 67 consecutive hip MR arthrograms were retrospectively reviewed independently by three musculoskeletal radiologists and one musculoskeletal fellow. IDEAL-SPGR images and the two-dimensional images, the latter from the routine MR arthrography protocol, were evaluated at separate sittings to grade each articular surface of the hip joint. By using arthroscopy as the reference standard, the sensitivity and specificity of the two techniques for detecting and grading cartilage lesions were determined. The McNemar test was used to compare diagnostic performance. Interreader agreement was calculated using Fleiss κ values.

Results.—For all readers and surfaces combined, the sensitivity and specificity for detecting cartilage lesions was 74% and 77%, respectively, for IDEAL-SPGR and 70% and 84%, respectively, for the routine MR arthrography protocol. IDEAL-SPGR had similar sensitivity ($P = .12$) to and significantly lower specificity ($P < .001$) than the routine MR arthrography protocol for depicting cartilage lesions. When analyzing the differences in sensitivity and specificity by reader, the two readers who had experience with IDEAL-SPGR had no significant difference in sensitivity and specificity for detecting cartilage lesions between the two sequences. For all readers and surfaces combined, IDEAL-SPGR had a higher accuracy in correctly grading cartilage lesion ($P = .012-.013$). Interobserver agreement for detecting cartilage lesions did not differ between the two techniques.

Conclusion.—IDEAL-SPGR had similar sensitivity and significantly lower specificity for detecting cartilage lesions and higher accuracy for grading cartilage lesions than did a routine MR arthrography protocol; the lower specificity of IDEAL-SPGR for detecting cartilage lesions was not seen in experienced readers.

▶ Evaluation of cartilage continues to grow in importance in musculoskeletal imaging. Although the diagnostic accuracy for ligament, meniscus, and other injuries by magnetic resonance (MR) imaging evaluation is high, cartilage lesions remain a challenge to detect and characterize in several joints, including the hip. In this article, Blankenbaker et al discuss the utility of iterative decomposition of water and fat with echo asymmetry and least-squares estimation (IDEAL-SPGR) compared with standard MR arthrographic sequences in the detection and grading of hip cartilage lesions. The IDEAL-SPGR proved similar in sensitivity, but exhibited lower specificity but higher accuracy in grading of lesions. It is interesting to note that experienced readers in the study fared better with the IDEAL-SPGR sequence. This likely reflects the greater experience with similar sequences at an academic institution with an active research enterprise in cartilage imaging. The inclusion of a less experienced reader adds external validity to the study.

One important detail to consider is the fact that arthrography had been performed before MR evaluation for both sets of sequences. Some authors have argued that direct arthrography of the hip may not be necessary, and the relative performance of the sequences in this study would be interesting to evaluate in patients not undergoing arthrography. Obtaining surgical correlation would be necessary, and surgeons (at least at our institution) request direct arthrography examinations before considering arthroscopy.

Early detection of cartilage lesions may help guide management aimed at slowing the progression of joint degeneration. As in many similar studies, normal and grade 1 cartilage lesions were combined for statistical analysis. From a study design, this makes sense given the difficulty of distinguishing the two with MR and arthroscopy, but one wonders how clinically important the distinction may be and in the future if differentiation may be accomplished and the results clinically relevant.

The theoretical advantage of cartilage evaluation with thin contiguous images is also discussed. As this study demonstrates, only through rigorous comparison with more widespread clinical sequences may we gauge the utility of new imaging approaches.

C. Strickland, MD

Presumed intraarticular gas microbubbles resulting from a vacuum phenomenon: visualization with ultrasonography as hyperechoic microfoci
Malghem J, Omoumi P, Lecouvet FE, et al (St Luc Univ Hosp — UCLouvain, Bruxelles, Belgium)
Skeletal Radiol 40:1287-1293, 2011

Objective.—Hyperechoic microfoci are sometimes visualized in normal joints. We hypothesized that these microfoci may correspond to gas microbubbles produced by a vacuum phenomenon. The purpose of our study was to demonstrate the possibility of generating intraarticular hyperechoic microbubbles by creating a vacuum phenomenon through traction on a metacarpophalangeal joint.

Materials and Methods.—We applied manual traction to the second metacarpophalangeal (MCP) joint of 22 volunteer subjects to separate articular surfaces with the aim of producing a vacuum. For one subject, the production of a vacuum was verified on a radiograph performed during the traction maneuver. For all subjects, ultrasonographic examination of the MCP joints was performed before, during, and after traction maneuvers. Two radiologists evaluated the presence of intraarticular hyperechoic microfoci and measured the widening of the joint space during traction.

Results.—In the first subject, the widening of the joint space and the production of an intraarticular gas-like cavity by traction was confirmed on the radiograph. In 10 out of the 22 volunteers, the widening of the joint space was immediately followed by the appearance of a large intraarticular hyperechoic band, which disappeared when the traction was stopped, followed by the appearance of hyperechoic microfoci that persisted several minutes. The widening of the joint during the traction maneuver was greater in the group where hyperechoic foci were produced than in the group with no hyperechoic foci (mean 2.5 vs. 1.2 mm and 2.2 vs. 0.8 mm, respectively, for observers 1 and 2; $P<0.05$, Mann-Whitney U test).

Conclusion.—Intraarticular hyperechoic microfoci may be produced and persist in normal joints after a traction maneuver. They are presumed to correspond to microbubbles created by a transient vacuum phenomenon (Fig 6).

▶ The use of ultrasound for musculoskeletal diagnoses remains a topic of interest in the United States and around the world. This article applies the technique to

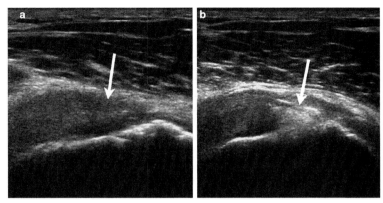

FIGURE 6.—Hyperechoic foci in a defect of a rotator cuff tendon. **a** A hypoechoic area is seen in the distal part of the supraspinatus tendon, compatible with a tear (*arrow*). **b** After mobilizing the shoulder, confluent hyperechoic foci appeared in the same area (*arrow*), possibly corresponding to a migration of articular microbubbles in the defect. (With kind permission from Springer Science+Business Media. Malghem J, Omoumi P, Lecouvet FE, et al. Presumed intraarticular gas microbubbles resulting from a vacuum phenomenon: visualization with ultrasonography as hyperechoic microfoci. *Skeletal Radiol.* 2011;40:1287-1293.)

evaluation of intraarticular gas in joints due to vacuum phenomenon. The presence of gas is frequently encountered in the interpretation of radiographs and MRI studies and may obscure or confuse pathology in direct arthrographic examinations. This study, which includes evaluation of metacarpophalangeal joints placed under traction and then observed at 15, 30, and 60 minutes, provides some interesting insights. First, the hyperechoic nondependent band that likely represents gas in the joint is immediately visible after the application of traction on the joint. Gas seems to persist for several minutes, which is an important fact to recognize when such a finding is encountered. If such a finding is a source of confusion, reimaging the patient after 30 minutes may help to exclude the presence other hyperechoic materials such as calcifications.

The authors describe some scenarios in which the use of maneuvers to create gas in the joint may actually aid in diagnosis. Fig 6 depicts a collection of small gas bubbles in a rotator cuff defect. Perhaps the use of gas produced by motions of the shoulder joint could help the interpreter to distinguish between rotator cuff tendinosis or tear.

The study includes patients with no known arthritis or history of significant injury. Whether the ability to produce vacuum phenomenon can be used to exclude an effusion or other pathology is interesting to consider and is a point raised by the authors. Several limitations are also described, including the lack of radiographic confirmation in all except the first subject. Whether the same phenomenon can be easily produced elsewhere and if loss of this finding has any clinical meaning remains unknown.

C. Strickland, MD

A Biomechanical Approach to MRI of Acute Knee Injuries

MacMahon PJ, Palmer WE (Harvard Med School, Boston, MA)
AJR Am J Roentgenol 197:568-577, 2011

Objective.—MRI is routinely performed to evaluate acute complex knee injuries. This article will review the fundamental biomechanical forces underlying the most important and common injuries and correlate MRI findings with specific traumatic mechanisms.

Conclusion.—MRI findings can reveal the traumatic mechanisms in many acute knee injuries. By applying a biomechanical approach in MRI interpretation, it is possible to use easily detected lesions, such as osseous contusion and ligament rupture, to predict subtle but important abnormalities that might otherwise be missed. This systematic focused analysis enables a more accurate and rapid interpretation of knee MR studies.

▶ This review provides a useful discussion of common biomechanical mechanisms of knee injury. Recognition of bone marrow edema and possible mechanism of injury is an important exercise to perform when interpreting magnetic resonance imaging (MRI) studies of any acutely injured joint. As the authors point out, specific patterns suggest injury in certain structures. In the interpretation of such studies, my colleagues and I certainly make note of specific patterns and use these to direct our attention (and the attention of our trainees) to likely sites of injury. Indeed, the pattern of edema often leads one to appropriately call a meniscus or ligament tear when the imaging appearance is equivocal but the mechanism highly suggestive.

This review also highlights the dangers of satisfaction of search. The anterior cruciate ligament injury is often obvious to the orthopedic surgeon by physical examination before ordering the MRI study. While the anterior cruciate ligament (ACL) injury is often clear by MRI as well, the utility of the imaging study is often to detect the more subtle secondary injuries such as those involving the posterolateral corner that may complicate a standard surgical repair.

Numerous imaging examples and clinical vignettes are included to reinforce the concepts described in the review. The high frequency of lateral collateral ligament injuries in the setting of acute ACL injury is also mentioned, which bears repeating. Residents early in training are well aware of the O'Donoghue triad from medical school and may overlook lateral collateral ligament injuries.

Mentioned obliquely is the importance of radiographs in the evaluation of knee trauma. A Segond fracture or deep lateral sulcus sign provides mechanistic information as well, and the diagnostic approach described here for MRI is also important to consider when evaluating radiographs.

C. Strickland, MD

MRI of the Pediatric Knee

Pai DR, Strouse PJ (Univ of Michigan Health System, Ann Arbor)
AJR Am J Roentgenol 196:1019-1027, 2011

Objective.—The purpose of this article is to describe findings on MRI in the evaluation of knee injury in pediatric patients.

Conclusion.—Injury patterns in the pediatric knee overlap and differ from adults. Differences include open physes, changing mechanics, and differences in ligamentous support. Awareness of normal variants, common incidental findings, and normal evolution of bone marrow aid in the interpretation.

▶ This review by Pai and Strouse serves to highlight several important considerations when using MRI to image the pediatric knee. Musculoskeletal radiologists spend the majority of their time interpreting images of the skeletally mature, so when pediatric cases appear on the work list, one needs to keep in mind the important differences in imaging findings and injury patterns described here.

Frequently injured structures such as the menisci simply have a different appearance in the skeletally immature. Increased signal on fluid-sensitive sequences seen in pediatric menisci may look degenerative to those more accustomed to reading images from adult patients. Residents will often confuse this point when seeing such images for the first time.

Discussion of the growth plate in the review is also helpful. Salter-Harris type fractures may masquerade clinically as soft-tissue derangements, and vigilance may be needed to detect them. Indeed, the physis demonstrates increased signal on fluid-sensitive sequences, and close scrutiny may be needed to detect a fracture, particularly if it is subacute. A recent case at our institution with a Salter-Harris type II injury at the femoral physis demonstrated the point nicely because the fracture was subacute and invisible on accompanying radiographs.

Avulsion injuries resulting in failure of the cruciate or other ligament complexes are also described. Residents interpreting pediatric radiographic examples of avulsion fractures benefit greatly when MRI examples can be shown that illustrate the associated soft-tissue injury. A posterior cruciate ligament bony avulsion may not look like a severe injury, although the MRI illustrates the injury fully.

The limitations of diagnostic accuracy when evaluating pediatric patients are also well discussed in the review. Specifically, the MRI criteria for assessment of osteochondritis dissecans stability are more problematic in pediatric patients. The treatment approach is also different (and frequently more conservative), which is important to consider when encountering a lesion that appears unstable by adult criteria. Recognition of cortically based lesions such as fibrous cortical defects is also particularly important and is described.

The review provides a concise guide to the important differences in evaluation of the adult and pediatric knee by MRI and serves as a helpful resource for those beginning to interpret such examinations.

C. Strickland, MD

Can Stress Radiography of the Knee Help Characterize Posterolateral Corner Injury?

Gwathmey FW Jr, Tompkins MA, Gaskin CM, et al (Univ of Virginia Health System, Charlottesville)
Clin Orthop Relat Res 470:768-773, 2012

Background.—Conventional MRI is limited for characterizing the posterolateral corner of the knee due to the region's anatomic variability and complexity; further, MRI is a static study and cannot demonstrate pathologic laxity. Stress radiography may provide additional information about instability.

Questions/Purposes.—We therefore (1) correlated varus stress radiography with MRI findings, (2) compared opening in patients who underwent surgical posterolateral corner stabilization versus those who did not, and (3) determined whether stress radiography findings could supplement MRI for making treatment decisions.

Patients and Methods.—We retrospectively studied 26 patients (27 knee injuries) and correlated lateral compartment opening on varus stress radiography with severity of posterolateral corner injury on MRI. We compared radiographic findings in 18 patients with complete injuries who underwent posterolateral corner stabilization with five who did not.

Results.—A complete posterolateral corner injury on MRI was associated with an average of 18.6 mm (10.0–36.5 mm) of varus opening versus 12.8 mm (7.5–17.0 mm) in partial injuries. Opening in operative cases that underwent stabilization was 16.5 mm (11.0–36.5 mm) versus 11.0 mm (7.5–13.5 mm) for those that did not. Ten of 15 partial injuries underwent stabilization, for which the varus opening was 13.6 mm (11.0–17.0 mm). Average varus opening in partial injuries that did not undergo stabilization was 11.0 mm (7.5–13.5 mm).

Conclusions.—Varus stress radiography correlated to MRI findings for posterolateral corner injury. The injuries we treated with reconstruction were associated with increased varus opening. In patients with partial posterolateral corner injury on MRI, we used degree of opening on varus stress radiography to aid the decision for stabilization.

Level of Evidence.—Level IV, diagnostic study. See Guidelines for Authors for a complete description of levels of evidence.

▶ Gwathmey et al address the utility of varus stress radiography in the evaluation of posterolateral corner injury of the knee in this retrospective review. Much effort has gone into description and identification of posterolateral corner injuries of the knee by MRI. As the authors mention, assessment of individual structures of the posterolateral corner is often difficult given their relatively small size and the anatomic variability at the location. Stress radiography presents an additional functional evaluation that complements the static anatomic imaging obtained by MRI when the knee is in neutral position.

The study demonstrates that widening of the lateral compartment is preferentially seen when varus stress is applied to patients who went on to have surgery compared with those who did not. This finding is important to consider but leaves the reader with several important questions: First, it is unclear how much additional information stress views provide that is not available with MRI and physical examination. It is possible that patients who demonstrate significant joint widening are clearly unstable upon physical examination and are headed to the operating room anyway. It would be interesting to study the effect of this single test on the decision of whether to operate.

As the authors point out, several confounding factors also deserve consideration: pain, swelling, and guarding likely directly influence the degree of joint widening depicted by radiographs. Comparison of radiographs obtained in clinic and under anesthesia would be an interesting study in itself.

Finally, the outcome of patients evaluated by stress radiography would be helpful. Perhaps stress radiographs are only helpful in cases that are equivocal by MRI and physical examination. Ongoing studies will be eagerly awaited as we attempt to improve interpretation of posterolateral corner injuries of the knee.

C. Strickland, MD

Other

Contrast-Enhanced Magnetic Resonance Imaging Positively Impacts the Management of Some Patients With Rheumatoid Arthritis or Suspected RA
Fox MG, Stephens T, Jarjour WN, et al (Univ of Virginia, Charlottesville; Ohio State Univ, Columbus)
J Clin Rheumatol 18:15-22, 2012

Objective.—Early diagnosis of rheumatoid arthritis (RA) is important given the availability of highly effective disease-modifying antirheumatic (DMARD) medications, including biologics. However, because of associated risks and cost, accurately assessing disease activity is critical. Because magnetic resonance imaging (MRI) can detect synovitis and bone marrow edema, both of which may precede erosion development, we sought to determine the impact of enhanced MRI on patient management in a group of patients referred for MRI by rheumatologists.

Materials and Methods.—After institutional review board approval, we evaluated all hand MRI examinations referred by the rheumatology department for synovitis evaluation between September 2007 and May 2009. The magnetic resonance images were classified as positive or negative and later reviewed by 2 musculoskeletal radiologists. A musculoskeletal radiologist and rheumatologist jointly reviewed the patients' medical records to determine the following: (1) Did the MRI findings alter treatment? (2) Were the treatment alterations beneficial?

Results.—The study included 48 patients (39 women and 9 men) with a mean age of 51 years (range, 18–79 years). Significant management changes initially occurred in 79% (23/29) of the positive (DMARDs added in 20) and in 11% (2/19) of the negative MR examinations with average follow-up of ~300 days. Eighty percent (16/20) of the patients with DMARDs added experienced symptom improvement, none of the patients whose medications were discontinued experienced symptom relapse, and 18% (4/22) of patients without initial therapeutic changes required delayed treatment modifications.

Conclusions.—Enhanced MRI significantly altered clinical management in 50% of these patients with RA or suspected RA. Therefore, when the clinical picture in a patient with RA or suspected RA is unclear, enhanced MRI can provide useful guidance for treatment modifications.

▶ This retrospective study seeks to get at an important question that comes up when evaluating cases of rheumatoid arthritis by MRI: do the findings demonstrated in the hand by MRI affect clinical management? In this study group, the answer is yes. Fifty percent of the patients included in the study had management changes made in the year following the MRI examination. This reinforces the notion that MRI imaging data are helpful in guiding management of an often confusing disease. As the authors point out, the high cost and potential side effects of disease-modifying antirheumatic drugs necessitates a reliable and reproducible way to measure disease status and progression. MRI seems uniquely suited to this role. MRI depicts synovitis and erosions well and shows soft-tissue abnormalities such as tenosynovitis. It also demonstrates the presence of bone marrow edema, which is important in predicting future development of erosions. MRI is expensive but less operator-dependent than ultrasound. Certainly ultrasound plays an important role, but MRI on a high-quality scanner with contrast and an optimized protocol potentially offers clinical information that cannot be obtained by other methods.

Importantly, the MRI examinations included in the study were initially evaluated for positivity or negativity using simple parameters. This provides some degree of external validity to the study because it parallels clinical practice. Still, discrimination of true synovitis from normal synovial enhancement in the interpretation of MRI is often difficult.

This study raises several questions. First, and most important, do the changes in management made on the basis of MRI findings improve patient outcomes? Certainly ongoing studies will be necessary to address this important question. It does seem that MRI provides important information to clinicians faced with contradictory lab values or a confusing clinical examination.

C. Strickland, MD

4   Pediatric Radiology

Introduction

We associate editors have greatly enjoyed and benefited from the enthusiasm, guidance, and comprehensive knowledge of our Editor-in-Chief of many years, Dr Anne Osborn of Utah. We take this opportunity to thank her and also extend many thanks on behalf of our readers.

This year we have chosen and commented once again on a wide variety of conditions (new, old, rare, common, and mimicking) as well as imaging technology. To highlight the value of such a range of selections, Dr Oestreich was consulted recently from Hungary on a patient with an unusual set of radiographic findings, who turned out to have an uncommon genetic syndrome that we abstracted last year,[1] the Stüve-Wiedemann syndrome. Despite having written the commentary, we did not make the prospective diagnosis in this child. One of Dr Oestreich's articles suggests the tide is turning against unneeded VCUGs. His coverage includes highlighting the use of eovist in tumor diagnosis; the question of ultrasound diagnosis for jejunal volvulus is debated; Lavy Moseley syndrome is split from Jarco Levin; and the cyamella is revealed.

Dr Offiah has no articles related to failed prospective diagnoses to boast about—not to say that missed diagnoses have not occurred! We must try to steer away from our favorite topic of child abuse, but we have yet again included articles on this: one, a brave attempt to set criteria for the objective dating of fractures, another in which the authors (to our obvious chagrin) suggest we eliminate some of the radiographs routinely performed as part of the skeletal survey, and second, an article in which MR spectroscopic brain imaging is used to predict outcome following nonaccidental head injury. On the subject of brain MRI, great advancements are being made and new biomarkers being developed such as measuring cortical thickness in ADHD (counterintuitively increased compared with normal controls). We have also included an article on the use of ultrasound in the pediatric emergency department by relatively untrained emergency department physicians in the United States, and here finally is our opportunity to boast, "UK radiologists have more control—it's not happening here…yet."

Alan E. Oestreich, MD
Amaka C. Offiah, BSc, MBBS, MRCP, FRCR, PhD

Reference

1. Jung C, Dagoneau N, Baujat G, et al. Stüve-Wiedemann syndrome: long-term follow-up and genetic heterogeneity. *Clin Genet.* 2010;77:266-272.

Gastrointestinal

Accurate localization of the position of the tip of a naso/orogastric tube in children; where is the location of the gastro-esophageal junction?

Cohen MD, Ellett MLC, Perkins SM, et al (Riley Hosp for Children, Indianapolis, IN; Indiana Univ School of Nursing, Indianapolis; Indiana Univ, Indianapolis, IN)
Pediatr Radiol 41:1266-1271, 2011

Background.—Abdominal radiographs are used to determine the location of the tip of a newly placed nasogastric tube. The precise location of the gastroesophageal junction has not been well described in the radiology literature.

Objective.—To improve interpretation of radiographs taken to evaluate the location of the tip of a nasogastric tube. Using UGI barium studies, we determined the anatomical location and variability of the position of the gastroesophageal (GE) junction and the pylorus.

Materials and Methods.—We reviewed 200 upper gastrointestinal barium studies (50 in each of 4 age groups). We measured the vertebral levels and distance of the gastroesophageal junction and the pylorus from the spine, the vertical distance of the gastroesophageal junction from the dome of the diaphragm and the distance from the gastroesophageal junction to the pylorus.

Results.—There is a constant location of the GE junction with no significant variation between age groups. There is a moderately constant location of the pylorus. The other measurements were very variable.

Conclusion.—The location of the GE junction is very constant, irrespective of age. Tube tips below the level of the vertebral disc between the 11th and 12th thoracic vertebra and/or more than 16 mm from the left side of the spine lie in the stomach and not the lower esophagus. Our results should help in accurate radiographic description of the location of the tip of an NG tube (Fig 1).

▶ That the location of the nasogastric or orogastric tube is clinically pertinent should be self-evident. That radiologists and pediatricians have not succeeded in using the hemidiaphragms or personal hunches to aid in the localizations might also be considered evident. The current authors propose using the relatively fixed vertebral column as a guideline to "hang one's hat on." From reading the article, I assume they are speaking of supine frontal radiographs in setting their standards (not prone) and that the presumption is that obese and cachectic subjects might also be evaluated under the same guidelines. Ultrasound imaging might alternately be used in cases of close calls as to whether the tube tip is above or below the gastroesophageal junction. They wisely exclude cases of hiatal hernia from their standards (one would have to know if such a hernia is present).

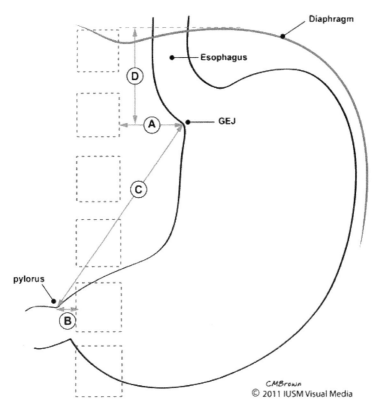

FIGURE 1.—Measurements made from the barium images. a The distance of the GE junction from the left side of the spine and the vertebral level of the GE junction. b The distance of the pylorus from the right margin of the spine and the vertebral level of the pylorus. c The distance from the GE junction to the pylorus. d The vertical distance from the apex of the left hemidiaphragm to the level of the GE junction. (Reprinted from Cohen MD, Ellett MLC, Perkins SM, et al. Accurate localization of the position of the tip of a naso/orogastric tube in children; where is the location of the gastro-esophageal junction? *Pediatr Radiol.* 2011;41:1266-1271, with kind permission from Springer Science and Business Media.)

The bothersome question of the Schatzki ring is also not raised. But, in the end, the authors have proposed a useful working guideline, illustrated in their Fig 1, for everyday use in radiographs of children.

A. E. Oestreich, MD

CT appearance of the duodenum and mesenteric vessels in children with normal and abnormal bowel rotation

Taylor GA (Harvard Med School and Children's Hosp Boston, MA)
Pediatr Radiol 41:1378-1383, 2011

Background.—Demonstration of the third duodenal segment (D3) in retroperitoneal location has been recently proposed as a method for excluding malrotation.

Objective.—This study was performed to determine whether a retroperitoneal third duodenal segment can reliably exclude malrotation.

Materials and Methods.—CTs of 38 patients with proven malrotation and 100 patients without malrotation were evaluated for the location of the duodenum/proximal small bowel, and the relationship of the superior mesenteric vein (SMV) to superior mesenteric artery (SMA).

Results.—The D3 segment was in normal retroperitoneal location in 100% of control patients, compared to 2.5% or (1 of 38) of patients with malrotation. Nine of 11 patients (91%) with malrotation imaged prior to surgery had the proximal bowel in an abnormal location, while all 100 control patients had it in a normal location. The SMV was in normal relationship to the SMA in 11/38 patients (29%) with malrotation, compared to 79% of normal controls. In 10 controls, a branch of the SMV was partially wrapped around the SMA, potentially mimicking partial mesenteric volvulus.

Conclusion.—A retroperitoneal location of the D3 segment makes the diagnosis of malrotation unlikely but not impossible. Additional imaging of the duodenojejunal junction or cecum may be necessary to reliably exclude intestinal malrotation.

▶ Well, well. Is this the exception that disproves the rule, or is it the exception that proves the rule? In last year's YEAR BOOK we cited and discussed Dr Yousefzadeh's potentially groundbreaking article on use of ultrasound scan to rule in or rule out malrotation that might be causing volvulus, especially in the infant.[1] Now comes Dr Taylor with a counterexample that would imply one cannot confidently exclude malrotation merely by a retroperitoneal position of the duodenum (on ultrasound scan). Dr Youzefzadeh attempts to strike back[2] by analyzing the level of imaging in the Taylor counterexample. But, the pertinent question in infants with (sudden) vomiting is "Is volvulus present?," which would imply immediate surgical intervention. If the duodenum third portion (D3) is correctly retroperitoneal, then it seems likely that duodenal-jejunal volvulus is not present, even if other parts of small bowel are malrotated. In any event, the Taylor article confirms that when a nonretroperitoneal position of D3 is found, volvulus is to be strongly suspected in the clinical setting, and the likelihood of volvulus is considerably lowered when D3 is retroperitoneal. A different helpful conclusion from Taylor's study is that the relative position of superior mesenteric artery and vein is not an absolute sign of malrotation or normal rotation (although it does change probabilities). Finally, Taylor's useful review of CTs clearly does not imply that CT is the first imaging method in suspected volvulus—it remains ultrasound scan or upper gastrointestinal fluoroscopy depending on how you react to his article.

A. E. Oestreich, MD

References

1. Yousefzadeh DK, Kang L, Tessicini L. Assessment of retromesenteric position of the third portion of the duodenum. an US feasibility study in 33 newborns. *Pediatr Radiol.* 2010;40:1476-1484.

2. Yousefzadeh DK. Regarding online publication of 'CT appearance of the duodenum and mesenteric vessels in children with normal and abnormal bowel rotation'. *Pediatr Radiol.* 2011;41:1481-1482.

Interloop fluid in intussusception: what is its significance?
Gartner RD, Levin TL, Borenstein SH, et al (Children's Hosp of Pennsylvania, Philadelphia; Montefiore Med Ctr, Bronx, NY; et al)
Pediatr Radiol 41:727-731, 2011

Background.—Sonography has been used to predict pneumatic reduction outcome in children with intussusception.

Objective.—To assess the prognostic significance of fluid between the intussusceptum and intussuscepiens with respect to reduction outcome, lead point or necrosis.

Materials and methods.—Sonograms of children with a discharge diagnosis of intussusception from four institutions were reviewed for interloop fluid and correlated with results of pneumatic reduction and surgical/pathological findings when available. Maximal dimension of interloop fluid on a transverse image and fluid complexity were evaluated.

Results.—Of 166 cases, 36 (21.7%) had interloop fluid. Pneumatic reduction was successful in 21 (58.3%) with fluid and 113 (87.6%) without. The average largest fluid dimension was 8.7 mm (range 5 mm—19 mm, median 8 mm) in cases with successful reduction and 12.8 mm (range 4 mm—26 mm, median 12.5 mm) in unsuccessful reduction ($p<0.05$). Fluid dimension equal to or greater than 9 mm correlated with failed reduction ($p<0.0001$; odds ratio 13:1). In 36 cases with interloop fluid that required surgery, there were four lead points and three necroses. In cases without fluid with surgical reduction, there was one lead point and one necrosis. Interloop fluid correlated with lead point ($p<0.04$) or necrosis ($p<0.03$). Its significance increased with larger amounts of fluid ($p<0.0001$). Patient age/fluid complexity did not correlate with reduction outcome ($p=0.9$).

Conclusion.—Interloop fluid was associated with increased failure of pneumatic reduction and increased likelihood of lead point or necrosis, particularly when the maximum dimension exceeded 9 mm (Fig 2).

▶ Life was simpler, albeit perhaps inappropriate, in the old days at Zürich Children's Hospital when P. P. Rickham MD was the professor of surgery. He insisted that no child with an intussusception be reduced by radiology, and surgery was always to be done. Thus, to reduce radiologically one had to do an "oops!" inadvertent reduction. Times (and pediatric surgeons) have changed. Whether fluoroscopically, most often with air, or under ultrasound (US) guidance, with fluid, the pediatric team usually has the radiologist attempting reduction, absent obvious peritonitis or free peritoneal gas. The metropolitan authors of this extensive study have looked into the finding of fluid between intussusceptum and intussuscipiens as a sign of caution for failure of reduction and increased likelihood of lead point or necrosis, especially when the greatest diameter

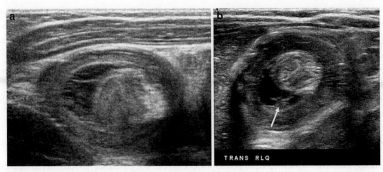

FIGURE 2.—Transverse sonographical images of an intussusception demonstrate septations (a) and debris (b) (*arrow*) within the interloop fluid. (Reprinted from Gartner RD, Levin TL, Borenstein SH, et al. Interloop fluid in intussusception: what is its significance? *Pediatr Radiol.* 2011;41:727-731, Copyright 2011, with permission from Springer-Verlag.)

measurement of the fluid was over 9 mm. Sometimes the interloop fluid demonstrated septations or debris on US, as shown on Fig 2. One can use the results of their study to decrease futile second and third attempts at reduction in some such patients. Meanwhile, beware of the double whammy: the rare child with perforated appendicitis (with appendicolith) in an intussusception.[1]

A. E. Oestreich, MD

Reference

1. Chang TP, Russell SA. Perforated appendicitis and appendicolith in a child presenting as intussusception: a case report. *Pediatr Emerg Care.* 2011;27:635-638.

Characterization of pediatric liver lesions with gadoxetate disodium

Meyers AB, Towbin AJ, Serai S, et al (Cincinnati Children's Hosp Med Ctr, OH)
Pediatr Radiol 41:1183-1197, 2011

Gadoxetate disodium (Gd-EOB-DTPA) is a relatively new hepatobiliary MRI contrast agent. It is increasingly used in adults to characterize hepatic masses, but there is little published describing its use in children. The purpose of this paper is to describe our pediatric MRI protocol as well as the imaging appearance of pediatric liver lesions using gadoxetate disodium. As a hepatocyte-specific MRI contrast agent, Gd-EOB-DTPA has the potential to improve characterization and provide a more specific diagnosis of pediatric liver masses (Fig 9).

▶ Nearly every week in the busy solid-tumor conference at our children's hospital, magnetic resonance imaging (MRI) studies with Eovist (also known as Primovist), the gadolinium-based MRI contrast agent, gadoxetate disodium, play a major role in the diagnostic imaging of children with liver tumors. This article gives an introduction to the use of this agent in children and then

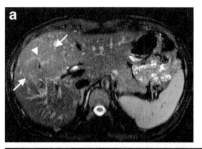

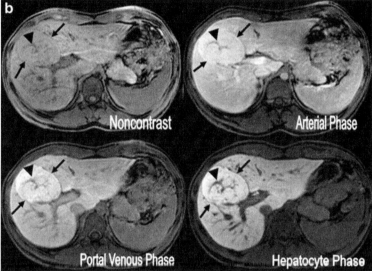

FIGURE 9.—Focal nodular hyperplasia in a 20-year-old woman. a Axial T2-weighted image with fat saturation shows a mass in the right lobe of the liver that is nearly isointense to the adjacent liver parenchyma (*arrows*). A hyperintense central scar is also seen (*arrowhead*). b Axial LAVA MR images before and after the administration of gadoxetate disodium. On the noncontrast image, the mass (*arrows*) is isointense and the central scar (*arrowhead*) is hypointense to the adjacent liver. During the late arterial phase of enhancement, the mass (*arrows*) is hyperintense to the adjacent liver and the central scar (*arrowhead*) remains hypointense. During the portal venous phase, the mass (*arrows*) is hyperintense to the adjacent liver and the central scar (*arrowhead*) remains hypointense. During the delayed hepatocyte phase, the tumor (*arrows*) is hyperintense to the adjacent liver parenchyma and the central scar (*arrowhead*) remains hypointense. (Reprinted from Meyers AB, Towbin AJ, Serai S, et al. Characterization of pediatric liver lesions with gadoxetate disodium. *Pediatr Radiol.* 2011;41:1183-1197, with kind permission from Springer Science and Business Media.)

highlights its pattern in all the major tumors or tumorlike entities involving the liver. This is great stuff! Please consider reading this article and studying its illustrations, such as Fig 9. The agent is not approved by the US Food and Drug Administration for children; the dose is modified from the adult usual dose. When administered to patients with normal liver and kidney function, about 50% is excreted via the hepatobiliary system, making the agent also useful to see the biliary tree. Delayed images at 20 (or more) minutes after injection (the hepatocyte phase, which follows earlier noncontrast, arterial, and portal venous phases) yield images often quite different from conventional gadolinium agents. Especially useful is a new ability to distinguish focal nodular hyperplasia (Fig 9) from liver metastases. In the 20-minute hepatocyte phase, focal nodular hyperplasia is hyperintense to normal liver, while metastases tend to be hypointense. Improved evaluation of a tumor's relationship to the biliary tree is also achieved on the new hepatocyte phase and often better characterization of the liver lesions.

A. E. Oestreich, MD

Transcapsular Arterial Neovascularization after Liver Transplantation in Pediatric Patients Indicates Transplant Failure

Herrmann J, Junge CM, Burdelski M, et al (Univ Med Ctr Hamburg-Eppendorf, Martinistrasse, Germany; Univ Clinic Schleswig-Holstein, Kiel, Germany; et al)
Radiology 261:566-572, 2011

Purpose.—To identify transcapsular arterial neovascularization with Doppler ultrasonography (US) in pediatric patients after liver transplantation and to assess the frequency of the finding, its underlying causes, and its relevance in terms of clinical outcome.

Materials and Methods.—The study was approved by the local ethics committee, with waived informed consent. All pediatric patients who underwent liver transplantation between January 2000 and December 2003 were retrospectively evaluated. Patients were followed up until June 2008, by using a predefined US protocol with prospective documentation. Of 182 consecutive liver transplantations performed in 162 patients (mean age, 4.5 years; range, 0.1−18.4 years) in this period, 25 patients with a total of 27 liver transplantations underwent US examinations conducted by multiple investigators and were primarily excluded. Student t tests and χ^2 tests were performed where appropriate. The Tarone-Ware test was used to compare transplant survival times.

Results.—Transcapsular arterial neovascularization was noticed in 13 of 137 patients (9.5%) and in 13 of 155 liver transplants (8.4%). The mean time until arterial neovessels appeared was 157 days after liver transplantation (median, 97 days; range, 19−477 days). Arterial neovascularization was associated with pronounced transplant malperfusion and inflammatory changes ($P < .001$). Patients with transcapsular arterial neovascularization had a significantly shorter mean transplant survival time (1426.4 days ± 244.5 [standard error], with 95% confidence interval: 947.23, 1905.23, vs 2526.4 days ± 92.1, with 95% confidence interval: 2345.84, 2706.97; $P = .008$) and a higher retransplantation rate (53.8% vs 19.7%, $P = .009$).

Conclusion.—Transcapsular arterial neovascularization, detected with color Doppler US, occurred in 9.5% (13 of 137) of pediatric patients and 8.4% (13 of 155) of liver transplants and was associated with underlying malperfusion and inflammation. The diagnosis of transcapsular arterial neovascularization was associated with reduced graft survival times

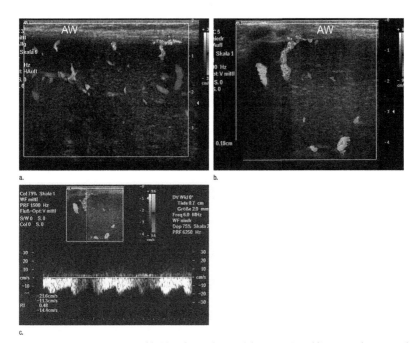

FIGURE 1.—Images in 6-year-old girl with extrahepatic biliary atresia and liver transplantation who developed postoperative hepatic artery thrombosis. Transcapsular arterial neovascularization was detected on day 246 after liver transplantation and can be seen in a—c. (a, b) Color Doppler US scans of the transplant periphery obtained with a high-resolution linear-array transducer show multiple transcapsular vessels bridging from the abdominal wall *(AW)* into the liver parenchyma. (c) Spectral Doppler scan demonstrates an arterial flow pattern directed toward the center of the liver. (Reprinted from Herrmann J, Junge CM, Burdelski M, et al. Transcapsular arterial neovascularization after liver transplantation in pediatric patients indicates transplant failure. *Radiology,* 2011;261;566-572. Copyright by the Radiological Society of North America.)

and a high retransplantation rate. The negative prognostic value of the sign may assist in a strategy of organ allocation (Fig 1).

▶ The title says it all (or at least most of it), but my comment is supposed to be at least 150 words long. As the authors point out, the neovascularization is locally of benefit to the transplanted liver, but unfortunately, the need for that neovascularity signals a dire prognosis for the liver. The neovessels, as nicely shown in Fig 1, bridge from the abdominal wall into the liver parenchyma with an arterial flow pattern on Doppler that is directed toward the central area of the liver. The Doppler pattern is best seen with a high-frequency linear transducer with low pulse repetition frequencies—and by an ultrasonographer experienced in this specialized demonstration. The majority of livers with this neovascularization showed inflammatory changes in the liver (hence a demand for more blood). Other imaging methods recently reported to allow evaluation of transplanted livers for danger signals include MRI elastography[1] and diffusion-weighted MRI.[2]

A. E. Oestreich, MD

References

1. Lee VS, Miller FH, Omary RA, et al. Magnetic resonance elastography and biomarkers to assess fibrosis from recurrent hepatitis C in liver transplant recipients. *Transplantation.* 2011;92:581-586.
2. Sandrasegaran K, Ramaswamy R, Ghosh S, et al. Diffusion-weighted MRI of the transplanted liver. *Clin Radiol.* 2011;66:820-825.

The positive color Doppler sign post biopsy: effectiveness of US-directed compression in achieving hemostasis

Alotaibi M, Shrouder-Henry J, Amaral J, et al (Univ of Toronto, Ontario, Canada; Georgetown Univ School of Medicine, Washington, DC)
Pediatr Radiol 41:362-368, 2011

Background.—Percutaneous biopsies of soft-tissue organs are frequently performed using US guidance. US permits visualization of blood flow on color Doppler imaging.

Objective.—To report the presence of color Doppler signal (positive color Doppler sign) along the biopsy tract after percutaneous needle biopsy of the liver and kidney as an indication of bleeding and to describe US-guided hemostasis.

Materials and Methods.—A case-control study of US-guided liver and kidney biopsies performed between January 2005 and September 2009 was undertaken. All pediatric patients with a positive color Doppler sign along the biopsy tract were included. Controls consisted of patients in whom no color Doppler sign was identified.

Results.—Fifty-three cases with positive color Doppler sign were identified. One hundred and six matched controls were selected. The average compression time was 9.2 min in kidney and 8.4 min in liver cases. US-guided compression achieved cessation of the positive color Doppler sign in all cases. There was no significant difference between the mean pre- and post-procedure hemoglobin and platelet levels between kidney cases and controls ($P=0.68$ and $P=0.63$, respectively) and between liver cases and controls ($P=0.45$ and $P=0.80$).

Conclusion.—Color Doppler US can detect bleeding post percutaneous liver and kidney biopsies. US-guided compression is effective in obliterating the color Doppler signal and achieving appropriate hemostasis (Fig 1).

▶ This article describes a highly practical technique that belongs in the everyday practice of pediatric ultrasound (US) yet is new information for most of us. Using US imaging to show the pathway of a hepatic or renal percutaneous biopsy needle is usual practice, including the color Doppler visualization of vessels to be avoided by the needle path. How simple and how ingenious, then, to use the color Doppler probe to demonstrate the presence or absence of bleeding at the needle-tip biopsy site at this point and then follow the site during compression to confirm the cessation of bleeding. (I compare it to the visual inspection of a small skin bleed after I have cut myself shaving.) As

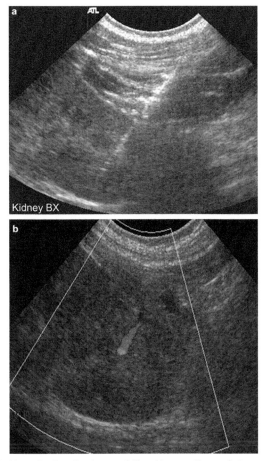

FIGURE 1.—Positive color Doppler sign post kidney biopsy. a Gray-scale image with needle is seen within the kidney parenchyma before removal. b Color Doppler image immediately after removal of the biopsy needle shows color flow in the needle tract with forming perinephric hematoma. (Reprinted from Alotaibi M, Shrouder-Henry J, Amaral J, et al. The positive color Doppler sign post biopsy: effectiveness of US-directed compression in achieving hemostasis. *Pediatr Radiol.* 2011;41:362-368, with kind permission from Springer Science and Business Media.)

the authors state, complications from needle biopsy are relatively uncommon but may be life-threatening if bleeding is uncontrolled. Fig 2 from the original article, for example, shows how color flow can show a jet of bleeding along a needle tract in the liver; Fig 3 of the original article nicely shows how compression can confirm from a renal biopsy that bleeding has stopped. To see is to believe, and to believe is to recommend this procedure.

A. E. Oestreich, MD

Pseudo Gallbladder sign in biliary atresia—an imaging pitfall

Aziz S, Wild Y, Rosenthal P, et al (Univ of California, San Francisco)
Pediatr Radiol 41:620-626, 2011

Background.—Ultrasound (US) is used to identify causes of neonatal cholestasis. We describe a potential sonographic pitfall, the "pseudo gallbladder," in biliary atresia (BA).

Objective.—To describe the *Pseudo Gallbladder sign (PsGB sign).*

Materials and Methods.—Sonograms/clinical records of 20 confirmed BA infants and 20 non-BA cases were reviewed retrospectively. For the BA group, preoperative sonography and surgical and pathological findings were examined. For the non-BA group, sonographic features and pathological findings were examined. The PsGB sign is defined as a fluid-filled

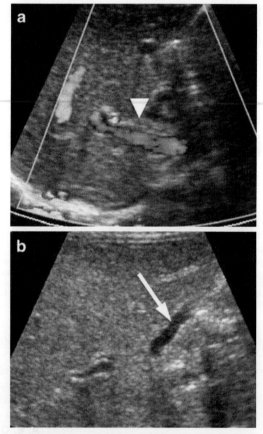

FIGURE 4.—The triangular cord sign (TC sign) in a BA patient. **a** The TC sign (*arrowhead*) measured 4.8 mm in this case of BA. **b** The PsGB sign in this case (*arrow*) is seen as a fluid-filled structure demonstrating an irregular contour but without a normal gallbladder wall. (Reprinted from Aziz S, Wild Y, Rosenthal P, et al. Pseudo Gallbladder sign in biliary atresia—an imaging pitfall. *Pediatr Radiol.* 2011;41:620-626, with kind permission from Springer Science and Business Media.)

structure, located in the expected region of the gallbladder, measuring ≤ 15 mm in length but without a well-defined or normal-appearing gallbladder wall.

Results.—A recognizable gallbladder and normal gallbladder wall were present in all non-BA infants. However, none of the BA infants had a sonographically normal gallbladder. Seventy-three percent of BA patients had a PsGB, and in 27% no gallbladder or gallbladder-like structure was detected.

Conclusion.—A gallbladder-like structure in BA is common and can be misinterpreted as a normal gallbladder, delaying diagnosis and therapy. Recognition of this imaging pitfall, described here as the pseudo gallbladder sign, will help avoid this error (Fig 4).

▶ How strange that when no gallbladder is present in an infant, one can often see on ultrasound scan a fluid-containing structure that mimics so closely a gallbladder yet lacks any echoic wall. It is not clear exactly what is being imaged, but not only should one not mistake the often wiggly entity for real gallbladder, but also one can use it to affirm the diagnosis of biliary atresia. Fig 4 shows not only the pseudo gallbladder sign but also the better-known triangular cord sign. Because the triangular cord takes some ultrasound sophistication to recognize, it is nice to have a companion pseudo gallbladder to help with the clinically important diagnosis in infants with neonatal cholestasis or, simply, jaundice. One other interesting vagary of the gallbladder about which I recently learned is intramural gallstones, recently reported in a relatively young adult with adenomyomatosis.[1] Thus, we have a sign with absent wall (pseudo) and a condition with too much wall (intramural stones).

A. E. Oestreich, MD

Reference

1. Apostolidis S, Zatagias A, Zevgaridis A. Intramural gallstones mimicking typical lithiasic cholecystitis. *South Med J*. 2011;104:59-60.

Spontaneous gall bladder perforation: a rare condition in the differential diagnosis of acute abdomen in children
Shukla RM, Roy D, Mukherjee PP, et al (Nil Ratan Sircar Med College and Hosp, Kolkata, India)
J Pediatr Surg 46:241-243, 2011

Gallbladder perforation is very rare in children and almost exclusively is a complication of cholecystitis, which accompanies severe inflammation of the gallbladder with or without cholelithiasis. Here we present 4 cases of spontaneous gall bladder perforation, which should be kept in mind as a condition for inclusion in the differential diagnosis of an acute abdomen in children.

▶ That the common cause of free peritoneal fluid in infants at several weeks/ months of age is perforation of the biliary tract[1] is well known. Much less well known in infancy or later in childhood is the entity of spontaneous gall bladder perforation, which accompanies severe gall bladder inflammation or other causes of local ischemia. The boys discussed in this article were 10, 8, and 6 years old and 4 months old. Each had nonspecific symptoms of acute abdomen, but generally also a rigid right upper abdomen or rebound tenderness in that region. Imaging was restricted to plain images that showed air-fluid levels in bowel but no free air. Because the perforation was of biliary contents, it is natural that no pneumoperitoneum was evident. Had sonography been the initial imaging method, as is typical in Europe, for example, fluid in the peritoneum and gall bladder inflammatory change might well have narrowed the diagnosis before surgery, and high detail sonography might have shown the discontinuity in the gall bladder wall. Therefore, for children with signs or symptoms similar to those in this article, high-detail ultrasound is to be strongly considered. Biliary nuclear imaging would likely have been revealing as well. As the authors aver, early diagnosis of gall bladder perforation and prompt surgical intervention are of crucial importance.

A. E. Oestreich, MD

Reference

1. Livesey E, Davenport M. Spontaneous perforation of the biliary tract and portal vein thrombosis in infancy. *Pediatr Surg Int.* 2008;24:357-359.

Multiple magnet ingestion: Is there a role for early surgical intervention?
Salimi A, Kooraki S, Esfahani SA, et al (Tehran Univ of Med Sciences, Iran)
Ann Saudi Med 32:93-96, 2012

Children often swallow foreign bodies. Multiple magnet ingestion is rare, but can result in serious complications. This study presents three unique cases of multiple magnet ingestion: one case an 8-year-old boy with multiple magnet ingestion resulting in gastric obstruction and the other two cases with intestinal perforations due to multiple magnet intake. History and physical examination are unreliable in children who swallow multiple magnets. Sometimes radiological findings are not conclusive, whether one magnet is swallowed or more. If magnets are not moved in sequential radiology images, we recommend early surgical intervention before gastrointestinal complications develop. Toy companies, parents, physicians, and radiologists should be warned about the potential complications of such toys (Fig 1).

▶ When will they ever learn? "They," as suggested in the article, include health care workers, including physicians, parents, and, for that matter, children and teachers. Much has been written in the past decade about the dangers of swallowing multiple magnets and allowing them to travel beyond the stomach. The current 3 cases include an uncommon example of a problem occurring (in an 8-year-old!) when magnetic, swallowed items remain in the stomach but form such a bulky bezoar-like mass in that stomach as to be considered gastric

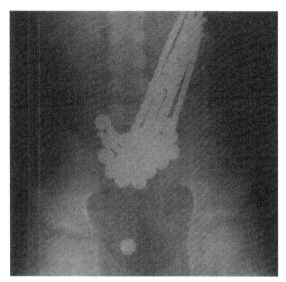

FIGURE 1.—A plain abdominal radiograph shows several bar-shaped and sphere-shaped magnets attached to each other. Together they mimic the shape of the stomach. One solitary magnet is seen far away in the intestine. (Reprinted from Salimi A, Kooraki S, Esfahani SA, et al. Multiple magnet ingestion: is there a role for early surgical intervention? *Ann Saudi Med.* 2012;32:93-96.)

obstruction. Their Fig 1 shows nearly a cast of the stomach from 35 magnetic toy bars, 22 tiny cylinder-shaped magnets, and 12 ball bearings (only 1 ball bearing had traveled into bowel beyond the stomach). The child reported, "Someone ordered me to eat several pieces of my toy." All 3 cases reemphasize the relatively benign clinical picture in this magnetopathy, and the ages of 8, 7, and 3 years are also representative. So once again, beware of multiple swallowed magnets in your patients, even without relevant history, peruse radiographs and ultrasound images carefully, and then alert pediatric or other surgeons that the patients are in jeopardy (of perforation, volvulus, intussusception, and other complications from magnets in adjacent bowel loops).

A. E. Oestreich, MD

Genitourinary

Sonography of renal venous thrombosis in neonates and infants: can we predict outcome?

Kraft JK, Brandão LR, Navarro OM (The Hosp for Sick Children, Toronto, Ontario, Canada)
Pediatr Radiol 41:299-307, 2011

Background.—The relationship between sonographic features of renal venous thrombosis (RVT) and outcome has not been described in a large series of patients.

Objective.—To analyze sonographic findings of RVT and their evolution in a large series of patients and to attempt to identify features that might predict outcome.

Materials and Methods.—Retrospective analysis of sonograms and medical records of neonates and infants diagnosed with RVT during the period 1998-2007.

Results.—Of 22 children (mean age: 3 days; age range: 0−107 days), RVT was bilateral in 12. Of 34 affected kidneys, thrombus in the main renal vein was seen in 17 and typical RVT sonographic findings without main renal vein thrombus were seen in the remaining 17. All children had US follow-up (range: 0.6−97.2 months). Three children with bilateral RVT died. Nine kidneys atrophied. Imaging findings associated with subsequent kidney atrophy included markedly reduced perfusion at diagnosis, subcapsular collections, patchy cortical echotexture and profoundly hypoechoic and irregular renal pyramids. Six patients (eight kidneys) presented with renal calcifications on initial sonogram before 7 days of life, suggesting antenatal RVT.

Conclusion.—Sonography is useful in neonatal and early infant RVT and might help predict renal atrophy. Antenatal RVT appears to be relatively common (Fig 3).

▶ One of the most important things to be learned from this article is that renal vein thrombosis can be initiated prenatally. The 8 kidneys with calcification of

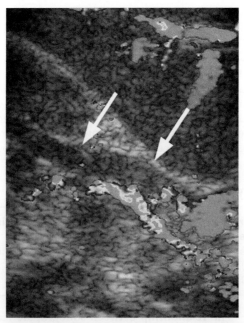

FIGURE 3.—Color Doppler transverse renal sonogram in a 1-day-old boy shows absence of color signal in the main renal vein, indicative of occlusive thrombus (*arrows*). (Reprinted from Kraft JK, Brandão LR, Navarro OM. Sonography of renal venous thrombosis in neonates and infants: can we predict outcome? *Pediatr Radiol.* 2011;41:299-307, with permission from Springer-Verlag.)

thrombus evident by 7 days of life described here provide the proof; according to the "10-day rule," it takes 10 days (or perhaps 9) for any process in the body at any age to calcify sufficiently to be visualized radiographically, and presumably also sonographically. Some of the stressful causes cited for renal vein thrombosis are clearly not antenatal, such as birth asphyxia, umbilical catheter placement, and postnatal infection. (I have recently discussed the vagaries of umbilical vein catheter placement elsewhere.[1]) The demonstration of main renal vein thrombosis, aided by Doppler color imaging (eg, Fig 3), is important to the outcome, because it predicts bad outcome.

A. E. Oestreich, MD

Reference

1. Oestreich AE. Umbilical vein catheterization—appropriate and inappropriate placement. *Pediatr Radiol.* 2010;40:1941-1949.

Ureteral triplication: A rare anomaly with a variety of presentations
Kokabi N, Price N, Smith GHH, et al (The Univ of Sydney, New South Wales, Australia)
J Pediatr Urol 7:484-487, 2011

Ureteral triplication remains a very rare congenital malformation of the urinary tract with a wide spectrum of presentation. The sporadic nature of this condition and its association with other anomalies makes evidence-based management difficult. We report two cases of triplication in association with the VACTERL syndrome, one developing pelvi-ureteric junction obstruction and the other vesico-ureteric reflux (Fig 2).

▶ Whereas duplication of an anatomic structure may be relatively commonplace, triplication, lying further from the norm, is relatively uncommon and can be instructive as well as pose more complex problems in treatment. Although well over 100 cases of ureteral triplication have been reported (hence, not a "very rare" entity), each has its individual associations, as emphasized in this article. Despite a female predominance, 1 of the 2 cases here reported was a male. He had an upper pole pelviureteric junction obstruction as suggested in Fig 2; it was treated with an upper pole pyeloplasty. Interestingly, the triplication of the upper ureter and its connections was not discovered (by imaging) until after 2 years of age. The female infant, with anorectal malformation, showed triplication of the upper ureter ipsilateral to a lower limb deformity with 9 metacarpals, each with corresponding digits. Not stated was if the 9 digits were mirror image (the only case we encountered with 9 toe digits was mirror image duplication with, for example, "little" toes at the medial and lateral sides and ulna duplication as well. (Similar mirror image nonadactyly has been reported in Sandrow syndrome,[1] but I digress.) Once triplication of a ureter has been discovered, detailed uroimaging, perhaps optimally with MRI, should be obtained.

A. E. Oestreich, MD

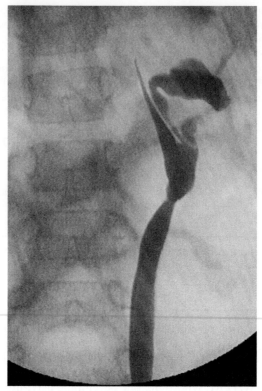

FIGURE 2.—RPG indicating Smith type III left ureteral triplication. Note tapered appearance of upper pole moiety, with an absence of filling, as a result of the PUJ obstruction. (Reprinted from Journal of Pediatric Urology. Kokabi N, Price N, Smith GH, et al. Ureteral triplication: a rare anomaly with a variety of presentations. *J Pediatr Urol.* 2011;7:484-487, Copyright 2011, with permission from Journal of Pediatric Urology Company.)

Reference

1. Kantaputra PN. Laurin-Sandrow syndrome with additional associated manifestations. *Am J Med Genet.* 2001;98:210-215.

Imaging the urinary tract in children with urinary tract infection

Hannula A, Venhola M, Perhomaa M, et al (Univ of Oulu, Finland)
Acta Paediatr 100:e253-e259, 2011

Aim.—To evaluate whether ultrasonography (US) alone is sufficient in imaging the urinary tract in 1185 children with urinary tract infection (UTI).

Methods.—The reports on US and voiding cystourethrography (VCUG) were reviewed.

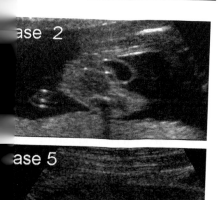

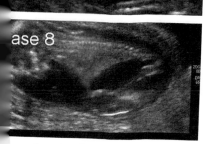

megalourethra diagnosed at 13—24 weeks'
the urethra as a cystic structure between the
tion of the urethra. Case 7 shows a distended
whole' bladder. (Reprinted from Amsalem H,
natal diagnosis and postnatal/autopsy findings
, with permission from ISUOG.)

an elongated and/or distended
anomalies (Fig 1).

can be diagnosed postnatally, it
tion can be diagnosed prenatally.
llow definitive diagnosis, demon-
ors state, a similar pattern may be
y state, the distinction becomes
ws the vessels in the cord. In all
ve uropathy, a distended prenatal
etal sonography of the region was
prune belly configuration of the
l megalourethra, as in 2 of their
of their cases, a previously unre-
ssociated with maternal diabetes

Results.—Initial US was normal in 861/1185 patients (73%). VCUG revealed abnormal findings in 285/861 (33%), of which grade III—V vesicoureteral reflux (VUR) comprised 97 cases (11%). During follow-up, VUR had resolved in 88/97 (91%) patients: in 50/57 (88%) patients without active treatment for VUR, in 27/29 (93%) with endoscopic and in 11/11 (100%) with open surgery for VUR. During follow-up, 11/97 patients (11%) had developed new renal scarring detectable in US, but no renal impairment occurred. Except for VUR, VCUG showed non-obstructive urethral valves in two infant boys with normal initial US. Thus, in 861 children with normal initial US, 40 patients with grade III—V VUR and two patients with significant nonreflux pathology may have benefited from surgical treatment, giving the total number of possibly missed pathological finding in 42/861 (4.9%) cases if VCUG had not been performed.

Conclusion.—We suggest that children with UTI could be examined using US alone and to use VCUG only after additional indications.

▶ The tide is turning. Voiding cystourethrography (VCUG) is known to involve unpleasantness for the patient and the family and to deliver considerable radiation to the patient (about 0.9 mSV, or the equivalent of 30 chest x-rays and indeed directed to the gonadal region). It can also be unpleasant for the health care team involved (radiology team). In this large retrospective review of results, especially of VCUGs performed in the face of normal ultrasound examinations of the kidneys, the number of possibly missed pertinent pathological findings if VCUG had not been performed was about 5% (2 cases of mild posterior urethral valves and 1 case of bilateral ureteroceles). This percent depends on the lack of hard data to support vesicoureteral reflux alone as a significant cause of renal scarring. Further, the authors quote a recent report that suggests abandoning routine use of VCUG because in a series of young infants with febrile urinary tract infection and normal ultrasound, no clinically significant urinary tract abnormality was found by VCUG.[1] Now, what are pediatric radiologist and their referring clinicians to do today? Shall we discomfort and radiate the many to discover the few who truly need an intervention to prevent renal damage and its consequences? The conclusion of the current article suggests that we "use VCUG only after additional indications." The problem is to wisely figure out those additional indications. "Because I want it" should no longer be considered a significant reason for VCUG.

A. E. Oestreich, MD

Reference

1. Ismaili K, Lolin K, Damry N, Alexander M, Lepage P, Hall M. Febrile urinary tract infections in 0- to 3-month-old infants: a prospective follow-up study. *J Pediatr.* 2011;158:91-94.

MRI of acquired posterior urethral diverticulum following su anorectal malformations

Podberesky DJ, Weaver NC, Anton CG, et al (Cincinnati Children's Ctr, OH)
Pediatr Radiol 41:1139-1145, 2011

Background.—Posterior urethral diverticulum (PUD) is one of common postoperative complications associated with anorecta mation (ARM) correction.

Objective.—To describe our MRI protocol for evaluating acqu following ARM surgery, and associated imaging findings.

Materials and Methods.—Two radiologists retrospectively rev pelvic MRI examinations performed for postoperative ARM identification and characteristics. Associated clinical, operative ar copy reports were also reviewed and compared to MRI.

Results.—An abnormal retrourethral focus suspicious for F identified at MRI in 13 patients. Ten of these patients underwe quent surgery or cystoscopy, and PUD was confirmed in five. A confirmed PUD cases appeared as cystic lesions that were at le in diameter in two imaging planes. Four of the false-positive ca punctate retrourethral foci that were visible only on a single ME One patient had a seminal vesical cyst mimicking a PUD.

Conclusion.—Pelvic MRI can be a useful tool in the posto assessment of suspected PUD associated with ARM. Radiologist have a high clinical suspicion for a postoperative PUD when a cyst posterior to the bladder/posterior urethra is encountered on two planes in these patients (Fig 1).

▶ Because posterior urethral diverticulum is a relatively common post complication after surgery for anorectal malformation and because, onc corrective surgery may be indicated, accurate imaging is important. T contrast (except for water in the Foley catheter placed into available r

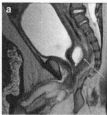 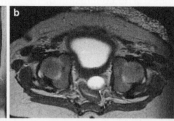 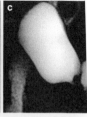

FIGURE 1.—A 6-month-old boy with high ARM initially treated by laparoscopically ass through with large postoperative PUD formed from a remnant of rectourethral fistula. The subsequently resected surgically. **a, b** Sagittal and axial T2-weighted MR images without fat demonstrate a round, cystic lesion posterior to the bladder base with dependent debris (*arro* 3-D reconstruction from an MRCP sequence shows the PUD (*arrow*). (Reprinted from Podb Weaver NC, Anton CG, et al. MRI of acquired posterior urethral diverticulum following surger rectal malformations. *Pediatr Radiol.* 2011;41:1139-1145, with kind permission from Spring and Business Media.)

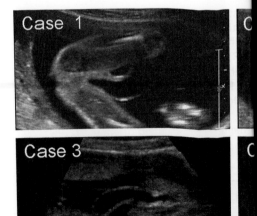

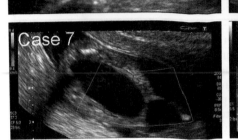

FIGURE 1.—Antenatal ultrasound images illustratin gestation. Cases 1, 2 and 5 show the penile portion of fetal legs. Case 3 shows the penile as well as the pelvic po bladder and dilated urethra and Case 8 has a classic 'ke Fitzgerald B, Keating S, et al. Congenital megalourethra: pr in 10 cases. *Ultrasound Obstet Gynecol.* 2011;37:678-68

fetal ultrasonography should look for phallic structure as well as any associate

▶ Although congenital megaloureth ra (CM seems fortunate when this unfortunate cond Detailed prenatal ultrasound scan seems to strated nicely in Fig 1. However, as the auth seen from a loop of umbilical cord —as th obvious with the use of Doppler, which sh their cases of this form of functional obstruc bladder was the initial finding, and detailed then performed, as it should have been. A abdomen has been associated with prenat cases. Anal atresia was also associated in 2 ported association. At least 3 cases of CM are known,[1] so that maternal diabetes and distended bladder are 2 reasons to search carefully in the male fetus for CM. Because ultrasound scan seems to diagnose CM so well, the additional use of prenatal magnetic resonance imaging might be reserved for evaluation of associated anomalies of the urinary tract and penile region.

A. E. Oestreich, MD

Reference

1. Vaux KK, Jones MC, Benirschke K, Bird LM, Jones KL. Megalourethra: a report of three cases associated with maternal diabetes and a review of the literature—is sonic hedgehog the common pathway? *Am J Med Genet A.* 2005;132A:314-317.

Testicular epidermoid cysts in children: sonographic characteristics with pathological correlation
Arellano CMR, Kozakewich HPW, Diamond D, et al (Children's Hosp Boston, MA)
Pediatr Radiol 41:683-689, 2011

Background.—Testicular epidermoid cyst is a rare benign tumor in children. Although this entity is widely described in adults in literature, there are no large series describing the pathological and radiological findings in children. Knowledge of the sonographic features seen in children may alter surgical treatment.

Objective.—To describe the specific US characteristics of testicular epidermoid cyst in children and to correlate these findings with pathology.

Materials and Methods.—All children with pathologically proven epidermoid cyst and preoperative sonograms diagnosed at a single children's hospital between 1978 and 2008 were included. For each child, the medical records, preoperative US and pathological specimens were reviewed and correlated.

Results.—Eleven patients (ages 1–17 years old) met our criteria. Nine cysts had characteristic target or onion ring appearances, the youngest patient had a simple cyst-like lesion, one cyst had a heterogeneous appearance, and more than 80% of the cysts presented daughter cysts attached along the periphery of the main cyst.

Conclusion.—In addition to the commonly described findings of the epidermoid cyst (the target and onion ring appearances), simple cysts and the presence of daughter lesions are newly described findings that point to the diagnosis of this benign entity in children (Fig 1).

▶ To distinguish the benign from the malignant is a worthy pursuit in any organ; and for guys, limiting surgery prospectively in testicular epidermoid cysts is a worthwhile achievement. This article, with pathologic correlation, nicely expands the diagnostic patterns associated with this lesion. The classical target and onion ring appearances demonstrated in Figure 1 cry out for the diagnosis,

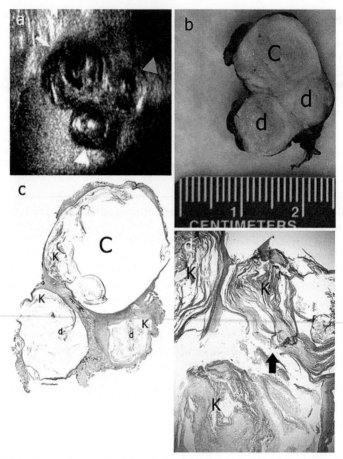

FIGURE 1.—Images of patient 11 of Table 1. Sonogram of the testicle in this 17-year-old shows (a) a multilobulated, well-circumscribed intratesticular mass, composed of daughter cysts, three lesions joined together. The main lesion of larger size (*white arrow*) and a small one adjacent (*gray arrowhead*) show the onion ring appearance. A second smaller lesion (*white arrowhead*) shows a target appearance. **b** A photograph of the cross-section of specimen shows three cysts, the main lesion *(C)* and two daughter cysts *(d)* with laminated configuration filled of white-yellow paste-like keratogenous material. **c** A low-power photomicrograph of the lesion shows the main large cyst *(C)* surrounded by two daughter cysts *(d)* filled with thin layers of keratin *(K)* (hematoxylineosin stain, original magnification, 20×). **d** A higher-power photomicrograph of the cyst's wall shows rupture of the capsule and communication between the main cyst and the daughter cyst *(black arrow)* filled with thin layers of keratin *(K)* (hematoxylin-eosin stain, original magnification 80×). (Reprinted from Arellano CMR, Kozakewich HPW, Diamond D, et al. Testicular epidermoid cysts in children: sonographic characteristics with pathological correlation. *Pediatr Radiol.* 2011;41:683-689, with kind permission from Springer Science and Business Media.)

but daughter cysts and simple-appearing cysts may be seen as well. Each boy had a nontender testicular mass on physical examination (and negative serum tumor markers). On ultrasound scan, the appropriate imaging modality, the largest cyst measured 2 cm in diameter. All cysts deformed the tunica albuginea. On pathology, with more than 80% of the cysts, small calcific densities were seen in the keratinizing squamous epithelium—foci of calcification could be recognized on ultrasound scan in 10 cases. None of their cases showed internal Doppler flow. All but 1 case in their series were removed by enucleation, sparing the remaining testis; good. The other testis was fully removed; not good, but this is the reason why this article is important for all ultrasound imagers, so we can advise against orchiectomy. Interestingly, recently reported, albeit in a 35-year-old, was an intrascrotal extratesticular epidermoid cyst with the onion skin ultrasound pattern (with a smaller daughter cyst, both surrounded by hydrocele, lying adjacent to the testis, and having no internal Doppler flow).[1]

A. E. Oestreich, MD

Reference

1. Agarwal A, Agarwal K. Intrascrotal extratesticular epidermoid cyst. *Br J Radiol.* 2011;84:e121-e122.

Laparoscopic excision of a rudimentary uterine horn in a child
Gaied F, Quiros-Calinoiu E, Emil S (McGill Univ Health Centre, Montreal, Quebec, Canada)
J Pediatr Surg 46:411-414, 2011

Unicornuate uterus with a rudimentary horn is the rarest congenital anomaly of the female genital system. It can result in a variety of gynecologic and obstetric complications. This case report is an acute presentation of a cavitated, noncommunicating, rudimentary horn in a premenarchal girl. Successful laparoscopic excision was performed. The full extent of the anomaly was diagnosed by a combination of operative findings and postoperative magnetic resonance imaging (Fig 3).

▶ Two somewhat related clinically important rare anomalies of the pediatric/adolescent uterus are cited here to alert imagers to their nature and imaging patterns. The Gaied article concerns a 12-year-old girl with colicky, intermittent, right lower quadrant pain for 3 months. Her abdominal ultrasound imaging revealed a 5.5-cm right solid paraovarian mass between the right ovary and the uterus. The dumbbell-sized mass along the broad ligament was excised, leaving the normal right ovary. The mass had both solid and hemorrhagic components. Postoperative MRI revealed a classic unilateral left unicornuate uterus. The second report[1] was of a Robert's uterus, which is an asymmetric septate uterus, in a 15-year-old symptomatic girl. In Robert's uterus, a blind hemiuterus is lined with endometrium, which causes menstrual bleeding that distends the blind cavity when, as in the reported case, it does not communicate with a fallopian tube. Surgical management cured the symptoms and is the appropriate treatment for Robert's uterus. The preoperative MRI and contrast CT contributed greatly to directing patient management, and the 3 figures of the article[1] are strongly recommended for our readers to learn about the condition. Fig 3 is here reproduced. The 2 rare conditions here reviewed have

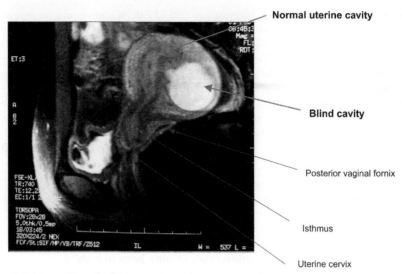

Normal uterine cavity

Blind cavity

Posterior vaginal fornix

Isthmus

Uterine cervix

FIGURE 3.—T2-weighted MRI: Median sagittal section of the pelvis. (Reprinted from Gaied F, Quiros-Calinoiu E, Emil S. Laparoscopic excision of a rudimentary uterine horn in a child. *J Pediatr Surg.* 2011;46:411-414, Copyright 2011, with permission from Elsevier.)

similarities despite their different natures, and both should be known to medical imagers who might encounter a similar case.

A. E. Oestreich, MD

Reference

1. Capito C, Sarnacki S. Menstrual retention in a Robert's uterus. *J Pediatr Adolesc Gynecol.* 2009;22:e104-e106.

Inguinal Hernia Containing Uterus and Uterine Adnexa in Female Infants: Report of Two Cases
Ming Y-C, Luo C-C, Chao H-C, et al (Chang Gung Univ College of Medicine, Taoyuan, Taiwan)
Pediatr Neonatol 52:103-105, 2011

We herein report two female cases, aged 1 and 1.5 months, of inguinal sliding hernias containing the uterus, fallopian tube, and ovary. The diagnosis of inguinal hernia with uterus and uterine adnexa was highly suspected preoperatively by ultrasonography and was confirmed during surgical correction. Freeing the attachment of fallopian tube and uterus from the sac and with reduction of the uterus, ovary, and fallopian tube back to the peritoneal cavity, high ligation of the hernia sac was performed in these cases. In conclusion, the hernia sac containing fallopian tube, ovary, and uterus in the female is very rare. We present our experience

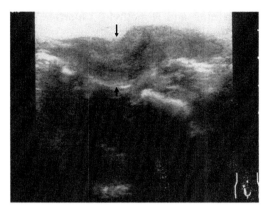

FIGURE 1.—Ultrasonography of the right groin reveals homogeneous structure with a central echoic line suspicious for herniation of uterus (black arrows) into the inguinal canal. (Reprinted from Ming Y-C, Luo C-C, Chao H-C, et al. Inguinal hernia containing uterus and uterine adnexa in female infants: report of two cases. *Pediatr Neonatol.* 2011;52:103-105, with permission from Taiwan Pediatric Association.)

of treatment with these rare cases and suggest that sonography be performed routinely in female infants with an inguinal hernia containing a palpable movable mass (Fig 1).

▶ The subject of this article is certainly not a common entity but one with so characteristic an image that it deserves to be among patterns recognized by pediatric medical imagers. Inguinal hernias with their own mesentery are defined as sliding hernias. In the female patient, a not inconsiderable number of such hernias contain ovary and sometimes fallopian tube as well. The alert ultrasound (US) imager should be able to recognize an ovary in the inguinal canal. The 2 subjects reported here presented with an irreducible mass in the groin. US revealed a structure in the hernia with a midline echogenic stripe that evoked the pattern of uterus, and, in 1 case, an ovarian cyst as well. Fig 1 nicely demonstrates a recognizable uterus in the inguinal canal. The female analog of the male processus vaginalis is the canal of Nuck (no pun, please). The authors found 5 previous case reports of uterus in the canal. The surgical situation involves the herniated uterus adhering to the wall of the Nuckian sac. The surgical procedure thus differs from that when only ovary is herniated, making the ultrasound recognition of uterus an important preoperative finding. The authors speculate that the only good explanation for the uterine herniation is an abnormality of the uterine suspensory ligaments. Preoperative US (or magnetic resonance) imaging of the female inguinal herniation and its proper interpretation is thus an important precaution.

A. E. Oestreich, MD

'Benign' ovarian teratoma and N-methyl-D-aspartate receptor (NMDAR) encephalitis in a child

Frawley KJ, Calvo-Garcia MA, Krueger DA, et al (Cincinnati Children's Hosp Med Ctr, OH)
Pediatr Radiol 42:120-123, 2012

N-methyl-D-aspartate receptor (NMDAR) encephalitis is a life-threatening paraneoplastic neuropsychiatric encephalitis that predominantly affects young women and has a strong association with ovarian teratomas. Removal of the ovarian teratomas improves the prognosis and decreases the risk of recurrence. We present an 11-year-old girl with NMDAR encephalitis with small bilateral teratomas not initially appreciated on abdominal CT or pelvic MRI. A 12-mm teratoma was identified in the right ovary and a 7-mm teratoma was identified in the left ovary on US follow-up at 5 months. Intraoperative sonography was used to localize the teratomas for excision. In NMDAR encephalitis, the ovarian teratomas can be very small, particularly in children, and easily missed on cross-sectional imaging. Awareness of the association of NMDAR encephalitis and ovarian teratomas will improve the diagnostic accuracy and imaging interpretation. Periodic sonography and MRI might be warranted in children if the initial study is negative (Fig 3).

▶ Severe psychotic and neurologic symptoms in a woman may well, albeit rarely, be related to ovarian teratomas. This association seems tenuous, but its consideration may be lifesaving. In the case reported here, the 11-year-old girl with no prior medical history presented with generalized tonic-clonic seizures and altered mental state, including headache, neck pain, and hypersomnia. MRIs revealed increased cortical signal in right superior frontal gyrus and both inferior medial cortical gyri. The key seemingly unrelated finding as eventually shown on ultrasound (Fig 3) was bilateral small ovarian teratomas.

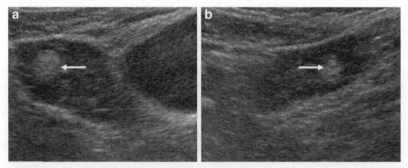

FIGURE 3.—US of the right and left ovaries demonstrates (a) a 12-mm well-defined echogenic lesion in the right ovary (*arrow*) and (b) a 7-mm well-defined echogenic lesion in the left ovary (*arrow*). The findings were concerning for small ovarian teratomas, given the patient's history of NMDAR encephalitis. (Reprinted from Frawley KJ, Calvo-Garcia MA, Krueger DA, et al. 'Benign' ovarian teratoma and N-methyl-D-aspartate receptor (NMDAR) encephalitis in a child. *Pediatr Radiol.* 2012;42:120-123, with permission from Springer Science and Business Media.)

This case beautifully illustrates this newly discovered association and how to investigate it! Although *N*-methyl-ᴅ-aspartate receptor (NMDAR) encephalitis represents only about 1% of encephalitis admissions in the intensive care unit, it has significant mortality, which is decreased if the frequently associated ovarian teratomas are removed. NMDAR is considered a paraneoplastic condition and is found more often in women than men. The message is clear: know this association and seek, if need be repeatedly, ovarian teratomata assiduously.

A. E. Oestreich, MD

Musculoskeletal

Clinical and radiological distinction between spondylothoracic dysostosis (Lavy-Moseley syndrome) and spondylocostal dysostosis (Jarcho-Levin syndrome)
Berdon WE, Lampl BS, Cornier AS, et al (Columbia Univ College of Physicians and Surgeons, NY; Hosp de la Concepcion, San German, Puerto Rico; et al)
Pediatr Radiol 41:384-388, 2011

In 1938, Saul Jarcho and Paul Levin from Johns Hopkins Hospital reported cases of thoracic insufficiency due to vertebral and rib anomalies. Nearly 30 years later, in 1966, Norman Lavy and associates from Indiana University reported a similar syndrome in a family from Puerto Rico. Lavy's description was followed by a report by John E. Moseley from New York City, where the name spondylothoracic dysplasia (dysostosis) was first used. For more than half a century, there has been confusion regarding the distinction between these two phenotypically similar syndromes that cause thoracic insufficiency. Spondylocostal dysostosis (SCD), or Jarcho-Levin syndrome, causes mild to moderate respiratory insufficiency, is pan-ethnic and has been linked to genes such as *DLL3*, which is known to be associated with the Notch pathway. In contrast, spondylothoracic dysostosis (STD), or Lavy-Moseley syndrome, results in more severe respiratory compromise, is largely linked to Puerto Rican cohorts and is thought to be associated to the *MESP2* gene, also a Notch pathway gene. Long-term studies of Puerto Rican cohorts with STD contradict the previously held belief that individuals affected with STD have markedly diminished life expectancy with as many as 25% surviving into later childhood and adult life (Fig 5).

▶ Here's one for the "splitters" as opposed to the "lumpers." When it comes to the dysostoses and dysplasias, it is satisfying when 2 previously separately described entities are shown to be the same (lumping); however, it is also important to "split" 2 disorders that have not been satisfactorily recognized as separate, when the splitting identifies clinically and genetically important differences. To recognize that the children with either of these dysostoses has an abnormal trunk is easy. This article explains why they should be distinguished from each other, if only because of the more severe respiratory compromise (due to thorax shape impairing lung volume and movement) in the Lavy-Moseley syndrome, as

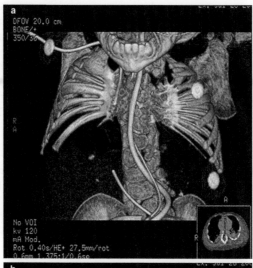

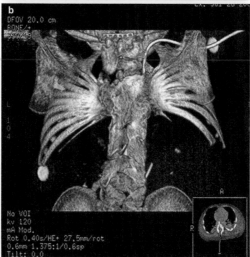

FIGURE 5.—Three-dimensional reconstruction of a chest CT scan in a child with STD. a Image shows an anteroposterior view and (b) shows a posteroanterior view. Note the malsegmentation and fusion of the spine with symmetrical posterior fusion of the ribs. (Reprinted from Berdon WE, Lampl BS, Cornier AS, et al. Clinical and radiological distinction between spondylothoracic dysostosis (Lavy-Moseley syndrome) and spondylocostal dysostosis (Jarcho-Levin syndrome). *Pediatr Radiol.* 2011;41:384-388, with kind permission from Springer Science and Business Media.)

demonstrated in their Fig 5. The diagnoses are also important because of the possibility of improving respiratory status through orthopaedic rib instrumentation, such as VEPTR.[1] After one recognizes that 1 of these 2 dysostoses is present, the current article is a good starting point for organizing the care and prognosis for the child.

A. E. Oestreich, MD

Reference

1. White KK, Song KM, Frost N, Daines BK. VEPTR™ growing rods for early-onset neuromuscular scoliosis: feasible and effective. *Clin Orthop Relat Res.* 2011;469: 1335-1341.

A symptomatic sesamoid bone in the popliteus muscle (cyamella)

Benthien JP, Brunner A (Univ of Basel, Switzerland; Cantonal Hosp Lucerne, Switzerland)

Musculoskelet Surg 94:141-144, 2011

Sesamoid bones of the popliteus muscle, also called cyamellae, are common in primates but rare in humans. They reside as accessory bones in the tendon itself or in the intersection between tendon and bone. They should be clearly distinguished from osteochondral flakes, periosseous calcifications, osteophytes and the fabella, a common sesamoid bone of the knee. In this case, we report a 25-year-old male with posterior lateral knee pain related to the popliteus tendon where a corresponding cyamella could be demonstrated on X-rays and MRI scans. The clinical findings may be related to the cyamella. Diagnosis and treatment of this rare pathology are discussed.

▶ Wow! A new bone that I have never knowingly seen in all my 45+ years in radiology! Admittedly it is rare, and any time I previously read about it in the literature, it did not reach my level of consciousness. Because it may be symptomatic, I want to cite it for you. A few days ago I saw this "new" sesamoid on radiographs of 1 knee of an 11-year-old boy with knee pain (see Figs of our case). My colleague Eric Crotty, MD, was able to cue me in on its name. The patella is near-universal; the fabella is not uncommon, but the cyamella in the popliteus tendon is most unusual. Benthien's article also features 2 characteristic MRI images of their case. The popliteus, to review, originates from the lateral condyle of the femur and inserts into the proximal dorsal tibia shaft. Eventually, a cyamella may perform a small articulation with the lateral dorsal femoral condyle that in adulthood may be symptomatic in osteoarthrosis. The patient discussed in the current article was active in recreational sport, and his pain resolved after physical therapy (not necessarily, however, as a consequence of it). The outer calcified margins of the cyamella in childhood, like that of the patella,[1] consists of a zone of provisional calcification of cartilage rather than a bony cortex. Hence, the cyalmella, which grows in childhood strictly by enchondral growth, has no periosteum.[1] Interestingly, Dr Benthien tells me he has seen additional cyamellae after submitting his article. So welcome to the cyamella and learn to recognize it the few times that it occurs, especially in the painful knee.

A. E. Oestreich, MD

Reference

1. Oestreich AE. Comment on Hedayati, et al. *Skeletal Radiol.* 2010;39:397.

Deficiency of interleukin-1-receptor antagonist syndrome: a rare auto-inflammatory condition that mimics multiple classic radiographic findings
Thacker PG, Binkovitz LA, Thomas KB (Mayo Clinic, Rochester, MN)
Pediatr Radiol 2011 [Epub ahead of print]

Deficiency of interleukin-1-receptor antagonist (DIRA) syndrome is a newly identified inflammatory disease of the skeleton and appendicular soft tissues presenting in early infancy that has yet to be reported in the

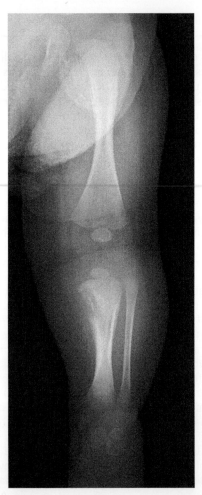

FIGURE 5.—Radiograph of the left lower extremity demonstrates cortical destruction and periostitis of the proximal tibial metaphysis. This appearance is similar to Wimberger's sign, which is associated with congenital syphilis. Additionally, there is a balloon-like periostitis of the medial proximal left femoral metaphysis. (Reprinted from Thacker PG, Binkovitz LA, Thomas KB. Deficiency of interleukin-1-receptor antagonist syndrome: a rare auto-inflammatory condition that mimics multiple classic radiographic findings. *Pediatr Radiol.* 2011;[Epub ahead of print], with kind permission from Springer Science and Business Media.)

radiology literature. The radiological manifestations of DIRA syndrome include multifocal osteitis of the ribs and long bones, heterotopic ossification and periarticular soft-tissue swelling. Thus, the pediatric radiologist should be made aware of this novel disease because its radiographic findings can mimic multiple other disease entities. With knowledge of the unique clinical presentation of DIRA syndrome and its multiple radiographic manifestations, the pediatric radiologist may be the first to suggest the correct diagnosis (Fig 5).

▶ If only because of the important mimics of the radiographic findings of this newly identified disease, one should carefully study this important article. The underlying genotypic abnormality involves a recessive mutation in IL1RN, which encodes for the interleukin-1-receptor antagonist. Even if you don't follow what that statement means, learn the manifestations of the disease, deficiency of interleukin-1-receptor antagonist (DIRA). The characteristic findings are appendicular soft-tissue swelling, pustular dermatitis, and sterile osteomyelitis beginning at birth or shortly thereafter. So you can tell the radiologist might be led astray into considering Caffey disease (infantile cortical hyperostosis), chronic recurrent multifocal osteomyelitis, syphilis, SAPHO (synovitis, acne, pustulosis, hyperostosis, and osteitis), child abuse, and metastatic neuroblastoma. Fig 5, for example, shows tibial metadiaphyseal destruction in their infant (disease course 1 to 2 months of age), sparing the metaphyseal collar, which resembles the Wimberger "bite" of congenital syphilis. The diagnosis of DIRA was confirmed, and the child showed excellent clinical response to anakinra (Biovitrum), an appropriate recombinant interleukin-1-receptor antagonist. DIRA can be life-threatening; it was classically described in 2009 by Aksentijevich and colleagues.[1] So here is a mimicking condition that has a specific genetic diagnostic confirmation, is dangerous, and can be confounded with several other important diagnoses in the same age group. By all means, learn about it and mention it in differential or primary diagnosis when appropriate.

A. E. Uestreich, MD

Reference

1. Aksentijevich I, Masters SL, Ferguson PJ, et al. An autoinflammatory disease with deficiency of the interleukin-1-receptor antagonist. *N Engl J Med*. 2009;360: 2426-2437.

The importance of conventional radiography in the mutational analysis of skeletal dysplasias (the TRPV4 mutational family)
Nemec SF, Cohn DH, Krakow D, et al (Cedars Sinai Med Ctr, Los Angeles, CA)
Pediatr Radiol 42:15-23, 2012

The spondylo and spondylometaphyseal dysplasias (SMDs) are characterized by vertebral changes and metaphyseal abnormalities of the tubular bones, which produce a phenotypic spectrum of disorders from the mild

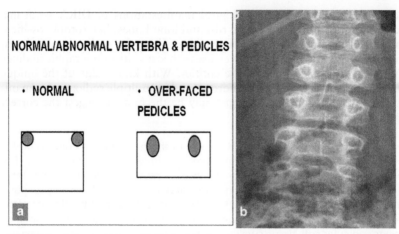

FIGURE 2.—A 4-year-old boy with brachyolmia (autosomal-dominant type) and vertebral involvement. a The diagram illustrates the characteristic appearance of over-faced pedicles associated with platyspondyly, compared to the normal appearance. b The anterior-posterior radiograph of the lumbar spine shows the overfacing of the enlarged pedicles and flattened vertebral bodies (also called open staircase). (Reprinted from Nemec SF, Cohn DH, Krakow D, et al. The importance of conventional radiography in the mutational analysis of skeletal dysplasias (the TRPV4 mutational family). *Pediatr Radiol.* 2012;42:15-23, with kind permission from Springer Science and Business Media.)

autosomal-dominant brachyolmia to SMD Kozlowski to autosomal-dominant metatropic dysplasia. Investigations have recently drawn on the similar radiographic features of those conditions to define a new family of skeletal dysplasias caused by mutations in the transient receptor potential cation channel vanilloid 4 (TRPV4). This review demonstrates the significance of radiography in the discovery of a new bone dysplasia family due to mutations in a single gene (Fig 2).

▶ Lumpers rejoice! A new family of dysplasias is identified, tied together with a TRPV4 mutation. The importance of such lumping is in gathering together disparate skeletal dysplasias in a genetically pertinent classification, aiding as well the recognition of children with characteristic intermediates between family members. It also gives grounding to dysplasia that affects the vertebral column without definite abnormality in epiphyses or metaphyses, namely, brachyolmia.[1] I have encountered 3 children likely to have brachyolmia in recent months. Additionally, I am always pleased that conventional radiography, my own subspecialty, is featured in a title of an important article. One problem I have is understanding the term over-faced pedicles seen in many brachyolmia cases and some others of the family members. Fig 2 shows this feature diagrammatically and mentions that the en face pedicles may seem large. Regardless of the term used, this is a nice contribution to pedicology, the recognition of the significance of abnormal pedicles on frontal radiographs. I recommend a close reading of the original article to refresh your knowledge of brachyolmia, metatropic dysplasia, and spondylometaphyseal dysplasia—type Kozlowski, all of which include some platyspondyly. The illustration of abnormal talus and calcaneus in metatropic dysplasia is a bonus of the review.

A. E. Oestreich, MD

Reference

1. Shohat M, Lachman R, Gruber HE, Rimoin DL. Brachyolmia: radiographic and genetic evidence of heterogeneity. *Am J Med Genet.* 1989;33:209-219.

Van Neck Disease: Osteochondrosis of the Ischiopubic Synchondrosis
Wait A, Gaskill T, Sarwar Z, et al (Pinnacle Health System, Harrisburg, PA; Duke Med Ctr, Durham, NC; Nemours Clinic, Jacksonville, FL; et al)
J Pediatr Orthop 31:520-524, 2011

Background.—Van Neck disease (VND) is a benign skeletal abnormality of children involving a hyperostosis of the ischiopubic synchondrosis (IPS) seen on radiographs. Patients typically complain of vague groin or buttock pain. Few descriptions of this disorder exist and it easily can be mistaken for other entities, particularly osteomyelitis or tumor. It is often considered a diagnosis of exclusion as laboratory values are usually normal and routine radiographic workup may be nonspecific. We present a series of patients with VND and we compare them with a similar cohort of patients with acute hematogenous ischiopubic osteomyelitis (IPOM). We also draw attention to a new magnetic resonance imaging (MRI) finding that seems to support the theory that VND results from an excessive pull of the hamstring tendon on the ischial tuberosity.

Methods.—All patients presenting to our institution for the evaluation of groin or buttock pain during an 8-year period (August 2001 to May 2009) were retrospectively identified. Twenty-five patients demonstrated enhancement of the ischiopubic area on MRI. Five patients were excluded for lack of sufficient laboratory data. Ten patients were diagnosed and treated with culture proven IPOM and 10 patients were diagnosed with VND and treated with observation. History, physical examination, laboratory values, plain films, and MRI were compared to identify the diagnostic differences between these 2 entities.

Results.—The age range for both groups was between 4 and 12 years old. The mean age was 7 years for the VND group and 7.6 years for the IPOM group. The VND group tended to have more distinct hyperostosis of the IPS on radiographs. The factors that were characteristic of IPOM were: fever, limp, pain with rotation of the hip, elevated erythrocyte sedimentation rate, elevated C-reactive protein (CRP), and positive blood culture. MRI showed obvious myositis, abscess, and free fluid surrounding the IPS in all patients with IPOM, but not in the VND patients. Enhancement was seen in the ischial tuberosity, near the hamstring origin, in nearly all Van Neck patients; this pattern of edema may support stress reaction and callus formation as a mechanism for IPS hypertrophy.

Conclusions.—VND is a little-known entity characterized by enlargement of the IPS and should be in the differential of groin or buttock pain in children from the age of 4 to 12 years. IPOM may present similar to VND. Absence of fever, limp, pain with rotation of the hip, elevated C-reactive protein/erythrocyte sedimentation rate, and negative blood culture can help to differentiate VND from IPOM. Presence of marrow edema around the IPS and in the ischial tuberosity, along with absence of surrounding myositis, abscess, and free fluid on MRI are reliable findings that can confirm the diagnosis of VND. The absence of these characteristics can eliminate the need for admission, aspiration, or biopsy. The treatment for VND is observation and the symptoms should abate over time with expectant management.

Level of Evidence.—Comparative Diagnostic, Level IV (Fig 2).

▶ Here we go again with Van Neck "disease" (VND)—this time with nice MRI differentiation from a clinical and sometimes plain image mimic, namely, acute hematogenous ischiopubic osteomyelitis. As the authors discuss, most times when the ischiopubic synchondrosis cartilage area fuses with a local widened bone bump, it is well recognized as a normal finding. However, when symptoms seem to be associated, such as groin or buttock pain, the entity is proclaimed to be VND. If MRI is performed, inflammation in adjacent muscles is not seen with VND and is seen in osteomyelitis in all 10 of their cases of each entity. As shown in Fig 2, enhancement of the ischiopubic synchondrosis region was seen in symptomatic VND on T2 axial images and T1 postgadolinium images and also seen in the children with osteomyelitis. Treatment of VND is "no treatment," as in the nonsymptomatic normal subjects. Curiously, the asymmetric Van Neck pattern of bulbous widening on images (plain images, MRI, or CT) has been strongly correlated with the footedness (foot dominance) of affected children in one study.[1] Van Neck "disease" or "configuration" (my preferred name), like "Sever disease" and similar entities, is most often a useful descriptor for

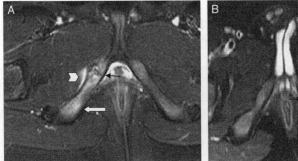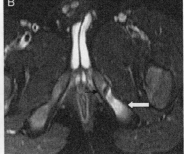

FIGURE 2.—Axial T2 images of two separate patients with Van Neck disease. Again note the assymetric appearance of the ischiopubic synchondrosis (black arrows). Each demonstrates enhancement of the ischium, near the hamstring attachment (white arrows), distinctive of Van Neck disease. Image A shows edema surrounding the synchondrosis and should not be confused with free fluid or abcess (white chevron). (Reprinted from Wait A, Gaskill T, Sarwar Z, et al. Van neck disease: osteochondrosis of the ischiopubic synchondrosis. *J Pediatr Orthop.* 2011;31:520-524, with permission from Lippincott Williams & Wilkins.)

those who like eponyms but raises questions when symptomatic. Wait et al's article contributes to the occasional need to distinguish from osteomyelitis.

A. E. Oestreich, MD

Reference

1. Herneth AM, Philipp MO, Pretterklieber ML, Balassy C, Winkelbauer FW, Beaulieu CF. Asymmetric closure of ischiopubic synchondrosis in pediatric patients: correlation with foot dominance. *AJR Am J Roentgenol.* 2004;182:361-365.

Dating fractures in infants
Halliday KE, Broderick NJ, Somers JM, et al (Nottingham Univ Hosps, UK; Paul O'Gorman Building, Bristol, UK)
Clin Radiol 66:1049-1054, 2011

Aim.—To document the timing of the appearance of the radiological features of fracture healing in a group of infants in which the date of injury was known and to assess the degree of interobserver agreement.

Materials and Methods.—Three paediatric radiologists independently assessed 161 images of 37 long bone fractures in 31 patients aged 0—44 months. The following features were assessed: soft-tissue swelling, subperiosteal new bone formation (SPNBF), definition of fracture line, presence or absence of callus, whether callus was well or ill defined, and the presence of endosteal callus.

Results.—Agreement between observers was only moderate for all discriminators except SPNBF. SPNBF was invariably seen after 11 days but was uncommon before this time even in the very young. In one case SPNBF was seen at 4 days.

Conclusion.—With the exception of SPNBF, the criteria relied on to date fractures are either not reproducible or are poor discriminators of fracture age (Table 3).

▶ Radiologists involved with the interpretation of radiographs in the context of suspected child abuse will be aware of both the difficulty in and the importance of providing an estimate of the age of any identified fracture(s). When faced with such a clinical dilemma, a usual recourse might be to practice "evidence-based medicine," that is, to review the current literature. Unfortunately, there are only a few peer-reviewed articles on the subject of the radiological dating of fractures, and between them these few studies include only a handful of patients of the relevant age group.

As the "true" age of any fracture included in any such study must be known, it is valid to ask whether treated "accidental" fractures heal at the same rate as untreated "abuse" fractures.

If we decide to ignore this hurdle on the basis that there is little or nothing we can do about it, a multitude of difficulties in designing a prospective study remain: ethical issues related to radiation exposure secondary to serial radiographs,

TABLE 3.—Summary of the Features of Fracture Healing From the Literature

Feature of Fracture Healing	Nottingham	O'Connor	First Author Islam	Yeo	Cumming
Resolution of soft tissue swelling	10 days	Late 10–21 days			
Earliest SPNBF	4 days	4 days	14 days	Mean 11.7 days	7 days
Loss of definition of fracture line	12–77 days	10–21 days	2–8 weeks		
Well-defined/hard callus	20–106 days	2–12 weeks			
Bridging callus		3–10 weeks	1.5–3.7 weeks		
Endosteal callus	8 days onwards		2 weeks onwards		

SPNBF, subperiosteal new bone formation.

practical issues related to the presence of casts and splints, and logistical issues related to the need for and cost of frequent (how frequent?) attendances to the imaging department are some hurdles that we cannot ignore. Given these problems, it is easy to understand why a retrospective design might be favored.

Although more straightforward, a retrospective study design will have many of its own problems, as illustrated by this present article by Halliday et al.

Despite the limitations of the study, the authors are to be commended for publishing the largest existing data set on the radiographic dating of fractures in infants. Unfortunately, many unanswered questions remain. For example, healing rate of fractures at different sites, healing rate of fractures in association with head injury, healing rate of fractures in relation to patient age, and healing of rib and metaphyseal fractures (this study was not designed to answer the latter), to list a few.

Table 3 in the article provides a summary of the current literature on radiographic dating of fractures. Clearly, the older the fracture, the less well we are able to date it.

A word of caution to readers of the article: take care in interpreting the authors' seemingly moderate interobserver reliability; it is not clear to me whether (to clarify terminology) a learning/consensus session was held with nonstudy radiographs, before commencement of the study proper; I think not. Although the authors' design probably represents the clinical situation (each of us assigning our own meanings to individual terms), the authors have published a research article, and it highlights the need (if research is to be robust) for researchers to establish and agree a priori the terminology and diagnostic categories to be used in their research; a "before and after training" design would work equally well.

This proviso aside, for the time being (until a robust prospective study allows us to truly practice evidence-based radiographic dating of fractures), the take-home message is that in infants and young children, subperiosteal new bone formation may be detected on radiographs as early as the fourth day, and is invariably present by the eleventh day, after the fracture was sustained.

A. C. Offiah, BSc, MBBS, MRCP, FRCR, PhD

The Prevalence of Uncommon Fractures on Skeletal Surveys Performed to Evaluate for Suspected Abuse in 930 Children: Should Practice Guidelines Change?

Karmazyn B, Lewis ME, Jennings SG, et al (Riley Hosp for Children, Indianapolis, IN; Joshua Max Simon Primary Care Ctr, Indianapolis, IN; Indiana Univ School of Medicine, Indianapolis)
AJR Am J Roentgenol 197:W159-W163, 2011

Objective.—The objective of our study was to evaluate the prevalence and site of fractures detected on skeletal surveys performed for suspected child abuse at a tertiary children's hospital and to determine whether any survey images may be eliminated without affecting clinical care or the ability to make a diagnosis.

Materials and Methods.—We identified all skeletal surveys performed for suspected abuse from 2003 to 2009 of children younger than 2 years. Repeated studies were excluded, as were studies not performed to evaluate for suspected abuse. From the reports, we documented the sites of all the fractures.

Results.—Nine hundred thirty children (515 boys and 415 girls) with a median age of 6 months met the entry criteria for the study. Fractures were detected in 317 children (34%), of whom 166 (18%) had multiple fractures. The most common sites for fractures were the long bones (21%), ribs (10%), skull (7%), and clavicle (2%). Ten children (1%) had fractures in the spine ($n = 3$), pelvis ($n = 1$), hands ($n = 6$), and feet ($n = 2$). All 10 children had other signs of physical abuse.

Conclusion.—In skeletal surveys performed for suspected child abuse, fractures limited to sites other than the long bones, ribs, skull, and clavicles are rare. The additional radiation exposure and cost of obtaining radiographs of the spine, pelvis, hands, and feet may outweigh their potential benefit. Given the rarity of fractures of the spine, pelvis, hands, and feet, consideration may be given to eliminating those views from routine skeletal surveys performed to evaluate for suspected child abuse (Tables 1 and 2).

▶ In the introduction to their article, the authors stress the importance of detecting fractures in a vulnerable child because recurrent episodes of increasing violence may end in that child's death. The authors then go on to identify fractures of the spinous process as being amongst those that have a high specificity for abuse. They emphasize the important role played by imaging, recounting the move away from the traditional "babygram" to high-quality skeletal surveys as recommended by US and UK guidelines. They perform a retrospective review of a large study population (960 children younger than 2 years), and, based on their detected prevalence of fractures of the pelvis, spine, and digits, they suggest that radiographs of the same might be omitted from routine skeletal survey.

This conclusion causes me some concern.

Yes, this may be the largest retrospective study on the subject. Yes, the low detection of spinal, pelvic, and digital fractures (Table 2) amongst a cohort with a relatively high prevalence of fractures at other sites (Table 1) does emphasize

TABLE 1.—Fractures in the Long Bones, Ribs, and Skull Identified on 930 Skeletal Surveys in Children Younger Than 2 Years

Site of Fracture	Fracture Detected on Survey		Equivocal Fracture Detected on Survey			
	Children	Fractures	Children	Equivocal Fractures	Follow-Up Imaging	Fractures Confirmed[a]
Long bones	202	375	50	82	79	19
Ribs	97	423	14	27	23	7
Clavicle	20	21	0	0	0	0
Scapula	3	3	2	1	1	0
Skull	67	75	2	2	2	1
Mandible	1	1	0	0	0	0
Nose	1	1	0	0	0	0
Total	309[b]	899	56[b]	112	105	27

[a]Fractures confirmed after follow-up imaging was performed.
[b]Some children had more than one fracture in more than one site.

TABLE 2.—Fractures in the Hands, Feet, Spine, and Pelvis Identified on Skeletal Surveys of 930 Children Younger Than 2 Years

Site of Fracture	Reported Fractures			Equivocal Fractures			Sum of All Fractures Confirmed[a]	
	Children	Fractures	Fractures Confirmed[a]	Children	Equivocal Fractures	Fractures Confirmed[a]	Children	Fractures
Hands								
Metacarpal	4	6	6	1	1	1	4	7
Proximal phalange	0	0	0	1	1	1	1	1
Feet								
Metatarsal	2	4	4	1	1	0	2	4
Spine	5	13	4	1	1	0	3	4
Pelvis	1	1	1	0	0	0	1	1
Total	12	24	15	3[b]	4	2	10[b]	17

[a]Confirmation of the fractures was based on review of the radiographs and follow-up imaging. Spinal fractures were excluded, based on negative follow-up CT scan or MRI.
[b]One child had fractures at two sites.

how uncommon such fractures are. However, merely because the prevalence of a finding is low does not diminish the importance of that finding when it does occur.

In fact, just the reverse. An isolated long bone fracture may be summarized as simply that. Add a hand radiograph, detect a healing metacarpal fracture, and the case for abuse is greatly strengthened. Or perhaps the hand radiograph is normal but the spine radiograph reveals multiple vertebral compression fractures. Then perhaps osteogenesis imperfecta should be considered.

The authors work in a tertiary referral center where the screening and referral process is robust, hence the high rate of fractures in their cohort. However, prevalence rates of fractures on skeletal surveys for abuse will vary according to the level of suspicion for abuse, local indicators for performing skeletal surveys, referral patterns, primary versus tertiary centres, and so forth. A quick review of skeletal surveys performed in my institution over the past 6 months reveals that 29 skeletal surveys (excluding post mortem surveys) were performed for suspected abuse (16 unexplained bruising, 10 long bone or skull fractures, 3 subdural hemorrhages with no skull fracture) of which none (0%) were positive for fractures at other sites. Therefore, to take the authors' argument to its logical conclusion, with a prevalence of any sort of additional fracture of 0%, in Sheffield perhaps we should be omitting the entire skeletal survey...okay I'm being facetious now, but I hope I make my point.

So we'd like to save time, costs, and radiation dose—and so we should, but the cost savings/losses related to expediting or delaying the diagnosis of abuse are not straightforward to calculate and require the input of health economists.

In the context of a skeletal survey, the radiation dose savings made from excluding the extremities are likely to be negligible. In the United Kingdom we do not perform a Towne view of the skull unless an occipital fracture is suspected. We do not perform dedicated anteroposterior views of the spine on the basis that most information on spinal fractures is best obtained from lateral projections and that anteroposterior views of thoracic and lumbar spine are available on the chest and abdominal radiographs, respectively. Perhaps such compromises should be encouraged rather than abolishing certain projections altogether.

Babygrams may have been of poor quality, but they did include the spine and usually the extremities. Let us not take a backward step.

To give the authors their due, at the end of both their abstract and their full article, they precede their suggestion of eliminating these views by one little word: may. Yes, it "may" be that eliminating these views will be cost effective, but until we have more robust data, I strongly advise that we all adhere to our national guidelines as they currently stand.

A. C. Offiah, BSc, MBBS, MRCP, FRCR, PhD

Immediate Treatment Versus Sonographic Surveillance for Mild Hip Dysplasia in Newborns
Rosendahl K, Dezateux C, Fosse KR, et al (Great Ormond Street Hosp for Children, London, UK; UCL Inst of Child Health, UK; Haukeland Univ Hosp, Bergen, Norway; et al)
Pediatrics 125:e9-e16, 2010

Objective.—We conducted a blinded, randomized, controlled trial to examine whether mildly dysplastic but stable or instable hips would benefit from early treatment, as compared with watchful waiting.

Patients and Methods.—A total of 128 newborns with mild hip dysplasia (sonographic inclination angle [α angle] of $43°-49°$) and stable or instable but not dislocatable hips were randomly assigned to receive either 6 weeks of abduction treatment (immediate-treatment group) or follow-up alone (active-sonographic-surveillance group). The main outcome measurement was the acetabular inclination angle, measured by radiograph, at 1 year of age.

Results.—Both groups included 64 newborns, and there was no loss to follow-up. With the exception of a small but statistically significant excess of girls in the active-sonographic-surveillance group, there were no statistically significant differences in baseline characteristics between the 2 groups. The mean inclination angle at 12 months was 24.2° for both groups (difference: 0.1 [95% confidence interval (CI): −0.8 to 0.9]), and all children had improved and were without treatment. The mean α angle was 59.7° in the treatment group and 57.1° in the active-surveillance group for a difference of 2.6° evaluated after 1.5 and 3 months (95% CI: 1.8 to 3.4; $P < .001$). At 1.5 months of age, the hips had improved in all treated children but not in 5 children under active surveillance ($P = .06$). Among the sonographic-surveillance group, 47% received treatment after the initial surveillance period of 1.5 months.

Conclusions.—Active-sonographic-surveillance halved the number of children requiring treatment, did not increase the duration of treatment, and yielded similar results at 1-year follow-up. Given a reported prevalence of 1.3% for mildly dysplastic but stable hips, a strategy of active surveillance would reduce the overall treatment rate by 0.6%. Our results may have important implications for families as well as for health care costs.

▶ The usual question surrounding ultrasound screening for developmental dysplasia of the hip (DDH) is whether it should be performed. Controversy surrounds the cost of the ultrasound itself, the costs of treatment, and the effectiveness and timing of treatment when DDH is diagnosed early. Different nations have different policies; for instance, in Germany and Austria, ultrasound screening is performed on all newborns within the first week of life; in Norway, it is performed in selected infants within the first week of life; in the United Kingdom, it is done in selected infants at approximately 6 weeks of age; the United States and, in particular, Canada, are somewhat less inclined toward ultrasound screening.

In this article, Rosendahl et al (from Norway) have shown that although universal treatment of infants with stable but mildly dysplastic hips from the time of birth resulted in more rapid normalization of the alpha angle, surveillance and treatment reconsideration at age 6 weeks did not result in more abnormal hips at 1 year of age. With a reported prevalence of 1.3% for mildly dysplastic but stable hips, a strategy of active surveillance would reduce the overall treatment rate by 0.6% with associated cost savings.

What the study did not (and was not designed to) look at was the rate of long-term complications (in particular, of avascular necrosis of the femoral head) in the immediate and delayed treatment groups.

All in all, results of this article will have more impact on those countries where ultrasound screening (whether selective or universal) is performed in the first week of life and (if I may say so, and you may disagree) go some way to justifying the UK approach of performing the screening ultrasound at 6 weeks in at-risk infants, as long as they had stable hips on clinical examination at birth.

For those of you wanting to follow the screening debate more closely, Tamai[1] provides a thought-provoking editorial to a more recent article by von Kries et al.[2]

A. C. Offiah, BSc, MBBS, MRCP, FRCR, PhD

References

1. Tamai J. Hip ultrasounds: where do we go from here? *J Pediatr.* 2012;160:189-190.
2. von Kries R, Ihme N, Altenhofen L, Niethard FU, Krauspe R, Rückinger S. General ultrasound screening reduces the rate of first operative procedures for developmental dysplasia of the hip: a case-control study. *J Pediatr.* 2012;160: 271-275.

Changes in quantitative ultrasound in preterm and term infants during the first year of life
Tansug N, Yildirim SA, Canda E, et al (Celal Bayar Univ, Manisa, Turkey)
Eur J Radiol 79:428-431, 2011

Since most of in utero bone mass accretion occurs during the third trimester and postnatal need for bone nutrients is increased, preterm infants have an increased risk of low bone mass. Early identification of the risk is of crucial importance. Quantitative ultrasound, which is a relatively inexpensive, portable, noninvasive, and radiation-free method, gives information about bone density, cortical thickness, elasticity and microarchitecture. The aim of this study was to obtain quantitative ultrasound measurements of tibial speed of sound of preterm and term infants and to assess clinical factors associated with these measurements during the first year of life.

Seventy-eight preterm and 48 term infants were enrolled in this study. Measurements were made on the 10th day of life in both groups, and were repeated on the 2nd, 6th and 12th months for preterm infants and on the 12th month for the term infants. Speed of sound on preterm infants was significantly decreased on the 2nd month but significantly increased on the 12th month ($P = 0.00$). Comparing speed of sound of term and preterm infants, 10th day measurements were significantly different ($P = 0.00$), but there was not any significant difference between the 12th month values ($P = 0.26$). There was not any relation between biochemical parameters and speed of sound.

The technique has potential clinical value for assessment of bone status. Further studies with long term follow up are needed to evaluate the value of quantitative ultrasound with other bone markers to predict the risk of fracture.

▶ The authors of this article list reliability, noninvasiveness, and relative low costs as requirements of any method of assessing bone strength in preterm infants. Their most persuasive arguments to support quantitative ultrasound

(QUS) over dual energy x-ray absorptiometry (DXA) are firstly that QUS avoids ionizing radiation and second that QUS is portable—the sick preterm infant does not have to be transported to the DXA room.

As with previous reports on the subject, this study confirms the decrease in bone speed of sound (SOS) that occurs in the first 2 months of life in preterm infants, which by age 12 months has "caught up" with SOS values of those born at term.

Like DXA, QUS has not been shown to correlate with biochemical markers of metabolic bone disease. It does, however, correlate with gestational age and (in the majority of studies) with birth weight, birth length, and head circumference. Is it therefore just an indication of bone size? We hope not, and indeed not all studies have shown a correlation between SOS and weight. Prospective longitudinal studies are required, correlating bone SOS with prevalence and incidence of fractures.

Noninvasiveness—check; relative low cost and portability—check; avoidance of ionizing radiation—check; but what are the positive and negative predictive values of bone SOS? What do the figures actually mean? In the final analysis, is this technique reliable?

A. C. Offiah, BSc, MBBS, MRCP, FRCR, PhD

Neurologic/Vertebral

Assessment of White Matter Microstructural Integrity in Children with Syndromic Craniosynostosis: A Diffusion-Tensor Imaging Study

Florisson JMG, Dudink J, Koning IV, et al (Sophia Children's Hosp, Rotterdam, The Netherlands)
Radiology 261:534-541, 2011

Purpose.—To assess whether architectural alterations exist in the white matter of patients with syndromic and complex craniosynostosis.

Materials and Methods.—The medical ethics committee approved this study. Written informed consent was obtained from parents or guardians before imaging. A prospective study was performed in children with syndromic and complex craniosynostosis aged 6–14 years. Forty-five patients were included: four had Apert syndrome, 14 had Crouzon-Pfeiffer syndrome, eight had Muenke syndrome, 11 had Saethre-Chotzen syndrome, and eight had complex craniosynostosis. In addition, seven control subjects were evaluated. For diffusion-tensor imaging, an echo-planar sequence was used with a diffusion gradient ($b = 1000$ sec/mm^2) applied in 25 noncollinear directions. Regions of interest (ROIs) were placed in the following white matter structures: pontine crossing tract, corticospinal tracts, medial cerebral peduncles, uncinate fasciculus (measured bilaterally), anterior commissure, frontal and occipital white matter (measured bilaterally), fornix, corpus callosum (measured in the genu and splenium), and corpus cingulum (measured bilaterally). Eigenvalues were measured in all ROIs and fractional anisotropy (FA) was calculated.

TABLE 2.—FA Values in White Matter Structures according to Syndrome and Genetic Background

Structure*	All Patients	Patients with Apert Syndrome (n = 4)	FGFR Group Patients with Crouzon-Pfeiffer Syndrome (n = 14)	Patients with Muenke Syndrome (n = 8)	TWIST Group (n = 11)†	Complex Craniosynostosis Group (n = 8)	Control Group (n = 7)	All Patients (n = 45)
PCT	0.32 (0.06)	0.32	0.32	0.31	0.3 (0.07)	0.32 (0.08)	0.31 (0.09)	0.31
CST	0.42 (0.06)	0.37	0.45	0.38	0.41 (0.07)	0.41 (0.07)	0.41 (0.12)	0.41
MCP	0.62 (0.08)	0.59	0.63	0.64	0.69 (0.04)	0.63 (0.05)	0.71 (0.07)	0.65
UNC	0.34 (0.09)	0.37	0.34	0.32	0.41 (0.08)	0.35 (0.06)	0.40 (0.03)	0.37
AC	0.23 (0.11)	0.4	0.26	0.25	0.31 (0.07)	0.26 (0.08)	0.30 (0.09)	0.28
FX	0.33 (0.08)	0.37	0.36	0.44	0.39 (0.04)	0.41 (0.09)	0.46 (0.07)	0.40
GCC	0.55 (0.09)	0.6	0.51	0.62	0.6 (0.05)	0.64 (0.09)	0.64 (0.07)	0.59
SCC	0.7 (0.08)	0.69	0.68	0.74	0.72 (0.10)	0.75 (0.06)	0.81 (0.04)	0.73
CG	0.5 (0.08)	0.51	0.53	0.51	0.48 (0.06)	0.49 (0.09)	0.55 (0.05)	0.51
MWM	0.42 (0.06)	0.41	0.39	0.44	0.44 (0.08)	0.41 (0.10)	0.47 (0.02)	0.43

Note.—Data are means; numbers in parentheses are standard deviations.
*PCT = pontine crossing tract, CST = corticospinal tract, MCP = medial cerebral peduncle, UNC = uncinate fasciculus, AC = anterior commissure, FX = fornix, GCC = genu of corpus callosum, SCC = splenium of corpus callosum, CG = corpus cingulum, MWM = mean white matter.
†The TWIST group was composed of patients with Saethre-Chotzen syndrome.

Results.—Across all measured ROIs, FA values were generally lower in all patients combined than in the control subjects ($P < .001$). There were no significant differences among subgroups of patients.

Conclusion.—Diffusion-tensor imaging measurements of white matter tracts reveal significant white matter integrity differences between children with craniosynostosis and healthy control subjects. This could imply that the developmental delays seen in these patients could be caused by the presence of a primary disorder of the white matter microarchitecture (Table 2).

▶ Children with craniosynostosis commonly (but not invariably) have mental deficiency. Raised intracranial pressure and/or hydrocephalus have traditionally been given as the explanation for this. However, some authors suggest the possibility of there being a primary congenital brain disorder. The authors of this paper have used diffusion tensor MRI in a bid to settle the matter. They found significantly lower white matter fractional anisotropy values for patients with craniosynostosis compared with normal controls (Table 2) and conclude that this finding (coupled with the fact that Muenke syndrome is almost never associated with raised intracranial pressure) supports there being a primary brain disorder secondary to the associated genetic mutations.

Because it is a significant clinical outcome of either hypothesis, it would have been useful had the authors documented how (if) intelligence differed between the groups and subgroups.

Some questions:

1. Are these white matter changes present in the brains of infants and neonates with craniosynostosis (an issue raised by the authors)?
2. If the answer to question 1 is no, then what is the explanation for white matter abnormality in Muenke syndrome?
3. If the answer to question 1 is yes, then what is the explanation for those children with craniosynostosis who have normal intelligence?

A. C. Offiah, BSc, MBBS, MRCP, FRCR, PhD

Biometry of the Corpus Callosum in Children: MR Imaging Reference Data
Garel C, Cont I, Alberti C, et al (Hôpital d'Enfants Armand-Trousseau, Paris, France; Hôpital Robert Debré, Paris, France)
AJNR Am J Neuroradiol 32:1436-1443, 2011

Background and Purpose.—The availability of data relating to the biometry of the CC in children that are easy to use in daily practice is limited. We present a reference biometry of the CC in MR imaging in a large cohort of children.

Materials and Methods.—Cerebral MR imaging studies of children with normal examination findings were selected retrospectively. Children born preterm and those with or at risk of developing cerebral malformations were excluded. The following parameters were measured: FOD, APD, LCC, GT, BT, IT, ST, and the S/T. Inter- and intraobserver agreement and sex effect were evaluated.

Results.—Six hundred twenty-two children were included (320 boys, 302 girls), ranging from 1 day to 15 years of age. Normal values (from the 3rd to 97th percentile) are provided for each parameter. All parameters showed rapid growth up to 3 years of age followed by slower (FOD, APD, LCC, GT and ST) or absent (S/T) growth. Growth of BT and IT was completed by 7—8 years. CC modeling (IT/ST) was completed by 3 years. FOD was larger in boys from the age of 1 year (statistically significant). The other parameters did not show any sex effect. Inter- and intraobserver agreement was excellent for all parameters except for IT.

Conclusions.—As measured, our data result in easy and reproducible MR imaging biometry of the CC in children (Fig 1, Table 3).

▶ As a pediatric radiologist with an interest in the musculoskeletal system, I am extremely familiar with tables, graphs, and atlases of normalcy. Growth charts,

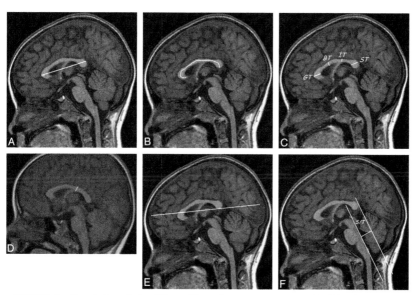

FIGURE 1.—Description of the different biometric parameters measured with MR imaging. *A*, Measurement of the APD of the CC, the distance between the anterior aspect of the genu and the posterior aspect of the splenium. *B*, Measurement of the true LCC, the curvilinear distance between the rostrum and the splenium at midthickness of the CC. *C*, Measurement of the thickness of the CC, at the level of the genu (GT), body (BT), isthmus (IT), and splenium (ST). *D*, measurement of the IT when the isthmus could not be identified because of insufficient CC modeling. IT was measured at the level where the fornix abuts the CC (CC-fornix junction). *E*, Measurement of the FOD, the distance between the extreme points of the frontal and occipital lobes. *F*, Evaluation of the position of the splenium. A line was drawn along the dorsal surface of the brain stem. Another line was drawn parallel to the first one and passing at the level of the most posterior point of the splenium. The S/T distance between those lines was measured at the level of the fastigium. (Reprinted from Garel C, Cont I, Alberti C, et al. Biometry of the corpus callosum in children: MR imaging reference data. *AJNR Am J Neuroradiol.* 2011;32:1436-1443, with permission from the American Society of Neuroradiology.)

TABLE 3.—Values of the Median, 3rd, and 97th Percentiles for the Different Parameters, as a Function of Age

Percentile	0	0.5	1	1.5	2	2.5	3	4	5	6	7	8	9	10	11	12	13	14	15
APD																			
3rd	36.8	43.7	47.9	50.6	52.4	53.6	54.4	55.5	56.2	56.8	57.4	57.9	58.5	59.1	59.7	60.4	61	61.7	62.5
Median	43.6	50.9	55.6	58.6	60.6	61.9	62.9	64.1	64.8	65.5	66	66.6	67.2	67.9	68.6	69.3	70.1	71	72
97th	62	63.9	66.8	69.1	70.6	71.7	72.5	73.5	74.2	74.8	75.4	76	76.6	77.3	78.1	79	79.9	81.1	82.3
LCC																			
3rd	47.6	60	66.9	70.7	72.7	73.8	74.4	75	75.3	75.6	76	76.5	77.1	77.7	78.4	79.2	80.1	81	82
Median	56.3	70.2	78.3	82.9	85.5	87	87.9	88.7	89.2	89.7	90.2	90.8	91.5	92.3	93.3	94.4	95.7	97.2	99
97th	81.7	89.1	95.3	99.1	101.3	102.6	103.3	104.1	104.5	105	105.6	106.3	107.1	108.2	109.4	110.9	112.7	114.8	117.5
GT																			
3rd	2.5	3.7	4.6	5.2	5.7	6	6.3	6.7	6.9	7	7.1	7.2	7.3	7.3	7.4	7.5	7.5	7.6	7.6
Median	4.3	5.8	6.9	7.7	8.3	8.8	9.1	9.6	9.9	10.1	10.2	10.3	10.4	10.5	10.6	10.6	10.7	10.8	10.8
97th	8.3	8.9	9.7	10.4	11	11.4	11.8	12.3	12.6	12.9	13	13.1	13.2	13.3	13.4	13.5	13.5	13.6	13.7
BT																			
3rd	1.3	1.8	2.2	2.6	2.9	3.1	3.3	3.5	3.7	3.8	3.9	3.9	4	4	4	4	3.9	3.9	3.7
Median	2.3	3	3.6	4.1	4.5	4.8	5	5.3	5.5	5.7	5.8	5.8	5.8	5.9	5.9	5.9	5.9	5.9	5.9
97th	5	5.3	5.7	6.1	6.5	6.8	7	7.4	7.6	7.7	7.8	7.9	7.9	8	8	8	8.1	8.2	8.4
IT																			
3rd	1.2	1.4	1.5	1.6	1.7	1.7	1.8	1.9	2	2.1	2.2	2.2	2.3	2.4	2.4	2.4	2.5	2.5	2.5
Median	1.9	2.2	2.5	2.7	2.8	3	3.1	3.2	3.4	3.5	3.6	3.7	3.8	3.8	3.9	4	4	4	4.1
97th	3.9	4.1	4.3	4.5	4.6	4.8	4.9	5.1	5.3	5.5	5.6	5.7	5.8	5.9	6	6	6.1	6.2	6.2
ST																			
3rd	1.9	3.4	4.4	5.1	5.6	6	6.2	6.7	6.9	7.2	7.4	7.5	7.6	7.7	7.7	7.7	7.5	7.1	6.3
Median	3.9	5.6	6.7	7.5	8.1	8.5	8.8	9.2	9.5	9.8	10	10.1	10.3	10.4	10.5	10.5	10.6	10.6	10.5
97th	9	9.2	9.9	10.5	10.9	11.3	11.5	11.9	12.2	12.5	12.7	12.8	13	13.1	13.3	13.5	13.7	14.1	14.8

Age (yr)

FOD boys																			
3rd	69.8	105.2	119.5	127.4	132.3	135.4	137.6	140.5	142.3	143.8	145.1	146.3	147.5	148.6	149.7	150.8	151.9	153	154
Median	116.3	133.9	143.3	148.9	152.5	154.9	156.6	158.8	160.3	161.5	162.5	163.4	164.4	165.3	166.2	167.1	168	168.9	169.7
97th	141	153.7	161.1	165.6	168.5	170.5	171.9	173.7	175	175.9	176.8	177.6	178.4	179.2	180	180.7	181.5	182.2	183
FOD girls																			
3rd	98.1	115.9	124.7	129.8	132.9	134.9	136.3	138.2	139.5	140.6	141.5	142.4	143.3	144.2	145	145.8	146.7	147.5	148.3
Median	109	128.5	138.7	144.8	148.7	151.2	152.9	155	156.3	157.3	158.1	158.9	159.6	160.4	161.1	161.8	162.5	163.2	163.9
97th	132.5	146.5	155.2	160.5	163.8	166.1	167.6	169.5	170.6	171.5	172.2	172.9	173.5	174.2	174.8	175.5	176.1	176.8	177.4
S/T																			
3rd	14	22.9	26.6	28.6	29.8	30.4	30.9	31.4	31.8	32.2	32.4	32.6	32.8	32.9	33	33	33	33	33.1
Median	22.6	28.9	32	33.8	34.8	35.4	35.8	36.4	36.8	37.1	37.4	37.6	37.8	37.9	38	38.1	38.1	38.1	38.1
97th	34.7	37.3	39	40	40.7	41.1	41.4	41.8	42.2	42.5	42.8	43.1	43.3	43.4	43.5	43.6	43.7	43.7	43.7
Ratio IT/ST																			
3rd	0.27	0.23	0.21	0.2	0.2	0.2	0.2	0.2	0.21	0.21	0.21	0.22	0.22	0.22	0.23	0.23	0.23	0.23	0.23
Median	0.49	0.42	0.38	0.36	0.35	0.35	0.35	0.35	0.35	0.36	0.36	0.37	0.37	0.37	0.38	0.38	0.38	0.38	0.38
97th	0.89	0.76	0.69	0.65	0.63	0.61	0.61	0.6	0.6	0.61	0.61	0.61	0.62	0.62	0.62	0.63	0.63	0.63	0.63
Ratio APD/FOD																			
3rd	0.34	0.34	0.35	0.35	0.35	0.35	0.36	0.36	0.36	0.37	0.37	0.37	0.37	0.37	0.37	0.37	0.38	0.38	0.38
Median	0.4	0.4	0.4	0.4	0.4	0.41	0.41	0.41	0.41	0.41	0.42	0.42	0.42	0.42	0.42	0.42	0.42	0.43	0.43
97th	0.45	0.45	0.45	0.45	0.46	0.46	0.46	0.46	0.46	0.46	0.46	0.47	0.47	0.47	0.47	0.47	0.47	0.48	0.48

the Greulich & Pyle bone age atlas, and Keat's atlas of normal variants are weapons used by me on a daily basis as I battle to reach clever diagnoses in short-statured children.

In this article, the authors provide standards for linear measurements (Fig 1) and reference values for these measurements (Table 3) from their assessment of 622 children aged from 1 day to 15 years. They also discuss 5 factors that influence the morphology of the corpus callosum (age, prematurity, genetics, sex, and handedness). Interestingly, ethnicity is not discussed—probably because (as with Greulich & Pyle's bone age atlas) it is not a major issue.

Because in my practice I am so used to (and dependent on) normal values, readers may accuse me of some prejudice in selecting this article as a must read; however, I should be surprised if the data do not prove useful in subtle clinical cases and as objective outcome measures for future research projects. Perhaps this article is not to the neuroradiologist what Greulich & Pyle and Keats are to the musculoskeletal radiologist, but nevertheless it is a useful tool.

A. C. Offiah, BSc, MBBS, MRCP, FRCR, PhD

Cortical Thickness in Fetal Alcohol Syndrome and Attention Deficit Disorder
Fernández-Jaén A, Fernández-Mayoralas DM, Quiñones Tapia D, et al (Hospital Universitario Quirón Madrid, Spain; Clínica Nuestra Señora del Rosario, Madrid, Spain; et al)
Pediatr Neurol 45:387-391, 2011

Fetal alcohol syndrome represents the classic and most severe manifestation of epigenetic changes induced by exposure to alcohol during pregnancy. Often these patients develop attention deficit hyperactivity disorder. We analyzed cortical thickness in 20 children and adolescents with fetal alcohol syndrome and attention deficit hyperactivity disorder (group 1), in 20 patients without fetal alcohol syndrome (group 2), and in 20 control cases. The first group revealed total cortical thickness significantly superior to those of the other two groups. In per-lobe analyses of cortical thickness, group 1 demonstrated greater cortical thickness in the frontal, occipital, and right temporal and left frontal lobes compared with the second group, and in both temporal lobes and the right frontal lobe compared with the control group. This study demonstrated greater cortical thickness in patients with attention deficit hyperactivity disorder and heavy prenatal exposure to alcohol, probably as an expression of immature or abnormal brain development.

▶ Emerson M. Pugh (1896–1981) said, "If the human brain were so simple that we could understand it, we would be so simple that we couldn't." Not that I wish to brand myself other than simple, but here's something I hadn't appreciated: cortical thickness *decreases* as a consequence of the normal development process. In fact (and I take this directly from the article), it has been shown that children with thinner cortices in the left parietal and frontal regions tend to perform better on verbal skill testing,[1] whereas older children, with thinner frontal and parietal cortices, perform better on tests of general intellectual function.[2]

Results of this study by Fernandez-Jaen et al further convince us of the complexity of the human brain; compared with normal subjects, whereas cortical thickness was increased in children with fetal alcohol syndrome plus attention-deficit/hyperactivity disorder (ADHD), it was reduced in those with ADHD without fetal alcohol syndrome. Complex indeed.

The authors suggest that based on their and others' results, MRI may be used in the future to classify subtypes of ADHD by etiology (or at least by comorbidity), perhaps influencing drug regimens and leading to an improved understanding of evolutionary patterns and prognoses in ADHD. Just think—we owe this exciting potential to the complexities of the human brain; I doubt it would be possible had the brain been simpler.

A. C. Offiah, BSc, MBBS, MRCP, FRCR, PhD

References

1. Sowell ER, Thompson PM, Leonard CM, Welcome SE, Kan E, Toga AW. Longitudinal mapping of cortical thickness and brain growth in normal children. *J Neurosci.* 2004;24:8223-8231.
2. Shaw P, Lerch J, Greenstein D, et al. Longitudinal mapping of cortical thickness and clinical outcome in children and adolescents with attention-deficit/hyperactivity disorder. *Arch Gen Psychiatry.* 2006;63:540-549.

Sensitive Diffusion Tensor Imaging Quantification Method to Identify Language Pathway Abnormalities in Children with Developmental Delay

Gopal SP, Tiwari VN, Veenstra AL, et al (Wayne State Univ School of Medicine, Detroit, MI)

J Pediatr 160:147-151, 2012

Objective.—To investigate whether abnormal regional white matter architecture in the perisylvian region could be used as an easy and sensitive quantitative method to demonstrate language pathway abnormalities in children with developmental delay (DD).

Study Design.—We performed diffusion tensor imaging in 15 DD subjects (age, 61.1 ± 20.9 months) and 15 age-matched typically developing (TD) children (age, 68.4 ± 19.2 months). With diffusion tensor imaging color-coded orientation maps, we quantified the fraction of fibers in the perisylvian region that are oriented in anteroposterior (AP) and mediolateral (ML) directions, and their ratio (AP/ML) was calculated.

Results.—The AP/ML ratio was more sensitive than tractography in characterizing perisylvian regional abnormalities in DD children. The AP/ML ratio of the left perisylvian region was significantly lower in DD children compared with TD children ($P = .03$). The ML component of bilateral perisylvian regions was significantly higher in DD children compared with TD children ($P = .01$ [left] and $P = .004$ [right]). No significant difference was found in the AP component in the two groups.

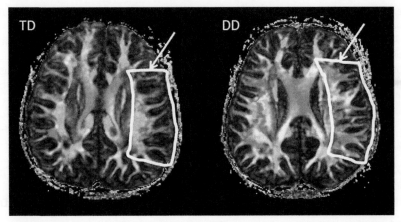

FIGURE.—Representative diffusion tensor color-coded orientation map of the left perisylvian area in children with TD and DD. In the region of interest (*shown in arrow*), proportion of *green* and *red components* of principal eigenvector are dramatically different in the two groups of children. For interpretation of the references to color in this figure legend, the reader is referred to web version of this article. (Reprinted from Journal of Pediatrics. Gopal SP, Tiwari VN, Veenstra AL, et al. Sensitive diffusion tensor imaging quantification method to identify language pathway abnormalities in children with developmental delay. *J Pediatr.* 2012;160:147-151, Copyright 2012, with permission from Elsevier.)

A significant negative correlation of the left ML component with Vineland communication skills was observed (r = −0.657, P = .011).

Conclusions.—The AP/ML ratio appears to be a sensitive indicator of regional white matter architectural abnormalities in the perisylvian region of DD children (Fig).

▶ Serendipity—I like that word; it has a way of rolling off the tongue.

Many medical discoveries were serendipitous, including (not in chronological order) the discoveries of penicillin, radioactivity, and of course our very own x-rays. Although the finding may be serendipitous, this does not, of course, imply an absence of hard work on the part of the finder.

In a diffusion tensor imaging (DTI) study of 7 children with Angelman syndrome, the authors of this article failed to identify the arcuate fasciculus (AF) in 6 of them. Perhaps by serendipity, the AF was identified in the seventh patient; however, it was not normal. Direct quantification of the color-coded DTI orientation map in this patient showed a significantly lower ratio of anteroposteriorly oriented fibers to mediolaterally oriented fibers in the perisylvian region compared with typically developing children. It was this observation that led to the hypothesis behind the current study. The figure demonstrates differences in orientation of the fibers in the perisylvian regions of delayed compared with typically developing children, thus proving the hypothesis correct.

This line of research may ultimately improve our understanding of the neurophysiology of developmental delay and associated language pathway abnormalities—and who knows, with this understanding, more hard work, and perhaps a little serendipity, one day researchers in the field may discover treatments that ameliorate the often devastating developmental delay seen in affected children.

A. C. Offiah, BSc, MBBS, MRCP, FRCR, PhD

Magnetic Resonance Spectroscopy Predicts Outcomes for Children With Nonaccidental Trauma

Aaen GS, Holshouser BA, Sheridan C, et al (Loma Linda Univ, CA)

Pediatrics 125:295-303, 2010

Objective.—We evaluated proton magnetic resonance spectroscopic imaging (MRSI) findings for children with traumatic brain injury attributable to nonaccidental trauma (NAT) early after injury, to determine whether brain metabolite changes predicted outcomes.

Methods.—Proton MRSI (1.5 T) was performed (mean: 5 days after injury [range: 1–30 days]) through the level of the corpus callosum for 90 children with confirmed NAT. Regional N-acetylaspartate/total creatine, N-acetylaspartate/total choline, and choline/creatine ratios and the presence of lactate were measured. Data on long-term outcomes defined at ≥6 months were collected for 44 of 90 infants. We grouped patients into good (normal, mild disability, or moderate disability; $n = 32$) and poor (severe disability, vegetative state, or dead; $n = 12$) outcome groups.

Results.—We found that N-acetylaspartate/creatine and N-acetylaspartate/choline ratios (mean total, corpus callosum, and frontal white matter) were significantly decreased in patients with poor outcomes ($P < .001$). A logistic regression model using age, initial Glasgow Coma Scale score, presence of retinal hemorrhage, lactate on MRSI scans, and mean total N-acetylaspartate/creatine ratio predicted outcomes accurately in 100% of cases.

Conclusions.—Reduced N-acetylaspartate levels (ie, neuronal loss/dysfunction) and elevated lactate levels (altered energy metabolism) correlated with poor neurologic outcomes for infants with NAT. Elevated lactate levels may reflect primary or secondary hypoxic-ischemic injury, which may occur with NAT. Our data suggest that MRSI performed early after injury can be used for long-term prognosis (Table 5).

▶ Nonaccidental injury, be it skeletal, neurologic, or other, remains topical; no year goes by without my selecting to comment on at least 1 article on child abuse, and this year is no different.

Faced with an infant or young child with traumatic head injury, the neuroradiologist plays both a diagnostic role—is this accidental or nonaccidental—and a prognostic role—what is the likely outcome for this child?

Traditional methods of determining severity of injury and therefore predicting outcome are discussed by van der Naalt et al.[1] Now, in this current article, Aaen et al introduce the prospect of using magnetic resonance spectroscopic imaging (MRSI) on early scans as a predictor of outcome. They give a clear and logical explanation as to why N-acetylaspartate/choline and N-acetylaspartate/creatine ratios are decreased while lactate levels are increased in nonaccidental

TABLE 5.—Prediction Models

Model	Variables Included	Correct Prediction of Good Outcome, %	Correct Prediction of Poor Outcome, %	Overall Outcome Prediction, %	−2 Log Likelihood
Base	Age Initial GCS score	94	67	86	26.64
1	Age Initial GCS score Retinal hemorrhage	94	75	89	26.4
2	Age Initial GCS score Retinal hemorrhage Lactate present	94	92	94	24.52
3	Age Initial GCS score Lactate present Mean total NAA/creatine ratio	97	92	96	10.72
4	Age Initial GCS score Retinal hemorrhage Mean total NAA/creatine ratio	97	92	96	7.47
5	Age Initial GCS score Retinal hemorrhage Lactate present Mean total NAA/creatine ratio	100	100	100	0.000

NAA indicates N-acetylaspartate.

head trauma and provide a prediction model for the various biomarkers (Table 5). They conclude that larger studies are required to confirm this predictive role of MRSI.

Because hypoxic ischemic injury (HII) is more common in nonaccidental than accidental head trauma, and because HII is associated with increased lactate, I wonder whether MRSI might not also have a diagnostic role in differentiating accidental from nonaccidental injury. Given all the complexities surrounding this topical subject, I think it would certainly be worth investigating.

A. C. Offiah, BSc, MBBS, MRCP, FRCR, PhD

Reference

1. van der Naalt J, Hew JM, van Zomeren AH, Sluiter WJ, Minderhoud JM. Computed tomography and magnetic resonance imaging in mild to moderate head injury: early and late imaging related to outcome. *Ann Neurol.* 1999;46:70-78.

State-of-the-Art Cranial Sonography: Part 1, Modern Techniques and Image Interpretation

Lowe LH, Bailey Z (Univ of Missouri-Kansas City)
AJR Am J Roentgenol 196:1028-1033, 2011

Objective.—In this era of radiation awareness, high-quality ultrasound is more important than ever. Although cranial sonography equipment has advanced greatly, application of modern techniques has not been utilized in a fashion commensurate to other cross-sectional modalities. This article will describe modern cranial sonography techniques, including the utility of linear imaging, use of additional fontanels, and screening Doppler imaging.

Conclusion.—When modern protocols are used, cranial sonography is highly accurate for the detection of cranial abnormalities (Fig 3).

▶ It is not always possible (or indeed necessary) to perform CT or MRI of the brain, particularly in the sick neonate. Often in these cases a cranial ultrasound scan, performed well, is all that is required. This article reminds us how to perform one well.

The article is in 2 parts; the first deals with techniques and image interpretation. The standard images to be obtained and common pathologies are illustrated. The review includes a demonstration of vascular anatomy and measurement and

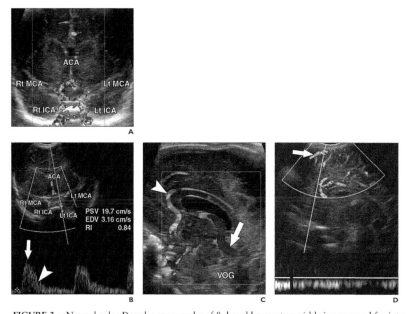

FIGURE 3.—Normal color Doppler sonography of 8-day-old premature girl being screened for intracranial hemorrhage. **A,** Sonogram obtained through circle of Willis illustrates right (Rt) and left (Lt) internal carotid arteries (ICA), right and left middle cerebral arteries (MCA), and anterior cerebral (ACA) arteries. Distinguishing between right versus left ACA is often difficult, but usually unnecessary. Thus, they are labeled together. **B,** Spectral Doppler tracing of circle of Willis obtained via anterior fontanel shows normal arterial flow pattern in MCA. Note continuous flow above baseline, including rapid systolic upstroke (*arrow*) followed by gradual decline in flow during diastole (*arrowhead*). Normal peak systolic velocity (PSV), end-diastolic velocity (EDV), and resistive index (RI) are indicated. **C,** Sagittal Doppler sonogram of venous system shows patent deep venous system, including vein of Galen (VOG) (*arrow*). Pericallosal branch of ACA (*arrowhead*) is noted. **D,** Sonogram of superficial venous system, including sagittal sinus (*arrow*), is shown. Observe normal venous spectrum showing continuous undulating venous flow. Incidentally noted is reversal of color map. (Reprinted from Lowe LH, Bailey Z. State-of-the-art cranial sonography: Part 1, Modern techniques and image interpretation. *AJR Am J Roentgenol.* 12011;96:1028-1033, with permission from the American Journal of Roentgenology.)

interpretation of the resistive indices of middle and internal cerebral arteries (Fig 3). Part 2 of the review discusses normal variants and common pitfalls of cranial ultrasound.[1]

In addition to the quality of the review, I have selected this article as a reminder that, particularly for less experienced radiologists and trainees, case reports, reviews, and the Continuing Medical Education articles that can be found in journals such as *Pediatric Radiology* all have a pragmatic if not an intellectual impact. They should not necessarily be shunned in favor of original research, just as cranial ultrasound should not necessarily be shunned in favor of CT or MRI.

A. C. Offiah, BSc, MBBS, MRCP, FRCR, PhD

Reference

1. Lowe LH, Bailey Z. State-of-the-art cranial sonography: Part 2, pitfalls and variants. *AJR Am J Roentgenol.* 2011;196:1034-1039.

Trainee Misinterpretations on Pediatric Neuroimaging Studies: Classification, Imaging Analysis, and Outcome Assessment
Guimaraes CVA, Leach JL, Jones BV (Cincinnati Children's Hosp Med Ctr, OH)
AJNR Am J Neuroradiol 32:1591-1599, 2011

Background and Purpose.—The scope of trainee misinterpretations on pediatric neuroimaging studies has been incompletely assessed. Our aim was to evaluate the frequency of trainee misinterpretations on neuroimaging exams in children, describe a useful classification system, and assess related patient management or outcome changes.

Materials and Methods.—Pediatric neuroimaging examinations with trainee-dictated reports performed without initial attending radiologist assessment were evaluated for discrepant trainee interpretations by using a search of the RIS. The frequency of discrepant trainee interpretations was calculated and classified on the basis of the type of examination on which the error occurred, the specific type and severity of the discrepancy, and the effect on patient management and outcome. Differences relating to examination type and level of training were also assessed.

Results.—There were 143 discrepancies on 3496 trainee-read examinations for a discrepancy rate of 4.1%. Most occurred on CT examinations (131; 92%). Most discrepancies (75) were minor but were related to the clinical presentation. Six were major and potentially life-threatening. Thirty-seven were overcalls. Most had no effect on clinical management (97, 68%) or resulted simply in clinical reassessment or imaging follow-up (43, 30%). There was no permanent morbidity or mortality related to the misinterpretations. The most common misinterpretations were related to fractures (28) and ICH (23). CT examinations of the face, orbits,

TABLE 1.—Categorization of Discrepant Trainee Interpretation

Type	Number of Discrepant Trainee Reports (Rate)[a]
1: Major, life-threatening	6 (0.17%)
1A: Finding not originally identified	5
1B: Finding identified, incorrectly characterized	1
2: Minor, related to clinical presentation	75 (2.1%)
2A: Finding not originally identified	56
2B: Finding identified, incorrectly characterized	19
3: Minor, unrelated to clinical presentation	8 (0.23%)
3A: Finding not originally identified	8
3B: Finding identified, incorrectly characterized	0
4: Possible abnormality	17 (0.49%)
4A: Confirmed on follow-up imaging	2
4B: Not confirmed on follow-up imaging	8
4C: No follow-up imaging performed	7
5: Abnormality called when none present (overcall)	37 (1.1%)
5A: Resulting in inappropriate therapy	2
5B: Not resulting in inappropriate therapy	35

[a] % of total exams interpreted (N = 3496).

TABLE 2.—Effect of Discrepant Trainee Interpretations on Clinical Management and Outcome

Type	Number of Discrepant Reports (% of Discrepancies)
1: No effect on clinical management/outcome	97 (68)
2: No direct treatment change but imaging or clinical follow-up performed related to the discrepancy	43 (30)
3: Direct treatment change, no sequelae	3 (2.1)
4: Direct treatment change (morbidity)	0 (0)
5: Death potentially related	0 (0)

and neck had the highest discrepancy rate (9.4%). Third- and fourth-year residents had a larger discrepancy rate than fellows.

Conclusions.—Trainee misinterpretations occur in 4.1% of pediatric neuroimaging examinations with only a small number being life-threatening (0.17%). Detailed analysis of the types of misinterpretations can be used to inform proactive trainee education (Tables 1 and 2).

▶ The pediatric hospital where I work (Sheffield Children's National Health Service Foundation Trust, United Kingdom) hopes in the not too distant future to take on the mantle of regional trauma center. Our trainees will first interpret much of the increased out-of-hours imaging that this will generate. This fact, coupled with my interest in teaching and training, meant that I was not able to overlook this article.

Similar work has been done in adults, but according to the authors, this is the first time misinterpretation by residents of pediatric neuroimaging has been reported. Categorization of the discrepancies found in the reports of trainees and residents compared with the final reports of board-certified neuroradiologists and the impact these discrepancies had on patient management are shown in Tables 1 and 2.

The 5 key points to note from this article and therefore areas to be emphasized in training programmes are:

1. The modality with the highest discrepancy rate was CT (in particular, of face, head, and neck).
2. The most common major misinterpretation was failure of recognition of diffuse brain edema.
3. Most discrepancies were related to fractures.
4. Most false-positives were related to accessory sutures being overcalled as fractures.
5. Third- and fourth-year residents fared less well than first- and second-year students, explained by the authors as being due to an element of false confidence in the more senior residents who therefore did not seek a second opinion from fellows.

The out-of-hours setup differs from department to department and country to country. For instance, typically in the United Kingdom, we do not have a radiology fellow on call at the same time as our trainees. However, emphasis could be placed on trainees (and fellows) having a lower threshold for seeking the opinion of the covering consultant (board-certified radiologist), and teleradiology plays an important role here.

Regardless of local setup, for anyone involved in the teaching and training of residents or the development of curricula, the results of this and other similar studies serve as useful indicators of how such curricula might be improved.

A. C. Offiah, BSc, MBBS, MRCP, FRCR, PhD

Thoracic/Airway/Vascular

Exogenous lipoid pneumonia. Clinical and radiological manifestations
Marchiori E, Zanetti G, Mano CM, et al (Fluminense Federal Univ, Rio de Janeiro, Brazil; Federal Univ of Rio de Janeiro, Brazil)
Respir Med 105:659-666, 2011

Lipoid pneumonia results from the pulmonary accumulation of endogenous or exogenous lipids. Host tissue reactions to the inhaled substances differ according to their chemical characteristics. Symptoms can vary significantly among individuals, ranging from asymptomatic to severe, life-threatening disease. Acute, sometimes fatal, cases can occur, but the disease is usually indolent. Possible complications include superinfection by nontuberculous mycobacteria, pulmonary fibrosis, respiratory insufficiency, cor pulmonale, and hypercalcemia. The radiological findings are nonspecific, and the disease presents with variable patterns and distribution. For this reason, lipoid pneumonia may mimic many other diseases.

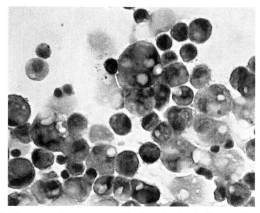

FIGURE 1.—Alveolar macrophages recovered by bronchoalveolar lavage. The cytoplasm is full of large rounded vacuoles that displace the nucleus to the periphery (oil red O stain, ×400). For interpretation of the references to color in this figure legend, the reader is referred to web version of this article. (Reprinted from Marchiori E, Zanetti G, Mano CM, et al. Exogenous lipoid pneumonia. Clinical and radiological manifestations. *Respir Med.* 2011;105:659-666, Copyright 2011, with permission from Elsevier.)

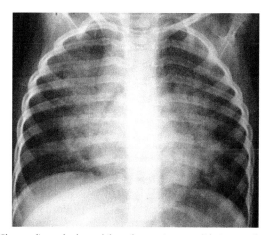

FIGURE 2.—Chest radiograph shows bilateral extensive consolidations predominantly in central zones of the lungs. (Reprinted from Marchiori E, Zanetti G, Mano CM, et al. Exogenous lipoid pneumonia. Clinical and radiological manifestations. *Respir Med.* 2011;105:659-666, Copyright 2011, with permission from Elsevier.)

The diagnosis of exogenous lipoid pneumonia is based on a history of exposure to oil, characteristic radiological findings, and the presence of lipid-laden macrophages on sputum or BAL analysis. High-resolution computed tomography (HRCT) is the best imaging modality for the diagnosis of lipoid pneumonia. The most characteristic CT finding in LP is the presence of negative attenuation values within areas of consolidation. There are currently no studies in the literature that define the best

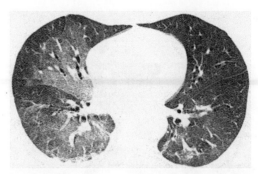

FIGURE 4.—HRCT demonstrates extensive ground-glass opacities in both lungs, predominantly seen on the right lung. (Reprinted from Marchiori E, Zanetti G, Mano CM, et al. Exogenous lipoid pneumonia. Clinical and radiological manifestations. *Respir Med.* 2011;105:659-666, Copyright 2011, with permission from Elsevier.)

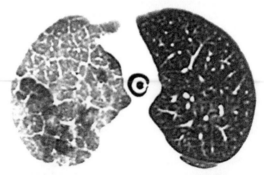

FIGURE 5.—HRCT shows areas of ground-glass attenuation in the right upper lobe, superimposed on interlobular septal thickening (crazy paving pattern). The left lung is normal. (Reprinted from Marchiori E, Zanetti G, Mano CM, et al. Exogenous lipoid pneumonia. Clinical and radiological manifestations. *Respir Med.* 2011;105:659-666, Copyright 2011, with permission from Elsevier.)

therapeutic option. However, there is a consensus that the key measure is identifying and discontinuing exposure to the offending agent. Treatment in patients without clinical symptoms remains controversial, but in patients with diffuse pulmonary damage, aggressive therapies have been reported. They include whole lung lavage, systemic corticosteroids, and thoracoscopy with surgical debridement (Figs 1, 2, and 4-8).

▶ This is an excellent review of lipoid pneumonia, covering its etiology, pathophysiology, clinical presentation and findings, features of bronchoalveolar lavage (Fig 1), radiological findings (Figs 2, 4-7), histological findings (Fig 8), complications, treatment and natural history, and outcome. There is an extensive list of causative agents, including laxatives, radiographic contrast media, some lipsticks, and even a certain occupation—of which more later.

Anyone with an interest in this topic could do worse than starting out by reading this article. I would also recommend a research paper by the same

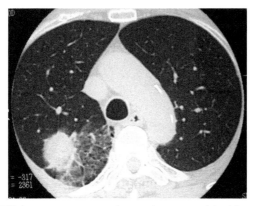

FIGURE 6.—HRCT demonstrates a mass on the posterior segment of the right upper lobe, with adjacent ground-glass opacities. (Reprinted from Marchiori E, Zanetti G, Mano CM, et al. Exogenous lipoid pneumonia. Clinical and radiological manifestations. *Respir Med.* 2011;105:659-666, Copyright 2011, with permission from Elsevier.)

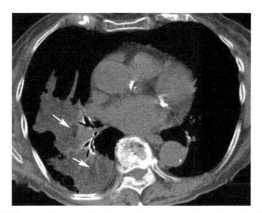

FIGURE 7.—HRCT scan at the level of the lower lobes with mediastinal window shows consolidation with superimposed areas of low attenuation (ranging from −31 to −116 HU) in the right lower lobe (arrows). (Reprinted from Marchiori E, Zanetti G, Mano CM, et al. Exogenous lipoid pneumonia. Clinical and radiological manifestations. *Respir Med.* 2011;105:659-666, Copyright 2011, with permission from Elsevier.)

authors in which they compare high-resolution CT scan findings in adults and children with lipoid pneumonia, concluding that although the crazy paving pattern is more commonly seen in adults, children more commonly present with consolidation.[1]

Speaking of consolidation, the most characteristic radiographic finding is the presence of areas of consolidation within which there are low attenuating (ie, fat-containing) foci with Hounsfield units of between −150 and −30. Having identified these on the CT scan of a (hypothetical) patient, you can bemuse

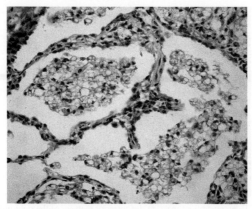

FIGURE 8.—Photomicrography shows the presence of lipid-laden macrophages that fill the alveolar airspaces. Note also macrophages inside the alveolar septa (original magnification, 40×; hematoxilin-eosin stain). (Reprinted from Marchiori E, Zanetti G, Mano CM, et al. Exogenous lipoid pneumonia. Clinical and radiological manifestations. *Respir Med.* 2011;105:659-666, Copyright 2011, with permission from Elsevier.)

your clinical colleagues with the casual enquiry, "Is fire-eating a hobby of his?" Imagine their renewed respect for you when they discover that yes, in fact, it is.

A. C. Offiah, BSc, MBBS, MRCP, FRCR, PhD

Reference

1. Marchiori E, Zanetti G, Mano CM, Irion KL, Daltro PA, Hochhegger B. Lipoid pneumonia in 53 patients after aspiration of mineral oil: comparison of high-resolution computed tomography findings in adults and children. *J Comput Assist Tomogr.* 2010;34:9-12.

Rupture of the left mainstem bronchus following endotracheal intubation in a neonate
Hawkins CM, Towbin AJ (Univ Hosp, Cincinnati, OH; Cincinnati Children's Hosp, OH)
Pediatr Radiol 41:668-670, 2011

Tracheobronchial rupture is a rare diagnosis with very high associated mortality in the neonatal population. Our case demonstrates the opportunity to diagnose this entity in a neonate via CT and introduces the utility of virtual bronchoscopy in clinical scenarios that preclude traditional bronchoscopy (Figs 1, 3, and 4).

▶ For most of us, this case report is the closest we will ever come to seeing tracheal rupture in a child from whatever cause, and almost certainly from endotracheal intubation (incidence 0.04%–0.012%). For this reason alone, it is worth reading the article. However, my opening statement notwithstanding,

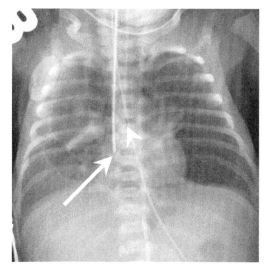

FIGURE 1.—Chest radiograph in a 1-day-old infant born at 25 weeks' gestational age shows an endo-tracheal tube with its tip (*arrow*) beyond the carina (*arrowhead*). In addition, there is a large volume of pneumomediastinum. There is diffuse ground-glass opacity within the right lung, consistent with surfac-tant deficiency syndrome. (Reprinted from Hawkins CM, Towbin AJ. Rupture of the left mainstem bron-chus following endotracheal intubation in a neonate. *Pediatr Radiol.* 2011;41:668-670, with permission from Springer Science and Business Media.)

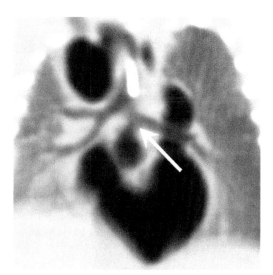

FIGURE 3.—Noncontrast CT of the chest in the same patient at 7 days of life. Coronal reformatted image shows a defect within the proximal left mainstem bronchus (*arrow*). This defect is continuous with the pneumomediastinum. Technique: kVp=100, mA=25, total mAs=56, slice thickness=3 mm, CTDI=2.1 mGy. (Reprinted from Hawkins CM, Towbin AJ. Rupture of the left mainstem bronchus following endotracheal intubation in a neonate. *Pediatr Radiol.* 2011;41:668-670, with permission from Springer Science and Business Media.)

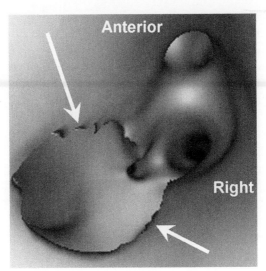

FIGURE 4.—Virtual bronchoscopy demonstrates a 2-mm tear within the posterior wall of the proximal left mainstem bronchus (*arrow*). The 3-D rendered image was obtained just beyond the bifurcation of the trachea. Virtual bronchoscopy was performed by performing axial-plane airway segmentation from MDCT data with Vitrea software (Vital Images, Inc.) allowing for intraluminal visualization similar to that obtained with traditional bronchoscopy. Airway segmentation can be performed manually by a trained technologist or automatically if appropriate software is available. (Reprinted from Hawkins CM, Towbin AJ. Rupture of the left mainstem bronchus following endotracheal intubation in a neonate. *Pediatr Radiol.* 2011;41:668-670, with permission from Springer Science and Business Media.)

because more neonates are being delivered alive at younger and younger gestational ages, you just never know.

We are used to seeing the high endotracheal tube (ETT) or the ETT with its tip in the right main bronchus; indeed one of the first things we teach our trainees when interpreting pediatric chest radiographs is to identify and comment on the position of all tubes and lines. This discipline should allow us to readily recognize if the ETT has perforated the trachea or bronchus (Fig 1). In this case, the tear itself was demonstrated on CT and CT virtual bronchoscopy (Figs 3 and 4).

Although the mortality rate in adults is only 9%, this rate is significantly higher in children (75%). Early diagnosis may prevent the development of mediastinitis, improving chances of survival. Perhaps not surprisingly, this particular neonate, born at 25 weeks' gestation with a weight of 680 g, did not survive. Her stormy course, the treatment options that were available, and why surgical intervention was not pursued are discussed in the article and reflect the day-to-day clinical dilemmas that we often face.

A. C. Offiah, BSc, MBBS, MRCP, FRCR, PhD

Quality assurance: using the exposure index and the deviation index to monitor radiation exposure for portable chest radiographs in neonates
Cohen MD, Cooper ML, Piersall K, et al (Indiana Univ School of Medicine, Indianapolis; et al)
Pediatr Radiol 41:592-601, 2011

Background.—Many methods are used to track patient exposure during acquisition of plain film radiographs. A uniform international standard would aid this process.

Objective.—To evaluate and describe a new, simple quality-assurance method for monitoring patient exposure. This method uses the "exposure index" and the "deviation index," recently developed by the International Electrotechnical Commission (IEC) and American Association of Physicists in Medicine (AAPM). The deviation index measures variation from an ideal target exposure index value. Our objective was to determine whether the exposure index and the deviation index can be used to monitor and control exposure drift over time.

Materials and Methods.—Our Agfa workstation automatically keeps a record of the exposure index for every patient. The exposure index and deviation index were calculated on 1,884 consecutive neonatal chest images. Exposure of a neonatal chest phantom was performed as a control.

Results.—Acquisition of the exposure index and calculation of the deviation index was easily achieved. The weekly mean exposure index of the phantom and the patients was stable and showed <10% change during the study, indicating no exposure drift during the study period.

Conclusion.—The exposure index is an excellent tool to monitor the consistency of patient exposures. It does not indicate the exposure value used, but is an index to track compliance with a pre-determined target exposure.

▶ The Fuji index of radiation exposure is called the sensitivity number, "S." In 2003, a colleague and I published an article in which we showed some correlation between S and image quality as assessed by the Commission of European Communities' Quality Criteria for the pediatric lateral spine radiograph.[1] Although S values were inversely proportional to radiation dose, just as Cohen and his team point out, S and other exposure indices of different manufacturers are not direct measures of radiation exposure.

For each machine and each imaged site, manufacturers provide a range of acceptable values for exposure indices. At the time of our article (2003) we were given a single (and relatively wide) S range for the pediatric lateral spine, with consideration for neither patient age nor size. By taking the 25th and 75th quartile ranges of those spine radiographs fulfilling a specific quality criterion, we were able to provide narrower age-specific ranges. These ranges were, however, only relevant to departments with Fuji computed radiography machines.

For this reason the development of standardized exposure and deviation indices is most welcome—values from the machines of different manufacturers can now be directly compared.

I reiterate the warning of these authors; these indices are not direct measures of radiation dose; rather, they are of value in quality assurance. Whether departments use the exposure index or the more recently developed deviation index, imaging parameters must be optimized to produce images of diagnostic quality at an acceptable radiation dose. Only after this should the deviation index be used to ascertain how close the actual radiation exposures are to the target values; clearly, the aim is to have a deviation index of zero. In this study, 95% of chest radiographs had a deviation index between −3 and 3 (a change in exposure ranging from twice to half the target value). The authors suggest that this variation may be related to the variation in weight of the imaged babies. The consistency of their exposure parameters has been confirmed; they now need to do what perhaps they should have done first, ie, set weight-specific target exposure indices.

A. C. Offiah, BSc, MBBS, MRCP, FRCR, PhD

Reference

1. Offiah AC, Hall CM. Evaluation of the Commission of the European Communities quality criteria for the paediatric lateral spine. *Br J Radiol.* 2003;76:885-890.

Evaluation of image quality and radiation dose at prospective ECG-triggered axial 256-slice multi-detector CT in infants with congenital heart disease
Huang M-P, Liang C-H, Zhao Z-J, et al (Guangdong General Hosp, Guangzhou, People's Republic of China; et al)
Pediatr Radiol 41:858-866, 2011

Background.—There are a limited number of reports on the technical and clinical feasibility of prospective electrocardiogram (ECG)-gated multi-detector computed tomography (MDCT) in infants with congenital heart disease (CHD).

Objective.—To evaluate image quality and radiation dose at weight-based low-dose prospectively gated 256-slice MDCT angiography in infants with CHD.

Materials and Methods.—From November 2009 to February 2010, 64 consecutive infants with CHD referred for pre-operative or post-operative CT were included. All were scanned on a 256-slice MDCT system utilizing a low-dose protocol (80 kVp and 60–120 mAs depending on weight: 60 mAs for ≤3 kg, 80 mAs for 3.1–6 kg, 100 mAs for 6.1–10 kg, 120 mAs for 10.1–15 kg).

Results.—No serious adverse events were recorded. A total of 174 cardiac deformities, confirmed by surgery or heart catheterization, were studied. The sensitivity of MDCT for cardiac deformities was 97.1%; specificity, 99.4%; accuracy, 95.9%. The mean heart rate during scan was 136.7 ± 14.9/min (range, 91–160) with a corresponding heart rate variability of 2.8 ± 2.2/min (range, 0–8). Mean scan length was 115.3 ± 11.7 mm (range, 93.6–143.3). Mean volume CT dose index, mean dose-length product and effective

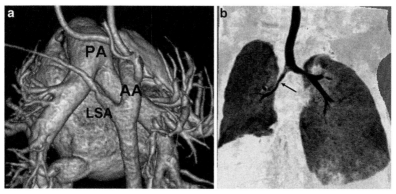

FIGURE 1.—Vascular ring and bronchial compression in a 2-month-old. The prospectively gated axial CT scan was performed at 80 kVp and 80 mAs after injection of 15 ml iodinated contrast medium (300 mg I/ml) at 1.2 ml/s (CTDI, 2.1 mGy; DLP, 21.71 mGy·cm; effective dose, 1.69 mSv). Mean heart rate during the scan was 129/min. a Volume rendered image shows an aberrant left subclavian artery (*LSA*), right aortic arch (*AA*) and pulmonary artery (*PA*) constituting a vascular ring, as the cause of the bronchial compression. b Minimum-intensity projection shows left bronchus isomerism and stenosis of the right main bronchus (*arrow*). (Reprinted from Huang M-P, Liang C-H, Zhao Z-J, et al. Evaluation of image quality and radiation dose at prospective ECG-triggered axial 256-slice multi-detector CT in infants with congenital heart disease. *Pediatr Radiol.* 2011;41:858-866, with permission from Springer Science and Business Media.)

dose were 2.1 ± 0.4 mGy (range, 1.5−2.8), 24.7 ± 5.9 mGy·cm (range, 14.7−35.8) and 1.6 ± 0.3 mSv (range, 1.1−2.5), respectively. Diagnostic-quality images were achieved in all cases. Satisfactory diagnostic quality for visualization of all/proximal/distal coronary artery segments was achieved in 88.4/98.8/80.0% of the scans.

Conclusion.—Low-dose prospectively gated axial 256-slice CT angiography is a valuable tool in the routine clinical evaluation of infants with CHD, providing a comprehensive three-dimensional evaluation of the cardiac anatomy, including the coronary arteries (Fig 1).

▶ It's heart-warming to read of the attempts made by radiologists in all subspecialties to minimize radiation dose, well illustrated by this article on cardiac CT. Advances in CT (and MR) technology have allowed such high-quality imaging that traditional fluoroscopic angiography is a thing of the past.

Although non-electrocardiogram (ECG)-synchronized scans are of better quality in children than might have been anticipated, adequate views of the coronary arteries (particularly in infants) requires ECG synchronization, which also has the advantage of improved overall image quality.

ECG synchronization may be performed by retrospective gating or prospective triggering. The former is associated with significantly higher radiation doses. Jin et al[1] were the first to report prospective ECG-triggered cardiac imaging in children, and others soon followed: the authors of this article and Pache et al,[2] for example. Pache et al discuss how technical refinements have allowed effective radiation doses from cardiac CT in children to be reduced from 28 to 1.3 mSv and reported a mean effective dose of 0.32 mSv. The mean effective dose in the current study was slightly higher at 1.6 mSv, perhaps related to the scanning techniques (Pache et al used a dual-source CT scanner). Even at these relatively low doses, diagnostic images are produced, as demonstrated by Fig 1 in an infant with a mean heart rate during the scan of 129 per min.

For a comprehensive review of the topic, interested readers are referred to the article by Goo.[3]

A. C. Offiah, BSc, MBBS, MRCP, FRCR, PhD

References

1. Jin KN, Park EA, Shin CI, Lee W, Chung JW, Park JH. Retrospective versus prospective ECG-gated dual-source CT in pediatric patients with congenital heart diseases: comparison of image quality and radiation dose. *Int J Cardiovasc Imaging.* 2010;26:63-73.
2. Pache G, Grohmann J, Bulla S, Arnold R, Stiller B, Schlensak C, Langer M, Blanke P. Prospective electrocardiography-triggered CT angiography of the great thoracic vessels in infants and toddlers with congenital heart disease: feasibility and image quality. *Eur J Radiol.* 2011;80:e440-e445.
3. Goo HW. State-of-the-art CT imaging techniques for congenital heart disease. *Korean J Radiol.* 2010;11:4-18.

Children Suspected Of Having Pulmonary Embolism: Multidetector CT Pulmonary Angiography—Thromboembolic Risk Factors and Implications for Appropriate Use
Lee EY, Tse SKS, Zurakowski D, et al (Children's Hosp Boston and Harvard Med School, MA; et al)
Radiology 262:242-251, 2012

Purpose.—To evaluate thromboembolic risk factors for pulmonary embolism (PE) detected by using computed tomographic (CT) pulmonary angiography in children and to determine whether such information could be used for more appropriate use of CT pulmonary angiography in this patient population.

Materials and Methods.—The institutional review board approved this HIPAA-compliant retrospective study and waived the need for patient informed consent. Two hundred twenty-seven consecutive CT pulmonary angiography studies in 227 pediatric patients who underwent CT pulmonary angiography for clinically suspected PE at a single large pediatric referral hospital between July 2004 and March 2011 were evaluated. Age, sex, referral setting, and D-dimer result, as well as seven possible risk factors, were compared between patients with and those without PE. Multiple logistic regression modeling was used to identify the independent risk factors of PE. Receiver operating characteristic curve analysis was applied to determine the optimal cutoff number of risk factors for predicting a positive CT pulmonary angiography result for PE in children.

Results.—Thirty-six (16%) of 227 CT pulmonary angiography studies were positive for PE. Five risk factors, including immobilization ($P < .001$),

TABLE 2.—Significant Independent Risk Factors for PE

Risk Factor	β Coefficient	Odds Ratio	95% CI	P Value
Immobilization	4.87	130.5	25.0, 681.8	<.001
Hypercoagulable state	3.06	21.4	3.5, 131.5	.003
Excess estrogen state	2.58	13.2	1.5, 123.7	.002
Indwelling CVL	3.28	26.4	5.5, 127.2	<.001
Prior PE and/or DVT	1.96	7.1	2.0, 27.2	<.001

Note.—The risk factors malignancy (P =.397) and underlying cardiac disease (P =.476) were tested but were not retained in the final multivariable model. The intercept term was −5.89.

TABLE 3.—Simplified Algorithm of Number of Risk Factors and Probability of PE

No. of Risk Factors*	Probability of PE (%)	95% CI (%)
None	0.5	0.1, 2
Any one	8	5, 15
Any two	62	46, 76
Any three or more	89	87, 99

*Risk factors were immobilization, hypercoagulable state, excess estrogen state, indwelling CVL, and prior PE and/or DVT.

hypercoagulable state ($P =.003$), excess estrogen state ($P =.002$), indwelling central venous line ($P < .001$), and prior PE and/or deep venous thrombosis ($P < .001$), were found to be significant independent risk factors for PE. With use of two or more risk factors as the clinical threshold, the sensitivity of a positive PE result was 89% (32 of 36 patients), and the specificity was 94% (180 of 191 patients).

Conclusion.—It is unlikely for CT pulmonary angiography results to be positive for PE in children with no thromboembolic risk factors. The use of risk factor assessment as a first-line triage tool has the potential to guide more appropriate use of CT pulmonary angiography in children, with associated reductions in radiation exposure and costs (Tables 2 and 3).

▶ None of us needs to be a genius to work out that maximum reduction in radiation dose to patients and minimum cost to our departments can be simultaneously achieved by not performing a given investigation at all! However, this model does not take into consideration the very reason for our (radiologists') existence: patient benefit.

The importance of this current article (and others like it) is that the investigators have provided evidence to support our decision making as to which children will benefit most from CT pulmonary angiography in the context of suspected pulmonary embolism. Furthermore, the data (Tables 2 and 3) might help strengthen our resolve when faced with bullish clinicians. I have said "might" rather than "will" because although a robust and well-conducted study, it is only single-center and retrospective. Most of us would be hard-pressed to refuse to perform CT pulmonary angiography on a child in whom clinical suspicion was high, despite the presence of only 1 risk factor. Sometimes clinicians do get it right; they don't need to be geniuses, sometimes it's a just matter of experience. Until results of prospective multicenter studies are available, despite the high quality of this present work, we, as radiologists, are likely to find the experience (and persistence) of our clinical colleagues more persuasive than the figures in the tables, but it's an excellent start to the provision of a robust evidence base.

A. C. Offiah, BSc, MBBS, MRCP, FRCR, PhD

Breathe In... Breathe Out... Stop Breathing: Does Phase of Respiration Affect the Haller Index in Patients with Pectus Excavatum?
Birkemeier KL, Podberesky DJ, Salisbury S, et al (Cincinnati Children's Hosp Med Ctr, OH)
AJR Am J Roentgenol 197:W934-W939, 2011

Objective.—The purpose of this article is to determine whether the phase of respiration at the time of imaging affects chest wall measurements and compression of internal structures in patients with pectus excavatum.

Materials and Methods.—Forty-seven patients (median age, 14 years) imaged for preoperative pectus excavatum underwent limited axial balanced steady-state free precession MRI of the chest at inspiration, expiration, and stop quiet breathing. Two radiologists, who were blinded to prior measurements, independently calculated the Haller index, asymmetry index, and sternal tilt in each phase of respiration. Compression of internal structures was recorded. Statistical comparison was performed.

Results.—The Haller index was significantly lower at inspiration, compared with stop quiet breathing and expiration, with medians (interquartile ranges) of 3.96 (3.27−4.61), 5.16 (4.02−6.48), and 5.09 (4.14−6.63), respectively ($p < 0.0001$ for both). No significant difference in Haller indexes was observed between expiration and stop quiet breathing ($p = 0.1171$). Of 11 patients with a Haller index less than 3.25 at inspiration, eight (72.7%) had an index greater than 3.25 on expiration and stop quiet breathing, which accounted for 17% (8/47) of all patients imaged. Compression of the liver or vascular structures was present in 24 (51%) patients. There was no significant difference in the asymmetry index, sternal tilt, or right heart compression between phases of respiration.

Conclusion.—Obtaining the Haller index at inspiration may result in a value significantly lower than that at expiration, potentially affecting surgical and financial decision making. Compression of the liver and vascular structures was observed in 51% of patients, but additional research is needed to determine the clinical significance of this finding.

▶ So there we have it; since the advent of multislice computed tomography (CT) scanners, as many as 17% of pectus patients may have had deferred or cancelled surgery or have had their medical insurance refused—all because they did as they were told and took a deep breath in for their CT scans. However (courtesy of the authors of this excellent article) we may all now begin to exhale.

The authors have shown that in patients with pectus, the Haller index (normal < 3.25) is significantly reduced in inspiration compared with both expiration and stop quiet breathing. In other words, are the inspiratory scans giving a true or a false picture of the severity of the pectus? By so elegantly highlighting the problem, Birkemeier et al have begun the debate that should stimulate relevant research studies culminating in standardization of the imaging technique.

Why has this not previously been an issue?

Because in the days when the Haller index was introduced, it was CT based; chest imaging could not be completed in a single breath hold, and the standard was to obtain scans during quiet breathing. However, with the advent of multi-slice CT scanners, most chest scans are now obtained at full inspiration (plus some images in expiration if it is required to exclude air trapping); hence, the current need to decide whether scans performed to calculate the Haller index should be performed in inspiration, expiration, or stop quiet breathing.

Henry Ford suggested that, "If you think of standardization as the best that you know today, but which is to be improved tomorrow, you get somewhere." All of us in the medical field are aiming for a place where patient outcomes are optimized. The getting there often takes longer than we would like, so in the meantime, don't hold your breath.

A. C. Offiah, BSc, MBBS, MRCP, FRCR, PhD

Congenital diaphragmatic hernia: lung-to-head ratio and lung volume for prediction of outcome

Alfaraj MA, Shah PS, Bohn D, et al (Univ of Toronto, Ontario, Canada)
Am J Obstet Gynecol 205:43.e1-43.e8, 2011

Objective.—The purpose of this study was to evaluate observed/expected (O/E) lung-to-head ratio (LHR) by ultrasound (US) and total fetal lung volume (TFLV) by magnetic resonance imaging as neonatal outcome predictors in isolated fetal congenital diaphragmatic hernia (CDH).

Study Design.—We conducted a retrospective study of 72 fetuses with isolated CDH, in whom O/E LHR and TFLV were evaluated as survival predictors.

Results.—O/E LHR on US and O/E TFLV by magnetic resonance imaging were significantly lower in newborn infants with isolated CDH who died compared with survivors (30.3 ± 8.3 vs 44.2 ± 14.2; $P < .0001$ for O/E LHR; 21.9 ± 6.3 vs 41.5 ± 17.6; $P = .001$ for O/E TFLV). Area under receiver-operator characteristics curve for survival for O/E LHR was 0.80 (95% confidence interval, 0.70–0.90). On multivariate analysis, O/E LHR predicted survival, whereas hernia side and first neonatal pH did not. For each unit increase in O/E LHR, mortality odds decreased by 11% (95% confidence interval, 4–17%).

TABLE 1.—Perinatal Factors and Risk of Mortality in 72 Fetuses with Isolated Congenital Diaphragmatic Hernia

Variable	Nonsurvivors (n = 25)	Survivors (n = 47)	P Value
Male sex, n (%)	11 (48)	20 (44)	.73
Gestational age at diagnosis, wk[a]	24.5 ± 6.4	24.3 ± 6.8	.89
Left-side congenital diaphragmatic hernia, n (%)	19 (76)	44 (94)	.03
Intrathoracic position of liver on ultrasound, n (%)	8 (32)	14 (30)	.89
Observed/expected lung-to-head circumference ratio on ultrasound[a]	30.3 ± 8.3	44.2 ± 14.2	< .01[b]
Observed/expected total fetal lung volume by magnetic resonance imaging[a,c]	21.9 ± 6.3	41.5 ± 17.6	< .01[b]
Gestational age at delivery, wk	37.3 ± 3.5	38.2 ± 1.7	.27
Birthweight, g[a]	2816 ± 717	3129 ± 520	.07
Apgar score[d]			
1-minute	4 (1–7)	6 (1–9)	< .01[b]
5-minute	6 (2–9)	8 (1–9)	< .01[b]
Umbilical artery cord pH[a]	7.20 ± 0.14	7.30 ± 0.07	.07
First neonatal arterial pH[a]	7.04 ± 0.15	7.14 ± 0.17	.02[b]
Extra corporeal membrane oxygenation use, n (%)	6 (26)	1 (2)	< .01[b]

[a]Data are given as mean ± SD.
[b]P < .05.
[c]Available in 26 fetuses: 10 nonsurvivors and 16 survivors.
[d]Data are given as median (range).

Conclusion.—In fetuses with isolated CDH, O/E LHR (US) independently predicts survival and may predict severity, allowing management to be optimized (Table 1).

▶ As we get better at diagnosing congenital disorders earlier and earlier in pregnancy, the question we ask ourselves, that we ask our colleagues, and that our patients ask us is, "Now what?" What does the identification of this or that condition in this pregnancy mean? Is an operation necessary? When? Will the baby survive? Should we terminate? We can more confidently answer these questions—in short give sound counseling and advice—if we are armed with robust predictors of survival.

This article concentrates on the power of prenatal lung volume calculations from ultrasound and MRI to predict postnatal outcome in fetuses with isolated congenital diaphragmatic hernia (CDH). Although there was no difference in mean gestational age at the time of diagnosis, there was a significant difference in lung volumes between survivors and nonsurvivors (Table 1).

Although prenatal MRI of the brain is generally accepted as being superior to prenatal ultrasound, the benefits of prenatal MRI over other systems is still argued, with some authors remaining convinced that prenatally, lung MRI has nothing to add over ultrasound. Results of this study will please both camps: although ultrasound did better at predicting outcome (note that both methods reached statistical significance), MRI was better at confirming the position of the liver. Another example of complementary rather than opposing technology. Although we await a large multicenter prospective study, the current results are promising in the context of isolated CDH.

Having an interest in the musculoskeletal system, and after reading this article, the question I ask myself is, "Now what?" In addition to that large multicenter prospective study of isolated CDH, perhaps another to investigate whether the techniques might prove similarly useful in other conditions associated with small lungs, such as certain constitutional bone disorders, is in order?

A. C. Offiah, BSc, MBBS, MRCP, FRCR, PhD

Miscellaneous

Childhood Cancer Risk From Conventional Radiographic Examinations for Selected Referral Criteria: Results From a Large Cohort Study

Hammer GP, Seidenbusch MC, Regulla DF, et al (Johannes Gutenberg Univ Mainz, Germany; Ludwig-Maximilians—Univ of Munich, Germany; German Res Ctr for Environmental Health, Neuherberg, Germany; et al)
AJR Am J Roentgenol 197:217-223, 2011

Objective.—Little is known about the long-term effects of exposure to diagnostic ionizing radiation in childhood. Current estimates are made with models derived mainly from studies of atomic bomb survivors, a population that differs from today's patients in many respects.

Materials and Methods.—We analyzed the cancer incidence among children who underwent diagnostic x-ray exposures between 1976 and 2003 in a large German university hospital. We reconstructed individual radiation doses for each examination and sorted results by groups of referral criteria for all cancers combined, solid tumors, and leukemia and lymphoma combined.

Results.—A total of 68 incidence cancer cases between 1980 and 2006 were identified in a 78,527-patient cohort in the German childhood cancer registry: 28 leukemia, nine lymphoma, six tumors of the CNS, and 25 other tumors. The standardized incidence ratio for all cancers was 0.97 (95% CI, 0.75—1.23). Dose-response relations were analyzed by multivariable Poisson regression. Although the cancer incidence risk differed by initial referral criterion for radiographic examination, a positive dose-response relation was observed in five patients with endocrine or metabolic disease.

Conclusion.—Overall, we observed no increase in cancer risk among children and youths with very low radiation doses from diagnostic radiation, which is compatible with model calculations. The growing use of CT warrants further studies to assess associated cancer risk. Our work is an early contribution of epidemiologic data for quantifying these risks among young patients.

▶ This very large study used a novel approach to estimate the cancer risk of diagnostic radiation in children. Strict exclusion criteria included an a priori definition of prevalent cancer (cancer on or within 6 months of first imaging), those at increased risk of malignancy (eg, children with Down syndrome), and those with high risk of mortality (eg, children with AIDS). An important consideration when evaluating the impact of the results is that radiation dose was prospectively recorded for each child; most studies on the subject have been retrospective and have therefore used estimates of radiation exposure. This article should be read by all.

The results are encouraging; the authors found no increased risk of diagnostic radiation-induced cancer. However, let us not be complacent; we need to be clear on one fact: this study deals with low individual effective radiation doses, that is, less than 5 microSv. Such doses are exceeded by most if not all CT examinations.

One final point: although low-dose radiation may not be associated with increased cancer risk, there are other issues to consider, such as cost-effectiveness. In this study, 8472 patients had 4 or more examinations with the most in a single patient being 85. Were all of these absolutely necessary?

We already do, and as pediatric radiologists we should continue to ask ourselves before every examination that we perform or supervise, "Is this study really necessary?"

A. C. Offiah, BSc, MBBS, MRCP, FRCR, PhD

Utilization of Emergency Ultrasound in Pediatric Emergency Departments
Chamberlain MC, Reid SR, Madhok M (Children's Hosps and Clinics of Minnesota, Minneapolis; Children's Hosps and Clinics of Minnesota, St Paul, MN)
Pediatr Emerg Care 27:628-632, 2011

Objectives.—This study aimed to determine the utilization of emergency ultrasound (EUS) in pediatric emergency departments (EDs) and in pediatric emergency medicine (PEM) fellowship training programs and to assess if PEM fellowship programs provided formal training in EUS.

Methods.—A Web-based survey was administered to pediatric emergency medical directors, fellowship directors, and graduating fellows.

Results.—A response was received from 60% of individuals and 68% of institutions. Of the responders, 27% reported that their institution had a EUS program. Also, 96% of the responders reported having a dedicated US machine in the ED, but only 61% reported using EUS for managing ED patients. Responders reported using EUS for the focused assessment by sonography for trauma examination (93%), abscess management (82%), vascular access (78%), bladder scanning (70%), cardiac activity confirmation (59%), and pericardial effusion detection (59%). For pediatric emergency staff physicians, 63% of the responders reported obtaining EUS training from general emergency physicians and 59% from a commercial ultrasound course and from pediatric emergency physicians. For PEM fellows, 34% reported having a standardized EUS training program. Of the responders, 69% reported receiving training from general emergency physicians during adult ED rotations and 38% reported receiving training from pediatric emergency physicians. Only 28% of programs reported using criteria established by the American College of Emergency Physicians for the number of scans performed to attain competence.

Conclusions.—In our study sample, there is wide variation in the uses of EUS and the training pediatric emergency physicians receive in its use (Fig 1, Table 3).

▶ None of the authors of this article on the use of emergency ultrasound (EUS) in pediatric emergency departments (EDs) is a radiologist. Not such a big deal; however, there are a large number of horrifying statistics presented here. You may take note of some of them by reading the abstract; for instance, only 27% of responders actually have an EUS training program at their institution (but 61% perform EUS), only 28% use criteria as published by the American College of Emergency Physicians for the number of scans performed to attain competence, and the majority received their training during adult ED rotations.

More horrifying statistics are to be found within the text of the article; for instance, only 44% of the scans performed in the ED are overread (double reported) by a radiologist. Not horrified yet? Then take a look at the data in Table 3 (44% of respondents had 8 or fewer hours of training). Next consider that the category of "other" in Fig 1 includes evaluation for testicular torsion and intussusception, consider the hours of training given to radiologists, and finally, with all this in mind, reflect on the difficulties trained radiologists and sonographers sometimes face when making these diagnoses.

If you are not horrified by now, then you are probably not a pediatric radiologist.

My aim, however, is not to horrify but to stimulate debate. The authors note that more than 50% of EDs have encountered resistance from their radiology departments when trying to start an EUS program. They suggest that this resistance might be generated by concerns regarding the accuracy of examinations

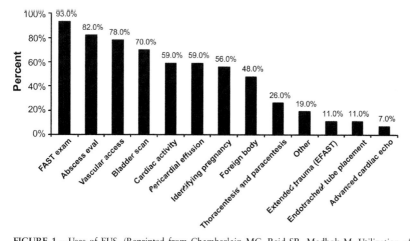

FIGURE 1.—Uses of EUS. (Reprinted from Chamberlain MC, Reid SR, Madhok M. Utilization of emergency ultrasound in pediatric emergency departments. *Pediatr Emerg Care.* 2011;27:628-632, with permission from Lippincott Williams & Wilkins.)

TABLE 3.—EUS Training Time and Required Scans

Response Selection	Result, %
Hours of training provided	
1–8 h	44
9–16 h	9
17–24 h	6
25–32 h	3
33–40 h	0
>40 h	38
Required scans to complete EUS training	
None required	31
<15 scans	19
16–25 scans	0
26–35 scans	0
36–45 scans	3
>46 scans	6
Use ACEP guidelines of 25–50 scans	28
Other	13

ACEP indicates American College of Emergency Physicians.

performed by pediatric emergency physicians and/or reimbursement. Any resistance that I feel is certainly related to the former, that is, diagnostic accuracy of ED physicians. However, is resistance the correct response? If 61% of institutions are already using EUS to manage ED patients, might we not better serve children by joining the 19% of radiology departments involved with EUS training for pediatric emergency medicine staff physicians, and should we not be involved in research such as that presented here?

A. C. Offiah, BSc, MBBS, MRCP, FRCR, PhD

5 Economics, Research, Education, and Quality

Introduction

As usual, this section of the YEAR BOOK OF DIAGNOSTIC RADIOLOGY contains a fascinating and diverse array of articles broadly spanning the realms of clinical practice, appropriateness, quality assurance, and safety. Notwithstanding the varied subject matter, all these papers are tied together by a common thread, constituting the core components needed to understand and deliver the highest quality service to our patients. Although all the articles are interesting, I suggest you make special effort to peruse the following:

First, there are several articles relating to cardiac CT imaging. The most important is on Appropriateness Criteria for Cardiac Computed Tomography. This is a carefully crafted document sponsored jointly by the American College of Radiology, the American Heart Association, and several other societies. It can even be downloaded for free from the Internet. After you review this article, you should also check the paper by van Kempen et al on the cost-effectiveness of calcium screening for coronary artery disease.

And while we are on the topic of cardiac imaging, you may not have heard that there are now MR-compatible pacemakers now approved for use in the United States. As such, you will probably want to review the article on the radiologist's role for scanning these MR-conditional pacemakers.

Finally, this section contains a couple of articles on the safety of gadolinium-based MR contrast agents. Over the last 3 to 5 years, the world has become attuned to the risk these agents pose for nephrogenic systemic sclerosis and has changed administration policies. The article by Wang et al shows that we have largely put the iatrogenic disease to rest.

Allen D. Elster, MD

Appropriate Criteria and Cost Effectiveness

ACCF/SCCT/ACR/AHA/ASE/ASNC/NASCI/SCAI/SCMR 2010 Appropriate Use Criteria for Cardiac Computed Tomography: A Report of the American College of Cardiology Foundation Appropriate Use Criteria Task Force, the Society of Cardiovascular Computed Tomography, the American College of Radiology, the American Heart Association, the American Society of Echocardiography, the American Society of Nuclear Cardiology, the North American Society for Cardiovascular Imaging, the Society for Cardiovascular Angiography and Interventions, and the Society for Cardiovascular Magnetic Resonance
Taylor AJ, Cerqueira M, Hodgson JM, et al (Official American College of Cardiology Foundation Representative; Official American Society of Nuclear Cardiology Representative; Official Society for Cardiovascular Angiography and Interventions Representative; et al)
Circulation 122:e525-e555, 2010

The American College of Cardiology Foundation, along with key specialty and subspecialty societies, conducted an appropriate use review of common clinical scenarios where cardiac computed tomography (CCT) is frequently considered. The present document is an update to the original CCT/cardiac magnetic resonance appropriateness criteria published in 2006, written to reflect changes in test utilization, to incorporate new clinical data, and to clarify CCT use where omissions or lack of clarity existed in the original criteria.

The indications for this review were drawn from common applications or anticipated uses, as well as from current clinical practice guidelines. Ninety-three clinical scenarios were developed by a writing group and scored by a separate technical panel on a scale of 1 to 9 to designate appropriate use, inappropriate use, or uncertain use.

In general, use of CCT angiography for diagnosis and risk assessment in patients with low or intermediate risk or pretest probability for coronary artery disease was viewed favorably, whereas testing in high-risk patients, routine repeat testing, and general screening in certain clinical scenarios were viewed less favorably. Use of noncontrast computed tomography for calcium scoring was rated as appropriate within intermediate- and selected low-risk patients. Appropriate applications of CCT are also within the category of cardiac structural and functional evaluation. It is anticipated that these results will have an impact on physician decision making, performance, and reimbursement policy, and that they will help guide future research.

▶ If you are involved in any way with the performance or interpretation of cardiac CT, this article is a must read. Nearly 70 pages in length, the list of coauthors reads like a "who's who" of cardiac imaging, incorporating the top experts from both the radiology and cardiology communities. The scope of the article is so broad that no brief summary can do it justice. The ultimate goal is to create an appropriateness rating on a scale from 0 to 10 as to whether a cardiac CT is indicated, given certain clinical conditions.

The complexity of this system is somewhat bewildering, especially compared with the perhaps more familiar American College of Radiology Appropriateness Criteria, in which each study (like spinal MRI) fits nicely on a single page or two. With cardiac disease, however, there are perhaps many more nuances to consider.

Specific subsections of the report deal with 1) detection of coronary artery disease (CAD) in symptomatic patients without known heart disease; 2) detection of CAD in asymptomatic individuals without known CAD; 3) detection of CAD in other clinical scenarios; 4) use of CT angiography in the setting of prior test results, including age, sex, electrocardiogram findings, and stress tests; and 5) use in pre- and postcardiac surgery evaluation and risk assessment.

A useful bibliography is included. The article is free and available on the Web at http://circ.ahajournals.org/content/122/21/e525.

A. D. Elster, MD

Comparative Effectiveness and Cost-Effectiveness of Computed Tomography Screening for Coronary Artery Calcium in Asymptomatic Individuals
van Kempen BJH, Spronk S, Koller MT, et al (Erasmus Med Ctr, Rotterdam, the Netherlands; Univ Hosp Basel, Switzerland; et al)
J Am Coll Cardiol 58:1690-1701, 2011

Objectives.—The aim of this study was to assess the (cost-) effectiveness of screening asymptomatic individuals at intermediate risk of coronary heart disease (CHD) for coronary artery calcium with computed tomography (CT).

Background.—Coronary artery calcium on CT improves prediction of CHD.

Methods.—A Markov model was developed on the basis of the Rotterdam Study. Four strategies were evaluated: 1) current practice; 2) current prevention guidelines for cardiovascular disease; 3) CT screening for coronary calcium; and 4) statin therapy for all individuals. Asymptomatic individuals at intermediate risk of CHD were simulated over their remaining lifetime. Quality-adjusted life years (QALYs), costs, and incremental cost-effectiveness ratios were calculated.

Results.—In men, CT screening was more effective and more costly than the other 3 strategies (CT vs. current practice: +0.13 QALY [95% confidence interval (CI): 0.01 to 0.26], +$4,676 [95% CI: $3,126 to $6,339]; CT vs. statin therapy: +0.04 QALY [95% CI: −0.02 to 0.13], +$1,951 [95% CI: $1,170 to $2,754]; and CT vs. current guidelines: +0.02 QALY [95% CI: −0.04 to 0.09], +$44 [95% CI: −$441 to $486]). The incremental cost-effectiveness ratio of CT calcium screening was $48,800/QALY gained. In women, CT screening was more effective and more costly than current practice (+0.13 QALY [95% CI: 0.02 to 0.28], +$4,663 [95% CI: $3,120 to $6,277]) and statin therapy (+0.03 QALY [95% CI: −0.03 to 0.12],

+$2,273 [95% CI: $1,475 to $3,109]). However, implementing current guidelines was more effective compared with CT screening (+0.02 QALY [95% CI: −0.03 to 0.07]), only a little more expensive (+$297 [95% CI: −$8 to $633]), and had a lower cost per additional QALY ($33,072/QALY vs. $35,869/QALY). Sensitivity analysis demonstrated robustness of results in women but considerable uncertainty in men.

Conclusions.—Screening for coronary artery calcium with CT in individuals at intermediate risk of CHD is probably cost-effective in men but is unlikely to be cost-effective in women.

▶ In the modern era, not only must a radiology study be effective in diagnosing a disease, it must be cost effective. Coronary artery calcium scoring is now in mainstream use, but its cost effectiveness has not yet been proven. This article from the cardiology literature attempts to address this issue.

Recent studies have found that the computed tomography (CT) calcium score is a strong predictor of cardiovascular disease independent of other risk factors.[1] More than half of individuals classified as intermediate risk from clinical factors are reclassified to high-risk or low-risk categories when calcium score is taken into consideration.

The authors conclude that screening for coronary artery calcium with CT is probably cost effective in men at intermediate risk of coronary heart disease (CHD). However, for women at intermediate risk for CHD, CT screening does not seem to be cost effective. These findings, if confirmed, have important policy as well as health-outcomes implications.

A. D. Elster, MD

Reference

1. Polonsky TS, McClelland RL, Jorgensen NW, et al. Coronary artery calcium score and risk classification for coronary heart disease prediction. *JAMA.* 2010;303:1610-1616.

Screening Cervical Spine CT in a Level I Trauma Center: Overutilization?
Griffith B, Bolton C, Goyal N, et al (Henry Ford Health System, Detroit, MI)
AJR Am J Roentgenol 197:463-467, 2011

Objective.—The objective of our study was to analyze the use of screening cervical spine CT performed after trauma and establish the opportunity of potentially avoidable studies when evidence-based clinical criteria are applied before imaging.

Materials and Methods.—All cervical spine CT examinations performed in the emergency department of a level 1 trauma center between January and December 2008 on adult patients with trauma were analyzed; 1589 studies were evaluated. Radiology reports and clinical data were reviewed for the presence of fracture or ligamentous injury and for the mode of injury. We also looked for documentation of clinical criteria used to perform the CT study. In particular, we looked for mention of posterior midline cervical tenderness, focal neurologic deficit, level of alertness, evidence of intoxication, and clinically apparent distracting injury. These five criteria were established by the National Emergency X-Radiography Utilization Study (NEXUS) to identify patients with a low probability of cervical spine injury who consequently needed no cervical spine imaging.

Results.—Of the 1589 studies reviewed, 41 (2.6%) were positive for an acute cervical spine injury and 1524 (95.9%) were negative. The remaining 24 studies (1.5%) were indeterminate on the initial CT examination but subsequent imaging and clinical follow-up failed to show acute injury. Of the 1524 examinations with no acute injury, 364 (23.9%) had no documentation of any of the five NEXUS low-risk criteria.

Conclusion.—The strict application of the NEXUS low-risk criteria could potentially reduce the number of screening cervical spine CT examinations in the setting of trauma in more than 20% of cases, thereby avoiding a significant amount of unnecessary radiation and significant cost.

▶ For more than a decade, radiologists and emergency physicians have tried to develop cost-effectiveness criteria for imaging the cervical spine in trauma patients. In 2000, the results of the National Emergency X-Radiography Utilization Study (NEXUS)[1] established low-risk criteria to identify patients with a low probability of cervical spine injury who consequently needed no cervical spine x-rays. To meet the NEXUS criteria, all of the following must be met: no tenderness at the posterior midline of the cervical spine; no focal neurologic deficit; normal level of alertness; no evidence of intoxication; and no clinically apparent, painful injury that might distract the patient from the pain of a cervical spine injury.

While the NEXUS investigators looked at the need for conventional radiography of the cervical spine in such patients, in recent years computed tomography (CT) has supplanted conventional x-ray as the method of choice for assessing cervical spine injury. The NEXUS criteria need to be reviewed in accordance with the new use of CT to see whether they are still valid and whether they might help reduce overuse of cervical CT in such patients.

In the current study, strict application of the NEXUS criteria would have decreased the number of negative cervical spine CT studies by 23.9%. Even applying more liberal criteria to include the presence or absence of pain, limited range of motion, or posterolateral cervical spine tenderness would have produced a 20.2% reduction.

A. D. Elster, MD

Reference

1. Hoffman JR, Mower WR, Wolfson AB, Todd KH, Zucker MI. Validity of a set of clinical criteria to rule out injury to the cervical spine in patients with blunt trauma. National Emergency X-Radiography Utilization Study Group. *N Engl J Med.* 2000;343:94-99.

Clinical Practice

"MR-Conditional" Pacemakers: The Radiologist's Role in Multidisciplinary Management

Colletti PM, Shinbane JS, Shellock FG (Univ of Southern California, Los Angeles, CA)
AJR Am J Roentgenol 197:W457-W459, 2011

Objective.—The recent approval of an "MR-conditional" pacemaker system by the U.S. Food and Drug Administration allows patients with that pacemaker system to undergo MRI examinations within specific conditions. These examinations must be attended by radiology health care professionals with training for the use of the pacemaker system.

Conclusion.—Radiologists should be knowledgeable of the specific limitations with regard to patient isocenter and coil positioning within the required 1.5-T MR system and the importance that the pacer be programmed before and after scanning (Fig 1).

▶ One of the major technical developments affecting magnetic resonance (MR) imaging in 2011 was the approval in February by the US Food and Drug Administration of the Revo MRI SureScan Pacing System (Medtronic; Minneapolis, MN) as "MR Conditional".[1] This pacemaker (Fig 1) as well as those from 2 other medical device companies (Biotronik, Berlin, Germany, and St. Jude Medical, St. Paul, MN) have previously been approved in Europe. Because it has been estimated that more than 1 million patients with pacemakers may have clinical indications for the use of MRI, the potential impact of this may be far reaching.

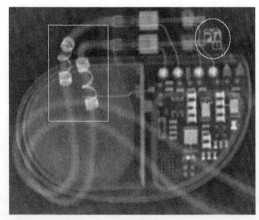

FIGURE 1.—Close-up radiograph of patient's pacemaker system shows wavy radiopaque markings for generator (*circle*) and leads (*rectangle*) confirming presence of Revo MRI SureScan System (Medtronic) [11]. (Courtesy of Burrows J, Medtronic, Inc.) *Editor's Note*: Please refer to original journal article for full references. (Reprinted from Colletti PM, Shinbane JS, Shellock FG. "MR-conditional" pacemakers: the radiologist's role in multidisciplinary management. *AJR Am J Roentgenol.* 2011;197:W457-W459, with permission from American Roentgen Ray Society.)

The conditions under which patients with SureScan pacers may safely undergo MR imaging are fairly rigorous. A cardiologist or other health care provider who has undergone SureScan training must first evaluate the patient and test several specifications concerning its impedance and voltage thresholds and, if correct, sets the pacemaker to the SureScan "on" mode.

MR imaging is permitted only at field strengths of 1.5 T. The body radiofrequency coil must not lie over the pacer, meaning that examinations of the thorax and upper abdomen are not possible. However, most other MR imaging scans are possible. There are strict limits on gradient slew rates and specific absorption rates. Following the MR procedure, the cardiologist resets the pacer to the SureScan "off" mode and retests its function.

A. D. Elster, MD

Reference

1. Mitka M. First MRI-safe pacemaker receives conditional approval from FDA. *JAMA.* 2011;305:985-986.

MRI of Patients With Cardiac Pacemakers: A Review of the Medical Literature
Zikria JF, Machnicki S, Rhim E, et al (Lenox Hill Hosp, NY)
AJR Am J Roentgenol 196:390-401, 2011

Objective.—Numerous studies testing the use of pacemakers with MRI have been published. Our aim was to analyze these trials to determine the safety of MRI for patients with cardiac pacemakers. We performed a systematic search of peer-reviewed databases. A total of 31 articles were reviewed.

Conclusion.—The data are heterogeneous with regard to MRI being considered for patients with pacemakers, and the benefits of the imaging should outweigh the risks.

▶ For many years, the presence of an implanted pacemaker has constituted a (nearly) absolute contraindication to MR imaging. Theoretical health risks to patients with pacemakers include movement of the pacemaker or leads due to the static magnetic field, damage to the pacemaker circuitry, and thermal injury to tissue arising from gradient-induced electrical currents in the leads. Since 2007, there have been at least 17 supposed MRI-associated deaths worldwide among patients with pacemakers.

Despite these limitations, in a number of situations, the benefit of MR scanning may outweigh the risk. At our medical center, and a number of others, we have successfully scanned a few patients with pacemakers after giving adequate informed consent and under careful cardiology supervision during the scan. In February 2011, the US Food and Drug Administration approved Medtronic's Revo MRI SureScan pacemaker, based on safety in 211 patients in a multicenter clinical trial. Other MRI-compatible pacemakers are also in development.

This article is a comprehensive review of the existing medical literature (31 papers cited) concerning the safety issues (theoretical and real) of scanning patients with pacemakers. It serves as a good guide to understanding the issues involved, which is still important even if one is scanning patients with one of the newer MR-compatible devices.

A. D. Elster, MD

National Trends in CT Use in the Emergency Department: 1995–2007
Larson DB, Johnson LW, Schnell BM, et al (Cincinnati Children's Hosp Med Ctr, OH; Yale Univ School of Medicine, New Haven, CT)
Radiology 258:164-173, 2011

Purpose.—To identify nationwide trends and factors associated with the use of computed tomography (CT) in the emergency department (ED).

Materials and Methods.—This study was exempt from institutional review board approval. Data from the 1995–2007 National Hospital Ambulatory Medical Care Survey were used to evaluate the numbers and percentages of ED visits associated with CT. A mean of 30 044 visits

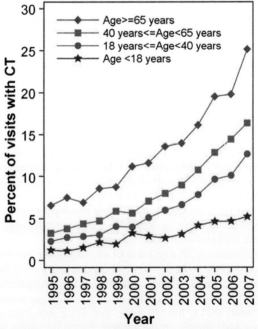

FIGURE 3.—Graph illustrates percentages of ED visits involving CT based on patient age. P < .01 for comparison among all years. (Reprinted from Larson DB, Johnson LW, Schnell BM, et al. National trends in CT use in the emergency department: 1995–2007. *Radiology.* 2011;258:164-173, Copyright by the Radiological Society of North America.)

were sampled each year. Data were also subcategorized according to multiple patient and hospital characteristics. The Rao-Scott χ^2 test was performed to determine whether CT use was similar across subpopulations. Data were evaluated according to exponential and logistic growth models.

Results.—From 1995 to 2007, the number of ED visits that included a CT examination increased from 2.7 million to 16.2 million, constituting a 5.9-fold increase and a compound annual growth rate of 16.0%. The percentage of visits associated with CT increased from 2.8% to 13.9%, constituting a 4.9-fold increase and a compound annual growth rate of 14.2%. The exponential growth model provided the best fit for the trend in CT use. CT use was greater in older patients, white patients, patients admitted to the hospital, and patients at facilities in metropolitan regions. By the end of the study period, the top chief complaints among those who underwent CT were abdominal pain, headache, and chest pain. The percentage of patient visits associated with CT for all evaluated chief complaints increased—most substantially among those who underwent CT for flank, abdominal, or chest pain.

Conclusion.—Use of CT has increased at a higher rate in the ED than in other settings. The overall use of CT had not begun to taper by 2007 (Fig 3, Table 2).

▶ If it seems to you that your radiology workload from the emergency room is continually increasing, you are not hallucinating. It is something everyone is experiencing as part of a national trend.

TABLE 2.—Chief Complaints Most Commonly Associated with CT Imaging

	1995		2001		2007	
Complaint Rank	Chief Complaint	Percentage of All CT-Associated Visits*	Chief Complaint	Percentage of All CT-Associated Visits*	Chief Complaint	Percentage of All CT-Associated Visits*
1	Headache	12.0	Headache	9.8	Abdominal pain	12.8
2	Head injury	11.5	Abdominal pain	8.3	Headache	7.5
3	Convulsions	5.8	Vertigo or dizziness	5.2	Chest pain	4.7
4	MVA	3.6	Head Injury	4.2	Side or flank pain	4.6
5	Accident	3.6	Side/flank pain	3.5	Head Injury	4.2
6	Vertigo or dizziness	2.8	Accident	3.4	Vertigo or dizziness	3.5
7	Abdominal pain	2.7	Convulsions	3.2	Accident	2.7
8	Unconscious	2.4	MVA	3.2	Convulsions	2.5
9	Cerebrovascular disease	2.3	Back pain	2.6	SOB	2.4
10	Loss of feeling	2.1	Loss of feeling	2.3	Back pain	2.0
No rank	All others	51.1	All others	54.2	All others	52.9

*Data are weighted percentages of ED visits in which CT was performed for the given chief complaint.

CT scanning seems to be the principal culprit. During the last year of the study (2007), about 14% of patients visiting an emergency room had a CT, an increase from 3.5% a decade before. Assuming the trend has continued, by 2012 we can predict that nearly 20% of emergency patients will receive CTs, amounting to over 20 million emergency visits with CTs annually.

As can be seen in Fig 3, the largest growth has been in the population age 65 and older. While only 5 years previously, the most common indication for CT was neurologic (principally headache or head trauma), by 2007 the principal indication was abdominal pain (Table 2).

The exponential growth of CT in the emergency room setting shows little evidence of slowing, and we must await future studies to demonstrate to what extent the cost and radiation exposure have been validated.

A. D. Elster, MD

Effect of Spinal Segment Variants on Numbering Vertebral Levels at Lumbar MR Imaging

Carrino JA, Campbell PD Jr, Lin DC, et al (Johns Hopkins Univ School of Medicine, Baltimore, MD; Booth Radiology, Woodbury, NJ; et al)
Radiology 259:196-202, 2011

Purpose.—To verify iliolumbar ligament (ILL) location, to evaluate magnetic resonance (MR) imaging morphologic features for detecting lumbosacral transitional vertebrae (TVs) (LSTVs), and to determine whether transitional situations are associated with anomalous vertebral numbering.

Materials and Methods.—Investigational review board approval was obtained for this HIPAA-compliant retrospective study. A review of 147 subjects was performed by using spine radiography as the reference standard to determine total and segmental vertebral count and transitional anatomy. Thoracolumbar TVs (TLTVs) and LSTVs were identified. The lumbosacral intervertebral disk angle (LSIVDA), defined as the angle between the end-plates, was measured, S1-2 disk morphology was rated according to the classification by O'Driscoll et al, and the ILL level was determined from MR images. Statistical analysis was performed by using χ^2 tests for dichotomous and ordinal variables and the t test for continuous variables.

Results.—An anomalous total number of vertebrae were present in 12 (8.2%) of 147 subjects. The ILL was identified in 126 (85.7%) of 147 subjects and was present at L5 in 122 (96.8%) subjects; the remaining four (3.2%) subjects had an anomalous total number of vertebrae. A complete S1-2 intervertebral disk was associated with LSTVs ($P = .004$); however, LSIVDA was not ($P = .2$). TLTVs were present in six (4.1%) and LSTVs were present in 22 (15.0%) of 147 subjects. Both were present in four (2.7%) subjects. The presence of a TLTV was associated with a higher incidence of a concomitant LSTV and vice versa ($P < .001$; odds ratio [OR], 13.7; 95% confidence interval [CI]: 2.7, 68.4]). A TLTV was not associated with an anomalous total number of vertebrae ($P = .46$), but an LSTV was ($P < .001$; OR, 7.4; 95% CI: 2.2, 24.8).

Conclusion.—The ILL denotes the lowest lumbar vertebra, which does not always represent L5. A well-formed, complete S1-2 intervertebral disk is associated with LSTVs, but alteration in LSIVDA is not. LSTVs are associated with anomalous vertebral numbering.

▶ This article serves to remind everyone about the potential pitfalls one might encounter in doing what seems to be a daily trivial workflow issue—number the segments of the lumbar spine on MRI for reporting purposes. There is appreciable anatomic variability at the lumbosacral junction and in the lumbar spine as a whole. Some people have 6 distinct lumbar vertebrae; others only 4. Many have transitional-type vertebrae that are part sacral, part lumbar.

The ramifications come principally when surgery is contemplated and one of these variant anatomies is encountered. This article gives some suggestions on how to identify and properly number these segments, or at least communicate to others the potential nomenclature difficulties encountered.

A. D. Elster, MD

The Radiologist as a Palliative Care Subspecialist: Providing Symptom Relief When Cure Is Not Possible

McCullough HK, Bain RM, Clark HP, et al (Wake Forest Univ Baptist Med Ctr, Winston-Salem, NC)
AJR Am J Roentgenol 196:462-467, 2011

Objective.—The purpose of this study was to determine the percentage of patients referred to an interventional radiology (IR) practice who need palliative care and to examine the training required for a diplomate of the American Board of Radiology (ABR) to qualify for the hospice and palliative medicine certifying examination.

Materials and Methods.—This retrospective study reviewed all patient referrals to an academic vascular and IR practice during the month of August 2009. The demographics, underlying diagnosis, and the type of procedures performed were ascertained from the electronic medical record. The requirements for a diplomate of the ABR to obtain certification as a hospice and palliative medicine subspecialist were evaluated and summarized.

Results.—Two-hundred eighty-two patients were referred to the IR service and underwent a total of 332 interventional procedures. Most of the patients (229 [81.2%]) had underlying diagnoses that would warrant consultation with a hospice and palliative medicine subspecialist; these patients were significantly older (58.5 vs 44.7 years; $p < 0.01$) and underwent more procedures (1.21 vs 1.02; $p < 0.01$). To obtain a subspecialty certification in hospice and palliative medicine, a radiologist needs certification by the ABR, an unrestricted medical license, 2 years of subspecialty training in hospice and palliative medicine, 100 hours of interdisciplinary hospice and palliative medicine team participation, active care of 50 terminally ill adult patients, and successful performance on the certification examination.

Conclusion.—Procedures related to palliative care currently compose the majority of our IR cases. Certification in hospice and palliative medicine can be achieved with a modest investment of time and clinical training.

▶ What an innovative and creative idea! Expanding the role of the radiologist far beyond the usual bounds as an interventionalist to become a "palliative care subspecialist." Just when it seems the boundaries of radiology are becoming encroached on by other specialties, radiologists seem to think outside the box and see possibilities where none existed before.

Such is the promise and opportunity of palliative care medicine. Many of the techniques needed are already well within the experience of interventional radiologists, including long-term central venous access, percutaneous drainage, percutaneous gastrostomy, and pain block procedures.

The American Board of Radiology now offers subspecialty certification in palliative care, which includes 2 years of subspecialty training in hospice and palliative medicine, 100 hours of interdisciplinary hospice and palliative medicine team participation, active care of 50 terminally ill adult patients, and successful performance on the certification examination. This pathway is not for everyone but will perhaps play a progressively important role in managing our chronically ill and dying patients in the long run.

A. D. Elster, MD

Influence of Annual Interpretive Volume on Screening Mammography Performance in the United States

Buist DSM, Anderson ML, Haneuse SJPA, et al (Group Health Res Inst, Seattle, WA; et al)
Radiology 259:72-84, 2011

Purpose.—To examine whether U.S. radiologists' interpretive volume affects their screening mammography performance.

Materials and Methods.—Annual interpretive volume measures (total, screening, diagnostic, and screening focus [ratio of screening to diagnostic mammograms]) were collected for 120 radiologists in the Breast Cancer Surveillance Consortium (BCSC) who interpreted 783 965 screening mammograms from 2002 to 2006. Volume measures in 1 year were examined by using multivariate logistic regression relative to screening sensitivity, false-positive rates, and cancer detection rate the next year. BCSC registries and the Statistical Coordinating Center received institutional review board approval for active or passive consenting processes and a Federal Certificate of Confidentiality and other protections for participating women, physicians, and facilities. All procedures were compliant with the terms of the Health Insurance Portability and Accountability Act.

Results.—Mean sensitivity was 85.2% (95% confidence interval [CI]: 83.7%, 86.6%) and was significantly lower for radiologists with a greater screening focus ($P = .023$) but did not significantly differ by total ($P = .47$), screening ($P=.33$), or diagnostic ($P=.23$) volume. The mean false-positive rate was 9.1% (95% CI: 8.1%, 10.1%), with rates significantly higher for radiologists who had the lowest total ($P=.008$) and screening ($P=.015$) volumes. Radiologists with low diagnostic volume ($P=.004$ and $P=.008$) and a greater screening focus ($P=.003$ and $P=.002$) had significantly lower false-positive and cancer detection rates, respectively. Median invasive tumor size and proportion of cancers detected at early stages did not vary by volume.

Conclusion.—Increasing minimum interpretive volume requirements in the United States while adding a minimal requirement for diagnostic interpretation could reduce the number of false-positive work-ups without hindering cancer detection. These results provide detailed associations between mammography volumes and performance for policymakers to consider along with workforce, practice organization, and access issues and radiologist experience when reevaluating requirements.

▶ Does practice make perfect? Or at least, do radiologists with high volumes perform better than those with lower volumes in screening mammography? The answer, as you might imagine, is not so clear-cut as we would like to believe. This study, looking at 120 mammographers, did show that radiologists with higher annual volumes had clinically and statistically significantly lower false-positive rates with similar sensitivities as their colleagues with lower volumes. Radiologists with a greater screening focus had significantly lower sensitivities and cancer detection rates and significantly lower false-positive rates. However, there was considerable variability in that performance across radiologists within volume levels had wide, unexplained variability, reinforcing the ideas that the volume-performance relationship is complex and may be influenced by several factors. Screening performance is unlikely to be affected by volume alone but rather by a balance in the interpreted examination composition.

A. D. Elster, MD

A Comparison of Follow-Up Recommendations by Chest Radiologists, General Radiologists, and Pulmonologists Using Computer-Aided Detection to Assess Radiographs for Actionable Pulmonary Nodules
Meziane M, Obuchowski NA, Lababede O, et al (Cleveland Clinic Foundation, OH)
AJR Am J Roentgenol 196:W542-W549, 2011

Objective.—The primary objective of our study was to compare the effect of a chest radiography computer-aided detection (CAD) system on the follow-up recommendations of chest radiologists, general radiologists, and pulmonologists.

Materials and Methods.—A chest radiography CAD system (Rapid-Screen 1.1) that has been approved by the U.S. Food and Drug Administration (FDA) and a second-generation version of the system (OnGuard 3.0) not yet approved by the FDA were applied to single frontal radiographs of 200 patients at high risk for lung cancer. One hundred patients had actionable nodules (mean size, 16.9 mm) and 100 patients did not. Six chest radiologists, six general radiologists, and six pulmonologists independently interpreted each image first without CAD and then with CAD during blinded reading sessions. The frequency with which readers correctly referred patients for follow-up tests was measured. Differential effects based on nodule size, shape, location, density, and subtlety were tested with multiple-variable logistic regression.

Results.—For patients without actionable lesions, pulmonologists showed an increase in their recommendations for follow-up from 0.46 unaided to 0.52 with CAD ($p = 0.001$), whereas chest and general radiologists had much lower average rates and were not affected by CAD's false marks (0.26 without CAD vs 0.25 with RapidScreen 1.1 and 0.26 with OnGuard 3.0, $p \geq 0.734$). CAD improved all readers' detection of moderately subtle lesions ($p = 0.013$) but did not significantly increase follow-up rates overall for patients with actionable nodules (0.63 unaided vs 0.63 with RapidScreen 1.1, $p = 0.795$; and 0.63 unaided vs 0.64 with OnGuard 3.0, $p = 0.187$).

Conclusion.—The effect of CAD on readers' clinical decisions varies depending on the training of the reader. CAD did not improve the performance of chest or general radiologists. Nonradiologists are particularly vulnerable to CAD's false-positive marks.

▶ Can a computer-assisted diagnosis (CAD) program allow a nonradiologist to perform as well as or better than a radiologist at correctly identifying pulmonary nodules? At least with the current version of technology, according to this article, the answer is no.

Previous studies have found that thoracic CAD improves the diagnostic accuracy of all radiology readers, with larger improvements for less-experienced readers. To my knowledge, this is the first study in which pulmonologists were included. What was interesting was that pulmonologists were negatively affected by CAD, succumbing to CAD's high propensity for identifying questionable lesions. Chest and general radiologists generally had no difficulty in dismissing false marks and maintaining their unaided follow-up rate.

A. D. Elster, MD

The Relative Effect of Vendor Variability in CT Perfusion Results: A Method Comparison Study
Zussman BM, Boghosian G, Gorniak RJ, et al (Thomas Jefferson Univ Hosp, Philadelphia, PA; et al)
AJR Am J Roentgenol 197:468-473, 2011

Objective.—There are known interoperator, intraoperator, and inter-vendor software differences that can influence the reproducibility of quantitative CT perfusion values. The purpose of this study was to determine the relative impact of operator and software differences in CT perfusion variability.

Materials and Methods.—CT perfusion imaging data were selected for 11 patients evaluated for suspected ischemic stroke. Three radiologists each independently postprocessed the source data twice, using four different vendor software applications. Results for cerebral blood volume (CBV), cerebral blood flow (CBF), and mean transit time (MTT) were recorded for the lentiform nuclei in both hemispheres. Repeated variables multivariate analysis of variance was used to assess differences in the means of CBV, CBF, and MTT. Bland-Altman analysis was used to assess agreement between pairs of vendors, readers, and read times.

Results.—Choice of vendor software, but not interoperator or intraoperator disagreement, was associated with significant variability ($p < 0.001$) in CBV, CBF, and MTT. The mean difference in CT perfusion values was greater for pairs of vendors than for pairs of operators.

Conclusion.—Different vendor software applications do not generate quantitative perfusion results equivalently. Intervendor difference is, by far, the largest cause of variability in perfusion results relative to interoperator and intraoperator difference. Caution should be exercised when interpreting quantitative CT perfusion results because these values may vary considerably depending on the postprocessing software (Fig 1A).

▶ This is a very important article, with both practical and philosophical implications. It teaches a lesson that sophisticated measurement software from different vendors may produce significantly different results.

We don't have to worry about simple measurements (such as distance, angles, or Hounsfield units). Here we can rest assured that the standard software from various CT vendors is quite consistent and reliable.

What we need to worry about are more complicated and sophisticated measurements such as perfusion, mean transit time, and cerebral blood volume, which are derived from complex models and may give dramatically different results.

Four software packages were used to compute 3 commonly used parameters in the assessment of stroke: Brain Perfusion, Extended Brilliance Workspace,

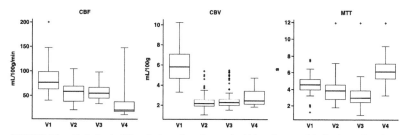

FIGURE 1A —Variation in CT perfusion values. Box-and-whisker plots graphically depict data; bottom and top of each box represent lower and upper quartiles, respectively, and band near middle of box is median. Ends of whiskers represent one SD above and below mean of data, and outliers are plotted as small dots. CBF = cerebral blood flow reported in mL/100 g/min, CBV = cerebral blood volume reported in mL/100 g, MTT = mean transit time reported in seconds, V = vendor, O = observer. A, Box-and-whisker plots show values obtained by vendor. (Reprinted from Zussman BM, Boghosian G, Gorniak RJ, et al. The relative effect of vendor variability in CT perfusion results: a method comparison study. *AJR Am J Roentgenol.* 2011;197:468-473, with permission from American Journal of Roentgenology.)

version 3.5, Philips Healthcare; CT Perfusion, version 4.3, GE Healthcare; Vitrea, version 2, Vital Images; and Aquarius Workstation, version 3.5, TeraRecon.

The results are shown graphically in Fig 1A. A large variation is easily appreciated, ranging from 50% to 300%. Because such measurements at many centers are now used to determine triage to intra-arterial thrombolysis, we should all think twice before relying just on the measurements we obtain from our workstations.

A. D. Elster, MD

T1 Pseudohyperintensity on Fat-Suppressed Magnetic Resonance Imaging: A Potential Diagnostic Pitfall
Huynh TN, Johnson T, Poder L, et al (Univ of California San Francisco)
J Comput Assist Tomogr 35:459-461, 2011

Magnetic resonance imaging findings in 2 patients with misleading T1 hyperintensity seen only on fat-suppressed images are presented; one with a renal cell carcinoma that was misinterpreted as a hemorrhagic cyst and the other with an ovarian serous cystadenocarcinoma that was misinterpreted as a complicated endometrioma. The apparent T1 hyperintensity on fat-suppressed images in these cases was likely due to varying perception of image signal dependent on local contrast, an optical effect known as the checker-shadow illusion. T1 pseudohyperintensity should be considered when apparently high T1 signal intensity is seen only on fat-suppressed images; review of non—fat-suppressed images may help prevent an erroneous diagnoses of blood-containing lesions (Figs 1 and 2).

▶ Although consisting of only a couple of case reports, this article deserves some mention because it points out how an interesting and little-known optical illusion, the "checker-shadow effect," (Fig 1) may lead to a spurious diagnosis

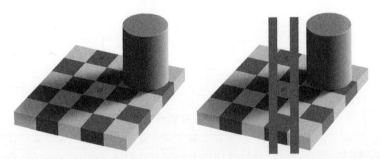

FIGURE 1.—Checker-shadow illusion. On the image to the left, the 2 squares marked A and B are the same shade of gray, although square B appears whiter. On the right, only after connecting the 2 squares does this become obvious. Images were reproduced from http://web.mit.edu/persci/people/adelson/checkershadow_illusion.html. Images may be reproduced and distributed freely. (Reprinted from Huynh TN, Johnson T, Poder L, et al. T1 pseudohyperintensity on fat-suppressed magnetic resonance imaging: a potential diagnostic pitfall. *J Comput Assist Tomogr.* 2011;35:459-461, with permission from Lippincott Williams & Wilkins.)

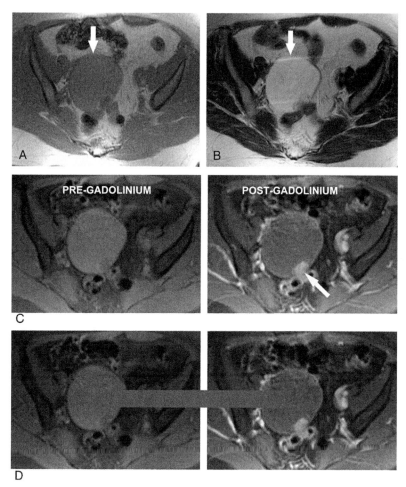

FIGURE 2.—A, Axial T1-weighted MR image in a 56-year-old woman with abdominal pain showing a cystic right ovarian mass (arrow) with mural nodularity. B, Axial T2-weighted MR image demonstrating a cystic mass (arrow) of fluid signal intensity with mural nodularity. C, Photomontage of axial fat-suppressed T1-weighted gradient echo images before (left side of montage) and after (right side of montage) the administration of gadolinium. The adnexal mass on pregadolinium imaging appears of high T1 signal intensity, although this is much less apparent on the postgadolinium image. A mural nodule (arrow) is visible, and the possibility of malignancy arising in a preexisting endometrioma was raised because of the combination of an apparently bright T1 cystic lesion with a mural nodule. D, Same photomontage as B but with the addition of a rectangle that is the same shade of gray as the adnexal mass on pregadolinium images. This demonstrates that the lesion is essentially the same color on both images, and the apparent high T1 signal intensity on pregadolinium imaging is artifactual. (Reprinted from Huynh TN, Johnson T, Poder L, et al. T1 pseudohyperintensity on fat-suppressed magnetic resonance imaging: a potential diagnostic pitfall. *J Comput Assist Tomogr.* 2011;35:459-461, with permission from Lippincott Williams & Wilkins.)

of hyperintensity on fat-suppressed magnetic resonance imaging scans. Potentially, this may lead to the erroneous diagnosis of hemorrhage.

In one case (an ovarian cystadenoma), the fluid content of the cyst appeared of moderately high T1 signal intensity on pregadolinium fat-suppressed

T1-weighted images (Fig 2), mimicking hemorrhage, not confirmed at autopsy. In retrospect, the "checker-shadow illusion" made the contents appear artificially hyperintense.

A. D. Elster, MD

Trends in the Utilization of CT Angiography and MR Angiography of the Head and Neck in the Medicare Population
Friedman DP, Levin DC, Rao VM (Jefferson Med College and Thomas Jefferson Univ Hosp, Philadelphia, PA)
J Am Coll Radiol 7:854-858, 2010

Purpose.—The aim of this study was to analyze trends in the utilization of CT angiography (CTA) and MR angiography (MRA) of the head and neck in the Medicare population over a 6-year interval.

Methods.—Nationwide Medicare Part B fee-for-service databases were reviewed. Current Procedural Terminology® codes for CTA and MRA of the head and neck were selected. MRA codes included studies without contrast, with contrast, and without and with contrast. Yearly and aggregate procedure volumes were compared for each Current Procedural Terminology code and modality. Data were also analyzed regarding contrast utilization and cost.

Results.—From 2002 to 2007, the volume of head CTA increased by 827%, and the overall volume of head MRA increased by 39%. The year-to-year percentage increase in overall volume of head MRA declined throughout the study period; almost all of the increase in the overall volume of head MRA occurred from 2002 to 2005. The volume of neck CTA increased by 1,074%, and the overall volume of neck MRA increased by 31%. An 18% decrease in the volume of neck MRA without contrast was offset by a 104% increase in the volume of neck MRA using contrast. The year-to-year percentage increase in the overall volume of neck MRA declined from 2002 to 2005; there was a decrease in volume of 3% from 2005 to 2007. From 2002 to 2007, when considering all study types, procedure volume increased by 71%; aggregate allowable charges increased by $181 million. Examinations using contrast increased by 235%. In 2002, 23% of examinations used contrast; in 2007, 46% of examinations used contrast.

Conclusions.—The rate of growth for head and neck CTA was dramatically higher than for MRA. Neck MRA using contrast also showed substantial growth. The Medicare population is now receiving more contrast material and radiation to noninvasively assess the arterial vasculature of the head and neck (Table 3).

▶ This article perhaps comes as no surprise to those involved in cerebrovascular imaging, who have witnessed their workload skyrocket over the last decade.

TABLE 3.—Aggregate Procedure Volumes, 2002 vs 2007

Study Type	Year 2002	2007	% Change 2002-2007
Head CTA	8,987	83,297	827%
All head MRA	272,387	377,820	39%
All head examinations	281,374	461,117	64%
Neck CTA	9,796	115,021	1,074%
All neck MRA	192,653	253,170	31%
All neck examinations	202,449	368,191	82%
All CTA	18,783	198,318	956%
Duplex ultrasound	2,533,820	3,038,905	20%
Catheter angiography	234,160	159,006	−32%

Technical advances have no doubt fueled the marked growth of neck CT angiography (CTA) and MR angiography (MRA). The images rival and may even surpass the very best catheter angiography by the 3-dimensional perspective they provide. Unfortunately, the database ends in 2007, but few would doubt that the trends continue into 2012. As shown in Table 3, carotid ultrasound scan also increased 20% in volume during the period, but catheter angiography declined by 32%.

The data also raise some interesting but unanswered questions, including whether this increase in advanced neurovascular imaging has resulted in improved patient outcomes, and how many fewer patients avoided complications because they did not need to undergo catheter angiography. At the same time, the increased dose of contrast needed may have subjected these patients to other complications, including contrast extravasation injuries and contrast-induced nephropathy. These questions and others will need to be addressed in the current economic climate as insurers and health care economists will demand to know what gains are being achieved for the increase in cost.

A. D. Elster, MD

Medical Economics

Medicare Payments for Noninvasive Diagnostic Imaging Are Now Higher to Nonradiologist Physicians Than to Radiologists

Levin DC, Rao VM, Parker L, et al (Thomas Jefferson Univ Hosp and Jefferson Med College, Philadelphia, PA; et al)
J Am Coll Radiol 8:26-32, 2011

Purpose.—Radiologists have always been considered the physicians who "control" noninvasive diagnostic imaging (NDI) and are primarily responsible for its growth. Yet nonradiologists have become increasingly aggressive in their performance and interpretation of imaging. The purpose of this study was to track overall Medicare payments to radiologists and nonradiologist physicians in recent years.

Methods.—The Medicare Part B files covering all fee-for-service physician payments for 1998 to 2008 were the data source. All codes for discretionary NDI were selected. Procedures mandated by the patient's clinical condition (eg, supervision and interpretation codes for interventional procedures, radiation therapy planning) were excluded, as were nonimaging radionuclide tests. Medicare physician specialty codes were used to identify radiologists and nonradiologists. Payments in all places of service were included. Overall Medicare NDI payments to radiologists and nonradiologist physicians from 1998 through 2008 were compared. A separate analysis of NDI payments to cardiologists was conducted, because next to radiologists, they are the highest users of imaging.

Results.—In 1998, overall Part B payments to radiologists for discretionary NDI were $2.563 billion, compared with $2.020 billion to nonradiologists (ie, radiologists' payments were 27% higher). From 1998 to 2006, payments to nonradiologists increased by 166%, compared with 107% to radiologists. By 2006, payments to nonradiologists exceeded those to radiologists. By 2008, the second year after implementation of the Deficit Reduction Act, payments to radiologists had dropped by 13%, compared with 11% to nonradiologists. In 2008, nonradiologists received $4.807 billion for discretionary NDI, and radiologists received $4.638 billion. Payments to cardiologists for NDI increased by 195% from 1998 to 2006, then dropped by 8% by 2008.

Conclusions.—The growth in fee-for-service payments to nonradiologists for NDI was considerably more rapid than the growth for radiologists between 1998 and 2006. Then, by the end of 2008, 2 years after the implementation of the Deficit Reduction Act, steeper revenue losses had been experienced by radiologists. The result was that by 2008, overall

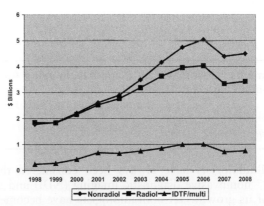

FIGURE 4.—Medicare Part B approved payments for discretionary noninvasive diagnostic imaging in outpatients; this includes both hospital outpatient facilities and private offices. Nonradiol = nonradiologist physicians, radiol = radiologists, IDTF/multi = independent diagnostic testing facilities and multispecialty groups. (Reprinted from Levin DC, Rao VM, Parker L, et al. Medicare payments for noninvasive diagnostic imaging are now higher to nonradiologist physicians than to radiologists. *J Am Coll Radiol.* 2011;8:26-32, Copyright 2011, with permission from American College of Radiology.)

Medicare fee-for-service payments for NDI were 4% higher to nonradiologists than they were to radiologists (Fig 4).

▶ The rapid growth in spending for diagnostic imaging over the past decade has captured the attention of not only insurance companies but government leaders and policy makers as well. It has tacitly been assumed or inferred that radiologists exert primary "control" over imaging, and their actions are driving this phenomenon. Conversely, many radiologists believe that self-referral by nonradiologist physicians is the major cause of the problem. This article by Levin and colleagues, part of a large corpus of work in health policy research, may help clarify certain trends and responsibilities in this debate.

The attached figure from their article (Fig 4) compares payments to radiologists and nonradiologist physicians over the 10-year study period. In 1998, the 2 groups started at comparable levels of reimbursement. These trend lines began to diverge and cross over in 2003, and by 2006, nonradiologists received 25% more reimbursement for outpatient diagnostic imaging than radiologists.

Additionally, after 2006, nonradiologists experienced proportionally less of a loss of revenue than radiologists (an 11% drop for the former and a 15% drop for the latter). This trend may be explained by the fact that the large majority of imaging examinations performed by nonradiologist physicians are done in their offices, for which they receive either a global or a technical component payment. Conversely, most examinations by radiologists are performed in hospital settings, for which they receive only the much lower professional component reimbursement.

It should be noted that during this period, the number of imaging studies performed at independent diagnostic testing facilities (IDTFs) markedly increased. Although the ownership of such entities cannot be determined by the Medicare database, evidence suggests that the majority of IDTFs nationwide have radiologist partners. Thus, allowing for IDTFs, it may be that radiologists may not have been quite so disadvantaged during the period as this study suggests.

A. D. Elster, MD

Radiation Safety

CT Radiation Dose: What Can You Do Right Now in Your Practice?
Coakley FV, Gould R, Yeh BM, et al (Univ of California San Francisco)
AJR Am J Roentgenol 196:619-625, 2011

Objective.—The purpose of this article is to review reasonable measures that community radiologists can realistically implement as a response to the current increased public concern regarding CT radiation risk.

Conclusion.—Potential measures include provision of patient information material, review of CT protocols and indications, promotion of alternative studies, use of decision support software, automatic tube current modulation, bismuth shields, improved image reconstruction algorithms, empowerment of technologists to adjust protocols, and calculation of radiation dose for possible reporting.

▶ This 6-page paper is an "easy read" and one that neatly summarizes several concepts about radiation dose at CT and what you can do to reduce exposure for your patients.

Most of the suggestions will come as no surprise, such as suggesting alternative imaging strategies such as MRI or ultrasound, employing decision support software (to reduce the number of unnecessary or poorly indicated exams), and reviewing CT protocols. At least 1 suggestion (employing bismuth shields) is highly controversial and not endorsed by many radiologists and physicists. The overall intent of the article is good, however.

From the technical dimension, reducing maximum tube potential (kVp) and using tube current (mA) modulation are important. Using better reconstruction algorithms (such as iterative methods) can reduce dose by up to 40% with little or no loss in image quality.

Finally, and perhaps most important, is the suggestion of empowering technologists to adjust the protocols dynamically as they monitor studies and record radiation exposure. Because technologists are at the front line of many technical decisions, their input and continued surveillance of the process of dose reduction is a key to success.

A. D. Elster, MD

Short-Term and Long-Term Health Risks of Nuclear-Power-Plant Accidents
Christodouleas JP, Forrest RD, Ainsley CG, et al (Univ of Pennsylvania, Philadelphia)
N Engl J Med 364:2334-2341, 2011

On March 11, 2011, A 9.0-magnitude earthquake struck the east coast of Japan. The total number of people who died in the earthquake and the tsunami that it generated is still being assessed, but the official estimation already exceeds 14,000. The natural disaster also caused substantial damage to the Fukushima Daiichi nuclear power plant, the consequences of which are still unclear. The purpose of this review is to put the emergency at the Japanese power plant, even as it is evolving, into the context of the extensive literature on nuclear reactor accidents by analyzing the mechanisms and major short-term and long-term health risks of radiation exposure. In addition, we briefly discuss the accidents at Three Mile Island in Pennsylvania in 1979 and at Chernobyl in Ukraine in 1986 because they illustrate the broad range of potential outcomes (Table 3).

▶ This is a short (8-page) review article concerning radiation injury and exposure of populations near 3 nuclear power plants where meltdowns or partial meltdowns have occurred: at the Fukushima Daiichi plant (Japan) in 2011, at Chernobyl (Ukraine) in 1986, and at Three Mile Island (US) in 1979.

TABLE 3.—Signs and Symptoms of Acute Radiation Sickness in the Three Phases after Exposure*

Prodrome, According to Exposure Level	Latency[†]	Illness[‡]
Mild (1 to 2 Gy)		
Vomiting; onset, 2 hr	Duration, 21–35 days; lymphocyte count, 800 −1500/mm^3	Fatigue, weakness; mortality, 0%
Moderate (2 to 4 Gy)		
Vomiting, mild headache; onset, 1–2 hr	Duration, 18–35 days; lymphocyte count, 500 −800/mm^3	Fever, infections, bleeding, weakness, epilation; mortality, ≤50%
Severe (4 to 6 Gy)		
Vomiting, mild diarrhea, moderate headache, fever; onset, <1 hr	Duration, 8–18 days; lymphocyte count, 300 to 500/mm^3	High fever, infections, bleeding, epilation; mortality, 20–70%
Very severe (6 to 8 Gy)		
Vomiting, severe diarrhea, severe headache, high fever, altered consciousness; onset, <30 min	Duration, ≤7 days; lymphocyte count, 100 to 300/mm^3	High fever, diarrhea, vomiting, dizziness, disorientation, hypotension; mortality, 50–100%
Lethal (>8 Gy)		
Vomiting, severe diarrhea, severe headache, high fever, unconsciousness; onset, <10 min	No latency; lymphocyte count, 0 to 100/mm^3	High fever, diarrhea, unconsciousness; mortality, 100%

Editor's Note: Please refer to original journal article for full references.
*Data are adapted from the International Atomic Energy Agency.[20]
[†]Lymphocyte counts in the latency phase represent the range of values that may be seen 3 to 6 days after radiation exposure.
[‡]Mortality estimates are for patients who do not receive medical intervention.

Three Mile Island was the mildest of the 3 disasters; the plant's containment structure fulfilled its purpose, and only a minimal amount of radiation was released. No definitive identifiable health effects have been identified. The Chernobyl reactor was built without a containment structure, and upon meltdown a giant plume of radioactive material was released into the atmosphere. At least 28 deaths related to radiation exposure occurred the year after the accident, and the long-term effects on the nearby populations with exposure to iodine-131 and cesium isotopes have shown an increase in thyroid cancers and leukemia. Data from Fukushima are not yet fully in but will likely result in a population exposure intermediate between Three Mile Island and Chernobyl. The radiation effects of Fukushima, however, are dwarfed by the loss of over 14 000 people from the tsunami itself.

The article contains a nice review of the stages of radiation sickness (Table 3) as well as a discussion about the differentiation between radiation dose, measured by the gray (Gy), and absorbed radiation dose, measured in the unit of the sievert (Sv).

A. D. Elster, MD

Risk of Radiation-induced Breast Cancer from Mammographic Screening

Yaffe MJ, Mainprize JG (Univ of Toronto, Ontario, Canada)

Radiology 258:98-105, 2010

Purpose.—To assess a schema for estimating the risk of radiation-induced breast cancer following exposure of the breast to ionizing radiation as would occur with mammography and to provide data that can be used to estimate the potential number of breast cancers, cancer deaths, and woman-years of life lost attributable to radiation exposure delivered according to a variety of screening scenarios.

Materials and Methods.—An excess absolute risk model was used to predict the number of radiation-induced breast cancers attributable to the radiation dose received for a single typical digital mammography examination. The algorithm was then extended to consider the consequences of various scenarios for routine screening beginning and ending at different ages, with examinations taking place at 1- or 2-year intervals. A life-table correction was applied to consider reductions of the cohort size over time owing to non-radiation-related causes of death. Finally, the numbers of breast cancer deaths and woman-years of life lost that might be attributable to the radiation exposure were calculated. Cancer incidence and cancer deaths were estimated for individual attained ages following the onset of screening, and lifetime risks were also calculated.

Results.—For a cohort of 100 000 women each receiving a dose of 3.7 mGy to both breasts and who were screened annually from age 40 to 55 years and biennially thereafter to age 74 years, it is predicted that there will be 86 cancers induced and 11 deaths due to radiation-induced breast cancer.

Conclusion.—For the mammographic screening regimens considered that begin at age 40 years, this risk is small compared with the expected mortality reduction achievable through screening. The risk of radiation-induced breast cancer should not be a deterrent from mammographic screening of women over the age of 40 years.

▶ This article is significant because it contradicts estimates made by Berrington de González and Reeves[1] from 2005 that mammographic screening of women before age 50 is not beneficial because of the risk of radiation-induced cancers generated. These earlier investigators from the United Kingdom calculated that such cancers would occur at the rate of about 50 in 100 000 women screened (vs 7.6 in 100 000 in the current article). Why such a difference in estimates? First, the earlier UK investigators had a higher dose per examination, reflecting film-screen mammography techniques. Second, they used an excessive relative risk model. Finally, in their analysis, survival for breast cancer was lower than that now being observed in North American women. This difference in survival may be related to differences in the size and stage of cancers detected: In the United Kingdom, a screening interval of 3 years is often used, whereas in North America, women are typically screened annually.

Perhaps this simply adds to the confusion of women and radiologists to know which guidelines to follow. However, for Yaffe and Mainprize (and for me), it appears the benefit of early screening mammography far exceeds the theoretical risks, or is at least beneficial enough to warrant its use.

A. D. Elster, MD

Reference

1. Berrington de González A, Reeves G. Mammographic screening before age 50 years in the UK: comparison of the radiation risks with the mortality benefits. *Br J Cancer.* 2005;93:590-596.

ACR Dose Index Registry

Morin RL, Coombs LP, Chatfield MB (Mayo Clinic Florida, Jacksonville; American College of Radiology, Reston, VA)
J Am Coll Radiol 8:288-291, 2011

The potential risks associated with radiation exposure from medical imaging have received considerable attention in the media recently. In a desire to improve safety, efforts to reduce radiation exposure to appropriate levels are being made by organizations and facilities across the country and the world. But what is the "appropriate" level of radiation for a given examination? In fact, what is the national average level of radiation that is currently being administered by imaging facilities for a particular examination, for example, a CT scan of the head? The answer to this question is not known; but this is precisely the type of question for which the ACR Dose Index Registry (DIR) soon hopes to provide insight.

▶ This report describes the design and testing of a new service/product for the American College of Radiology (ACR), the ACR Dose Index Registry (DIR). The phase II portion of the pilot project reported herein is now complete, and the ACR DIR was rolled out officially in May 2011. The idea is simple and potentially very useful—to allow facilities to compare their CT dose indices with those of peer facilities and to national standards. Information related to dose indices for all CT examinations will be collected, anonymized, transmitted to the ACR, and stored in a database. Institutions will then be provided with periodic feedback reports comparing their results by body part and examination type with aggregate results.

The overall success of this project will require facilities to take the time to interface their equipment and send data to the national registry. ACR's Peer-View started out in a similar fashion, and if this will serve as the prototype, we can expect it will take a few years before there is enough momentum to make the database usable and sustainable. It is an excellent project of which all institutions should consider becoming a part.

A. D. Elster, MD

Adult patient radiation doses from non-cardiac CT examinations: a review of published results

Pantos I, Thalassinou S, Argentos S, et al (Univ of Athens, Greece)
Br J Radiol 84:293-303, 2011

Objectives.—CT is a valuable tool in diagnostic radiology but it is also associated with higher patient radiation doses compared with planar radiography. The aim of this article is to review patient dose for the most common types of CT examinations reported during the past 19 years.

Methods.—Reported dosimetric quantities were compared with the European diagnostic reference levels (DRLs). Effective doses were assessed with respect to the publication year and scanner technology (*i.e.*, single-slice *vs* multislice).

Results.—Considerable variation of reported values among studies was attributed to variations in both examination protocol and scanner design. Median weighted CT dose index (CTDIw) and dose length product (DLP) are below the proposed DRLs; however, for individual studies the DRLs are exceeded. Median reported effective doses for the most frequent CT examinations were: head, 1.9 mSv (0.3—8.2 mSv); chest, 7.5 mSv (0.3—26.0 mSv); abdomen, 7.9 mSv (1.4—31.2 mSv); and pelvis, 7.6 mSv (2.5—36.5 mSv).

Conclusion.—The introduction of mechanisms for dose reduction resulted in significantly lower patient effective doses for CT examinations of the head, chest and abdomen reported by studies published after 1995. Owing to the limited number of studies reporting patient doses for multislice CT examinations the statistical power to detect differences with single-slice scanners is not yet adequate.

▶ This is a nice review of concepts in dosimetry as well as a survey of expected doses patients receive when undergoing noncardiac CT scans in modern facilities. I particularly liked the introductory section, which gave a good review (with a few equations, but not terrible ones) about the ways dose is measured.

In the modern era, with emphasis on radiation dose and cancer risk, all radiologists need to be familiar with these terms. Radiation exposure in CT is calculated differently and has a meaning different from radiation exposure in conventional radiography. So, if you don't know the difference between the CTDI (CT dose index) and the DLP (dose-length product), or between the "organ dose" and the "effective dose," you need to read this article.

A. D. Elster, MD

Frequent Body CT Scanning of Young Adults: Indications, Outcomes, and Risk for Radiation-Induced Cancer
Zondervan RL, Hahn PF, Sadow CA, et al (Massachusetts General Hosp, Boston)
J Am Coll Radiol 8:501-507, 2011

Purpose.—The aims of this study were to define the magnitude of frequent body CT scanning of young adults and to determine associated patient diagnoses, examination indications, short-term outcomes, and estimated radiation-induced cancer risk.

Methods.—Patients aged 18 to 35 years who underwent chest or abdominopelvic CT between 2003 and 2007 at any of 3 hospitals were identified and categorized by total number of scans per body part as rarely (<5), intermediately (>5 and <15), or frequently (>15) scanned. Medical records of the frequently scanned were reviewed. Cumulative radiation exposure, calculated from typical effective doses, was used to estimate cancer risk. Cancer incidence and mortality were estimated using the Biological Effects of Ionizing Radiation method.

Results.—A total of 25,104 patients underwent 45,632 scans, of whom 23,851 (95%) and 70 (0.3%) were rarely and frequently scanned, respectively. Among frequently scanned patients, the most common diagnoses were cancer (19 of 36 [52.8%]) and cystic fibrosis with lung transplantation (11 of 36 [30.5%]) for chest CT and cancer (25 of 34 [73.5%]) for abdominopelvic CT. During the mean 5.4 years (range, 0.9-7.6 years) of follow-up, 46% of frequently scanned patients (32 of 70) died. Of the 47 cancers predicted in the entire cohort, 36 (77%) and 2 (3%) were expected in the rarely and frequently scanned.

Conclusions.—The majority of CT-induced cancers are predicted to result from sporadic rather than frequent scanning. Frequent scanning confers a significant cancer risk but occurs in severely ill patients, a large proportion of whom die before any radiation-induced cancer would be a factor in their health (Fig 1).

▶ Reducing the exposure of patients to ionizing radiation from imaging procedures, especially CT, has been a major focus of the radiology community for the last several years. Special and justifiable attention has been directed to the pediatric population, but all age groups are at risk. This article focuses on a special group of young adult patients who may be at particular risk—those between 18 and 35 years who receive multiple/repeated CTs of the chest, abdomen, and pelvis over a limited time period.

In the 25 000 + patient cohort studied, the number of patients and number of multiple examinations were staggering. Fig 1 shows these results, and you will be amazed at the number of patients receiving 10, 15, or even 20 CT examinations over the study period.

The majority of young adults who undergo frequent body CT scanning (average, 0.3 examinations per year) carry a diagnosis of locally advanced or metastatic cancer, have undergone transplantation, or both. About half of this

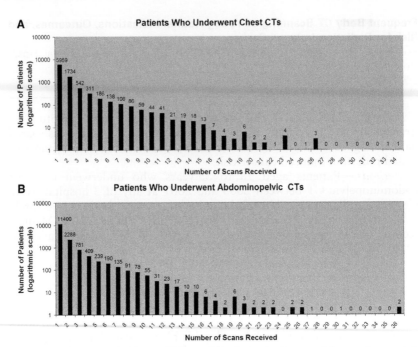

FIGURE 1.—Frequency distribution of CT scans obtained per patient in young adults over a 5-year period for the chest (A) and abdominopelvic (B) regions. (Reprinted from Zondervan RL, Hahn PF, Sadow CA, et al. Frequent body CT scanning of young adults: indications, outcomes, and risk for radiation-induced cancer. *J Am Coll Radiol.* 2011;8:501-507, Copyright 2011, with permission from American College of Radiology.)

population will die of their primary disease within a 5-year period. For those who survive, however, the lifetime risk of induced cancer may be at least 2%. Although this is a large percentage, considering the severity of these patients' diseases, and factoring in benefit versus risk, that may not be unreasonable.

Personally, I am more concerned about the less-ill subgroup of patients that are included in this study—those with urinary tract calculi who appear at our emergency room on a regular basis and undergo CT stone studies. Such patients can easily have a dozen or more CTs over a 5-year period, and though we use the lowest possible dose, they may still be at risk long term.

A. D. Elster, MD

Contrast Agents

Incidence of Nephrogenic Systemic Fibrosis after Adoption of Restrictive Gadolinium-based Contrast Agent Guidelines
Wang Y, Alkasab TK, Narin O, et al (Massachusetts General Hosp, Boston; et al)
Radiology 260:105-111, 2011

Purpose.—To retrospectively determine the incidence of nephrogenic systemic fibrosis (NSF) in a large academic medical center after the adoption of restrictive gadolinium-based contrast agent (GBCA) administration guidelines.

Materials and Methods.—For this retrospective HIPAA-compliant study, institutional review board approval was obtained and the requirement for informed consent was waived. Restrictive GBCA guidelines were adopted in May 2007. The guidelines *(a)* require a recent serum creatinine level measurement in any patient who is aged 60 years or older and/or at risk for renal disease, *(b)* limit the maximal weight-based GBCA dose administered to any patient with an estimated glomerular filtration rate (eGFR) lower than 60 mL/min/m^2 to 20 mL, and *(c)* prohibit the administration of any GBCA in patients who have an eGFR lower than 30 mL/min/m^2 and/or are undergoing chronic dialysis treatment (except in emergency situations). The electronic medical records were searched for all contrast material—enhanced magnetic resonance (MR) imaging examinations performed during the post—guidelines adoption period between January 2008 and March 2010 and the pre—guidelines adoption and transitional period between January 2002 and December 2007. Separate pathology records were searched for biopsy-confirmed cases of NSF during the same study periods. The incidences of NSF during the pre—guidelines adoption and transitional period and post—guidelines adoption period were compared by using the paired Z test.

Results.—A total of 52 954 contrast-enhanced MR examinations were performed during the post—guidelines adoption period. Of these 52 954 examinations, 46 464 (88%) were performed in adult patients with an eGFR of 60 mL/min/m^2 or higher or presumed normal renal function and 6454 (12%) were performed in patients with an eGFR of 30—59 mL/min/m^2. Thirty-six patients with an eGFR lower than 30 mL/min/m^2 underwent contrast-enhanced MR imaging for emergent indications. Review of the pathology records for January 2008 to September 2010 revealed no new cases of NSF resulting from GBCA exposure.

Conclusion.—After restrictive guidelines regarding GBCA administration were instituted, no new cases of NSF were identified among 52 954

TABLE 1.—GBCA Guidelines for Imaging Adult Patients, Based on Renal Disease Severity

Renal Disease Severity	Guideline
eGFR $\geq$ 60 mL/min/m^2	GBCA can be administered as indicated.
eGFR 30—59 mL/min/m^2	Weight-based dose of GBCA (0.2 mL/kg) can be administered, with maximal dose of 20 mL allowed within 24 hours.
eGFR < 30 mL/min/m^2	GBCA cannot be administered, except in cases of medical necessity. Informed patient consent is required.
	Nephrology consultation is required, preferentially before requested examination is performed.
	Hemodialysis should be considered; for patients already receiving dialysis treatment, dialysis should be performed promptly after the GBCA injection.

Note.—GBCA administration guidelines developed and used at the authors' institution are listed.

contrast-enhanced MR examinations, including those performed in patients with an eGFR lower than 60 mL/min/m² (Table 1).

▶ Nephrogenic systemic fibrosis (NSF) was perhaps the hottest topic for the YEAR BOOK OF RADIOLOGY for 2009. It was a disease largely created by radiologists and their zealous use of gadolinium-based contrast agents. Although the relationship between gadolinium exposure and NSF was first reported in 2006, it was not until May 2007 that the US Food and Drug Administration ordered a "black box warning" notifying physicians of the risk of this disorder. Many radiology departments had already modified their protocols before this warning, and the rest did shortly thereafter.

Fortunately, because of the response of the radiology community, this horrible disease is now largely history. In the current article, adoption of the American College of Radiology guidelines (Table 1) has effectively eliminated the disorder. Continued vigilance is required, but it looks as though we have nipped this one in the bud.

A. D. Elster, MD

Incidence of Immediate Gadolinium Contrast Media Reactions

Prince MR, Zhang H, Zou Z, et al (Cornell and Columbia Univs, NY)
AJR Am J Roentgenol 196:W138-W143, 2011

Objective.—Our objective was to determine the incidence of immediate adverse events for gadolinium-based contrast agents.

Materials and Methods.—All gadolinium-based contrast agent adverse events reported to radiology quality assurance committees were graded according to American College of Radiology criteria and divided by the total number of injections to determine incidence during the past 10 years. For each event, an age- and examination-matched control patient was identified to compare sex, weight, creatinine, eosinophil count, allergic history and gadolinium-based contrast agent dose differences. The U.S. Food and Drug Administration (FDA) Adverse Event Reporting System (AERS) database was analyzed to compare local experience to national trends.

Results.—Abdominal MRI had the highest rates of adverse events, 0.013% compared with brain (0.0045%, $p < 0.001$) or spine (0.0034%, $p < 0.001$). Adverse events were more likely in women, with a female to male ratio of 3.3, and in patients with history of prior allergic reactions ($p < 0.001$). Immediate adverse events rates were 0.2, 0.5, 1.2, and 3.3 per 1,000 injections for gadodiamide, gadopentetate dimeglumine, gadobenate dimeglumine, and gadoteridol, respectively. Gadobenate dimeglumine had more severe patient reactions, including three patients who arrested (defined as the patient becoming unresponsive and the code team being called), one of whom died. From 2004 to 2009, the FDA received reports on 40 gadolinium-based contrast agent U.S. deaths unrelated to nephrogenic systemic fibrosis, with an incidence per million doses of 0.15, 0.19,

TABLE 4.—Adverse Events in U.S. Reported to Food and Drug Administration from 2004 to 2009 (Excluding Nephrogenic Systemic Fibrosis)

Type of Chelate	GBCA Name	Doses in Millions	Events[a]	Excluding NSF (i.e., Anaphylaxis) Events[a]/Million	Deaths	Deaths/Million
Nonionic linear	Gadodiamide	13.5	63	4.7	2	0.15
	Gadoversetamide	5.4	45	8.3	1	0.19
	Gadopentetate dimeglumine	26	1616	62	25	0.97
Ionic linear	Gadoxetate	—	14	—	0	—
	Gadobenate	3.4	1097	322	9	2.7
Macrocyclic	Gadoteridol	2.8	139	49	2	0.70
Unspecified	Unspecified		75		1	
Total		51	3049	60	40	0.9

[a]Includes events with outcomes coded as death, life-threatening, disability, hospitalized, congenital, intervention required, and other. GBCA = gadolinium-based contrast agent. Dash (—) indicates not available.

0.97, 2.7, and 0.7 for gadodiamide, gadoversetimide, gadopentetate dimeglumine, gadobenate dimeglumine, and gadoteridol, respectively.

Conclusion.—This limited retrospective analysis shows that gadolinium-based contrast agents are very safe, with only rare reports of death, and raises the possibility that nonionic linear gadolinium-based contrast agents and gadopentetate dimeglumine may have fewer severe immediate adverse events compared with gadobenate dimeglumine (Table 4).

▶ Over the last five years, safety issues surrounding gadolinium have largely focused on reducing the incidence of nephrogenic systemic sclerosis, a potentially lethal skin and multiorgan disease associated with use of gadolinium-based contrast agents in patients with renal insufficiency. Because of vigilance of the radiologic community, nephrogenic systemic sclerosis has been largely eliminated and is no longer a cause of death or disability in patients undergoing contrast-enhanced magnetic resonance examinations. This causes us to refocus our attention to hypersensitivity reactions from these agents, which result in approximately 7 deaths in the United States each year.

This retrospective review of the 6 major gadolinium contrast agents in use in the United States tabulates the major adverse events reported to the US Food and Drug Administration over the period 2002 to 2007 (Table 4). These data show some very suggestive trends and differences among the agents. Perhaps the most telling statistic is the number of deaths per million doses, which ranges from a high of 2.7 for gadobenate to 0.15 for gadodiamide. The relatively higher death rate for gadobenate compared with gadopentetate confirms results from an article by Abujudeh et al from 2010.[1]

A. D. Elster, MD

Reference

1. Abujudeh HH, Kosaraju VK, Kaewlai R. Acute adverse reactions to gadopentetate dimeglumine and gadobenate dimeglumine: experience with 32,659 injections. *AJR Am J Roentgenol.* 2010;194:430-434.

Assessment of Adverse Reaction Rates during Gadoteridol-enhanced MR Imaging in 28078 Patients

Morgan DE, Spann JS, Lockhart ME, et al (Univ of Alabama at Birmingham)
Radiology 259:109-116, 2011

Purpose.—To determine adverse reaction rates in a tertiary care clinical setting after adoption of gadoteridol as the institutional routine magnetic resonance (MR) imaging contrast agent.

Materials and Methods.—With institutional review board approval, informed consent waiver, and HIPAA compliance, a prospective observational study of 28 078 patients who underwent intravenous gadoteridol-enhanced MR imaging from July 2007 to December 2009 was performed. Reactions were recorded by technologists who noted types of reactions, method of injection, and treatment. Reactions were classified as mild, moderate, or severe per American College of Radiology definitions. Comparisons of reaction rates with dose and method of injection were analyzed with the Fisher exact and χ^2 tests.

Results.—Overall reaction rate was 0.666% (187 patients), including 177 mild, six moderate, and four severe reactions. Treatment was given in 27 patients (14.4%). The most frequent reaction was nausea (and/or vomiting) in 149 patients (79.7% of patients with any adverse reaction, 0.530% of overall population). Method of injection did not affect reaction rate or severity. There was no difference in type or severity of reactions in comparison of patients receiving half the dose versus patients receiving the standard dose ($P = .33-.75$).

Conclusion.—The observed adverse reaction rate to gadoteridol was lower than previously reported. Specifically, the rate of nausea (0.530%) was less than half the rate (1.4%) in clinical trials of 1251 patients, leading to FDA approval in 1992. Rates of adverse reactions for this macrocyclic contrast agent are comparable to those published for linear gadolinium-based contrast agents.

▶ Gadolinium-based contrast agents have excellent safety profiles and are well tolerated by patients. Minor adverse reactions (such as nausea, vomiting, dizziness, or injection-site pain) occur with frequencies ranging from 0.07% to 2.4%. "Allergic-type" responses with rash, hives, urticaria, and/or bronchospasm occur at rates of 0.004% to 0.7%. Severe, life-threatening non-immunoglobulin E—mediated anaphylactic reactions are exceedingly rare, occurring less than 0.01% of the time.

Any time a newer contrast agent comes out, there is always a look-back period to see whether the reaction rates in practice correspond to those of the premarketing and postmarketing surveillance surveys. Often, the reported reaction rates are lower in this follow-up period. The "Weber effect" may explain this phenomenon, in that shortly after a new drug is introduced, considerable attention is directed to it and reactions may be overreported; years later, as interest fades, the adverse reaction rate may be underreported.

So, in this case, we have gadoteridol (which, by brand name is ProHance, made by Bracco Diagnostics), doing quite well on its late postmarketing surveillance survey. Although one can never be sure of the accuracy of the exact numbers reported, it does appear that this agent is well tolerated with an adverse reaction rate similar to most other gadolinium-containing agents.

A. D. Elster, MD

Incidence of Contrast-Induced Nephropathy in Patients With Multiple Myeloma Undergoing Contrast-Enhanced CT

Pahade JK, LeBedis CA, Raptopoulos VD, et al (Harvard Med School, Boston, MA)
AJR Am J Roentgenol 196:1094-1101, 2011

Objective.—The purpose of this article is to evaluate the incidence of contrast-induced nephropathy (CIN) and the effects of associated risk factors in patients with multiple myeloma undergoing contrast-enhanced CT (CECT) with IV administration of nonionic iodinated contrast agent.

Materials and Methods.—This retrospective review of medical records identified patients with a diagnosis of myeloma who underwent a CECT examination of the chest, abdomen, or pelvis between January 1, 2005, and December 1, 2008. Analysis for CIN, as defined by an increase in creatinine level after the CECT examination of 25% or more, or of 0.5 mg/dL, compared with the level before the CECT examination, both within 48 hours and within 7 days, was performed. Statistical correlations between the development of CIN and creatinine level before CECT examination, patient location, type and amount of contrast agent, blood urea nitrogen—creatinine ratio, history of diabetes, hypercalcemia, Bence Jones proteinuria, β_2-microglobulin level, albumin level, International Myeloma Staging System stage, and history of myeloma provided at the time the CT examination was ordered were calculated.

Results.—Forty-six patients who completed 80 unique examinations were included; their average creatinine level before CECT examination was 0.97 mg/dL. There was no significant difference in the average creatinine levels before CT examination between patients without and those with CIN. Four (5%) and 12 (15%) patients developed CIN within 48 hours and 7 days, respectively. Only serum β_2-microglobulin level showed a statistically significant ($p = 0.03$) correlation with the development of CIN.

Conclusion.—The incidence of CIN in patients with multiple myeloma with a normal creatinine level is low and correlates with β_2- microglobulin levels. The administration of contrast agent in this patient population is safe but should be based on the potential benefit of the examination and the expected low risk of developing CIN.

▶ Multiple myeloma has long been considered a relative contraindication to the administration of iodinated contrast secondary to the risk of contrast-induced nephropathy (CIN). However, nearly all of the studies documenting this risk were performed before the mid-1980s and were based on administration of high-osmolar contrast material. Does this risk still exist in the age of low-osmolar agents? And if so, what is this risk? If the risk still exists, can we possibly stratify the multiple myeloma population into lower- and higher-risk groups? Those are the critically important concepts this article seeks to answer.

Although there are a number of serious limitations of this study (retrospective review, no way to assess patient hydration status or concurrent infection, restriction of patient population to those with normal or minimally elevated creatinine levels precontrast), the overall rate of CIN was relatively low and compatible with the risk in patients with other forms of renal insufficiency.[1] The intriguing result that the risk of CIN in these patients correlates with serum β_2-microglobulin levels may be the most reliable indicator of whether a myeloma patient with normal or mildly impaired renal function should undergo an iodine-contrast enhanced procedure. Further research will be needed to confirm this finding, which could be quite useful in assessing risk.

A. D. Elster, MD

Reference

1. Cheruvu B, Henning K, Mulligan J, et al. Iodixanol: risk of subsequent contrast nephropathy in cancer patients with underlying renal insufficiency undergoing diagnostic computed tomography examinations. *J Comput Assist Tomogr.* 2007; 31:493-498.

Quality

Characteristics of Falls in a Large Academic Radiology Department: Occurrence, Associated Factors, Outcomes, and Quality Improvement Strategies
Abujudeh H, Kaewlai R, Shah B, et al (Massachusetts General Hosp, Boston, MA)
AJR Am J Roentgenol 197:154-159, 2011

Objective.—The objective of our study was to describe the characteristics of falls in a radiology department.

Materials and Methods.—The departmental incident report database was retrospectively searched for fall incidents that occurred from March 2006 through October 2008. During that period, 1,801,275 radiologic examinations were performed in our department and there were 82 falls, yielding an incidence of 0.46 per 10,000 examinations. We collected patient information, associated factors, specific circumstances surrounding each incident, the location of each incident, and patient outcome.

Results.—Eighty-two falls occurred involving 82 patients (35 males, 47 females; mean age, 58.2 years; range, 3—92 years): 66 falls (80%) involved outpatients; 11, inpatients; and five, visitors accompanying a patient. Radiography and CT-MRI units were the top two most common locations of falls (45/82, 55%). Thirty-six events (36/82, 44%) were directly related to a radiologic examination. Most falls were witnessed (61/82, 74%) and unassisted (50/82, 61%), and a majority occurred while the patient was standing or ambulating (59/82, 72%). Most patients (70/82, 85%) had at least one predisposing factor for falling. Sixteen patients (16/82, 20%) had fallen within the previous 3 months. Twenty-four falls (24/82, 29%) resulted in a documented injury (17 minor, seven moderate or severe) with one patient dying. Patients were more likely to be injured if they fell while ambulating ($p = 0.0257$, univariate analysis) or if they were taking antihypertensive medication ($p = 0.02$, multivariate analysis).

Conclusion.—Falls were uncommon in the radiology department studied; however, they can result in significant morbidity and mortality.

▶ Falls in a hospital are considered serious sentinel events and in recent years have attracted considerable scrutiny by the Joint Commission and other health care accrediting organizations. Most research about falls has been conducted in hospitalized or nursing home populations, so it is welcome that the authors of this study chose to review radiology department falls in both hospitalized and ambulatory patients.

The fall rate of 0.46 per 10 000 examinations is on par with our own experience, meaning that a busy department may easily have a dozen or more falls per year. About 29% of the radiology falls resulted in injury, 41% of which were considered moderate or severe.

There were no major surprises in who fell, as the same populations at risk identified in other inpatient studies were seen. These included advanced age, altered mental status, history of falls, and the use of certain medications (cerebral nervous system-acting, antihypertensives, and analgesics). The authors can only suggest that better communications among health care providers and identification of patients at risk for falls as methods for lowering the fall rate in radiology departments.

A. D. Elster, MD

Comparing the accuracy of initial head CT reporting by radiologists, radiology trainees, neuroradiographers and emergency doctors
Gallagher FA, Tay KY, Vowler SL, et al (Addenbrooke's Hosp, Cambridge, UK; Cancer Res UK Cambridge Res Inst, Cambridge; et al)
Br J Radiol 84:1040-1045, 2011

Objectives.—Demand for out-of-hours cranial CT imaging is increasing and some departments have considered addressing this shortfall by allowing non-radiologists to provisionally report imaging studies. The aim of this work was to assess whether it is appropriate for non-radiologists to report head CTs by comparing the misreporting rates of those who regularly report head CTs with two groups of non-radiologists who do not usually report them: neuroradiographers and emergency doctors.

Methods.—62 candidates were asked to report 30 head CTs, two-thirds of which were abnormal, and the results were compared by non-parametric statistical analysis.

Results.—There was no evidence of a difference in the score between neuroradiographers, neuroradiologists and general consultant radiologists. Neuroradiographers scored significantly higher than senior radiology trainees, and the emergency doctors scored least well.

Conclusion.—The results of this preliminary study show that appropriately trained neuroradiographers are competent at reporting the range of abnormalities assessed with this test and that their misreporting rates are similar to those who already independently report these studies.

▶ With increasing numbers of after-hours emergency head computed tomography (CT) scans, there is a natural concern regarding patient quality and safety as to the level of training appropriate to reliably diagnose the most common abnormalities. These authors set out to compare the abilities of neuroradiologists, general radiologists, senior-level radiology trainees, and emergency department physicians.

Each group of physicians reviewed 30 head CTs, 20 of which were abnormal. Typical abnormal cases included such diagnoses as isodense subdural hematomas, subarachnoid hemorrhage, acute cerebral infarction, dense middle cerebral artery sign, and neoplasm. The maximum possible score was 30. Fig 2 in the original article shows the results in graphical form.

No significant difference was noted among the general radiologists and neuroradiologists, but both scored somewhat higher than radiology trainees. The radiology trainees, in turn, scored better than the emergency medicine physicians. The findings confirm a widely held concept that general radiologists can perform at nearly an equivalent level to dedicated neuroradiologists when only a limited range of emergency diagnoses are considered.

A. D. Elster, MD

Distress in the Radiology Waiting Room

Flory N, Lang EV (Beth Israel Deaconess Med Ctr-Harvard Med School, Boston, MA)
Radiology 260:166-173, 2011

Purpose.—To assess the level of distress in women awaiting radiologic procedures.

Materials and Methods.—In this institutional review board–approved and HIPAA-compliant study, 214 women between 18 and 86 (mean, 47.9) years of age completed the State Trait Anxiety Inventory (STAI), Impact of Events Scale (IES), Center for Epidemiologic Studies Depression Scale (CES-D), and Perceived Stress Scale (PSS) immediately prior to their procedures. One hundred twelve women awaited breast biopsy; 42, hepatic chemoembolization for cancer; and 60, uterine fibroid embolization. Data were analyzed with multivariate analysis of variance and post hoc Tukey tests. Results are reported as means and 95% confidence intervals (CIs).

Results.—All three patient groups experienced abnormally high mean PSS, IES, and CES-D scores, but only the breast biopsy group had highly abnormal anxiety levels. Breast biopsy patients had a significantly higher mean STAI score of 48 (95% CI: 45, 50) than did women awaiting hepatic chemoembolization (mean score, 26; 95% CI: 22, 29; $P < .001$) and fibroid embolization (mean score, 24; 95% CI: 21, 27; $P < .001$). IES ratings did not differ significantly among the groups, with a mean score of 26 (95% CI: 23, 29) for breast biopsy patients, 23 (95% CI: 18, 28) for hepatic chemoembolization patients, and 23 (95% CI: 18, 27) for fibroid embolization patients. The CES-D score did not differ significantly among breast biopsy (mean score, 15; 95% CI: 13, 17), hepatic chemoembolization (mean score, 14; 95% CI: 11, 18), and fibroid embolization (mean score, 12; 95% CI: 9, 15) patients. PSS ratings of breast biopsy patients were significantly higher (mean score, 18; 95% CI: 16, 19) than those of hepatic chemoembolization patients (mean, 15; 95% CI: 13, 17; $P < .01$), but they were not significantly different from those of women awaiting fibroid embolization (mean, 16; 95% CI: 14, 18; $P = .23$).

Conclusion.—Uncertainty of diagnosis can be associated with greater stress than is awaiting more invasive and potentially risky treatment.

▶ It is, unfortunately, not too often that we radiologists think long and hard about the emotional distress our patients may be experiencing as they wait for an examination or the result of a test. Perhaps this article will remind us that in certain situations, patients become extraordinarily distressed, and this may affect their ultimate outcome. I think it is no coincidence that the article is authored by 2 women.

Although the study group was confined to women, we should not be surprised if the results would extend to men as well.

A surprising result was that breast biopsy, a procedure with often relatively little objective pain, elicited the most distress among women patients. Conversely, hepatic embolization and uterine fibroid embolization, both potentially highly painful procedures, were met with relatively less anxiety.

The implications of this work are several. First, health care providers should set aside their own notions about "minor" and "major" procedures and appreciate more the distress associated with uncertainty of diagnosis. Secondly, there is no such thing as a "simple" diagnostic procedure. Finally, radiology personnel should be specifically trained in offering emotional support to all patients experiencing such distress.

A. D. Elster, MD

6 Cardiac Imaging

Introduction

This has been an exciting year in cardiac imaging. The accuracy of coronary CT angiography to exclude obstructive coronary artery disease and the accuracy of cardiac MRI delayed enhancement to identify myocardial infarction or scarring have been established and are generally accepted. However, physiologic imaging today is still dominated by radionuclide imaging. Myocardial ischemia, the consequence of some but not all higher grade coronary stenoses, is of clinical importance, and traditionally SPECT or PET myocardial perfusion imaging were the tests of choice to determine the physiologic significance of coronary artery stenoses. In the past year, several remarkable trials have been published that evaluate vasodilator stress and rest perfusion imaging with CT and MRI and compare them with radionuclide imaging—and the results are stunning! A study on the use of delayed enhancement MRI on patients after cardiopulmonary resuscitation for sudden cardiac death or sustained monomorphic ventricular tachycardia showed that 50% more patients would have a new alternate diagnosis after MRI compared with the standard workup using other imaging modalities. These include otherwise undetected acute myocardial infarcts that likely would have significant impact on patient management. New data have emerged that tell us that downstream utilization after CT-based workup of acute chest pain in the emergency department results in no change of resources used, but allows for increased diagnosis of coronary artery disease and, as a result, significantly decreases recurrences and rehospitalization over a 90-day period. Overall these have been very important advances in the field. I truly hope that YEAR BOOK readers will find the selected articles informative and will enjoy reading them.

Suhny Abbara, MD

Patient Management After Noninvasive Cardiac Imaging: Results From SPARC (Study of Myocardial Perfusion and Coronary Anatomy Imaging Roles in Coronary Artery Disease)
Hachamovitch R, for the SPARC Investigators (Cleveland Clinic Foundation, OH; et al)
J Am Coll Cardiol 59:462-474, 2012

Objectives.—This study examined short-term cardiac catheterization rates and medication changes after cardiac imaging.

Background.—Noninvasive cardiac imaging is widely used in coronary artery disease, but its effects on subsequent patient management are unclear.

Methods.—We assessed the 90-day post-test rates of catheterization and medication changes in a prospective registry of 1,703 patients without a documented history of coronary artery disease and an intermediate to high likelihood of coronary artery disease undergoing cardiac single-photon emission computed tomography, positron emission tomography, or 64-slice coronary computed tomography angiography.

Results.—Baseline medication use was relatively infrequent. At 90 days, 9.6% of patients underwent catheterization. The rates of catheterization and medication changes increased in proportion to test abnormality findings. Among patients with the most severe test result findings, 38% to 61% were not referred to catheterization, 20% to 30% were not receiving aspirin, 35% to 44% were not receiving a beta-blocker, and 20% to 25% were not receiving a lipid-lowering agent at 90 days after the index test. Risk-adjusted analyses revealed that compared with stress single-photon emission computed tomography or positron emission tomography, changes in aspirin and lipid-lowering agent use was greater after computed tomography angiography, as was the 90-day catheterization referral rate in the setting of normal/nonobstructive and mildly abnormal test results.

Conclusions.—Overall, noninvasive testing had only a modest impact on clinical management of patients referred for clinical testing. Although post-imaging use of cardiac catheterization and medical therapy increased in proportion to the degree of abnormality findings, the frequency of catheterization and medication change suggests possible undertreatment of higher risk patients. Patients were more likely to undergo cardiac catheterization after computed tomography angiography than after single-photon emission computed tomography or positron emission tomography after normal/nonobstructive and mildly abnormal study findings. (Study of Perfusion and Anatomy's Role in Coronary Artery [CAD] [SPARC]; NCT00321399).

▶ This study is an open-label, multicenter, sequentially sampled observational registry study that aimed to compare stress perfusion imaging with single-photon emission computed tomography (SPECT) or positron emission tomography (PET) to coronary CT angiography with respect to their posttest resource utilization. There were 40 international sites that enrolled patients. It is remarkable that the sites would perform routine clinical imaging protocols that may differ from site to site and that all patients were referred to the respective modalities based on clinical indications. Enrollment in the study was performed only after patients were referred to the respective imaging tests. This may of course introduce substantial bias but does reflect real-world clinical management. The study found that the impact of imaging on posttest medical management was only modest and that in the CT group use of invasive angiography was greater after the test in patients who showed "mildly abnormal" results on CTA (coronary atherosclerotic plaque but no significant obstruction).

S. Abbara, MD

Utility of Cardiovascular Magnetic Resonance in Identifying Substrate for Malignant Ventricular Arrhythmias
White JA, Fine NM, Gula L, et al (Univ of Western Ontario, London, Ontario, Canada)
Circ Cardiovasc Imaging 5:12-20, 2012

Background.—Sudden cardiac death (SCD) and sustained monomorphic ventricular tachycardia (SMVT) are frequently associated with prior or acute myocardial injury. Cardiovascular magnetic resonance (CMR) provides morphological, functional, and tissue characterization in a single setting. We sought to evaluate the diagnostic yield of CMR-based imaging versus non−CMR-based imaging in patients with resuscitated SCD or SMVT.

Methods and Results.—Eighty-two patients with resuscitated SCD or SMVT underwent routine non-CMR imaging, followed by a CMR protocol with comprehensive tissue characterization. Clinical reports of non-CMR imaging studies were blindly adjudicated and used to assign each patient to 1 of 7 diagnostic categories. CMR imaging was blindly interpreted using a standardized algorithm used to assign a patient diagnosis category in a similar fashion. The diagnostic yield of CMR-based and non−CMR-based imaging, as well as the impact of the former on diagnosis reclassification, was established. Relevant myocardial disease was identified in 51% of patients using non−CMR-based imaging and in 74% using CMR-based imaging (P=0.002). Forty-one patients (50%) were reassigned to a new or alternate diagnosis using CMR-based imaging, including 15 (18%) with unsuspected acute myocardial injury. Twenty patients (24%) had no abnormality by non-CMR imaging but showed clinically relevant myocardial disease by CMR imaging.

Conclusions.—CMR-based imaging provides a robust diagnostic yield in patients presenting with resuscitated SCD or SMVT and incrementally identifies clinically unsuspected acute myocardial injury. When compared with non CMR-based imaging, a new or alternate myocardial disease process may be identified in half of these patients (Fig 5).

▶ This is a very interesting prospective cohort study that aims to evaluate the diagnostic usefulness of cardiac MRI (CMR) in patients who have been resuscitated due to sudden cardiac death (SCD) or sustained monomorphic ventricular

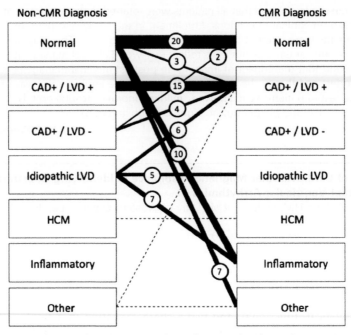

Non-CMR Diagnosis   CMR Diagnosis

FIGURE 5.—Change in diagnosis category after performance of cardiovascular magnetic resonance (CMR) imaging. Weighted lines represent number of patients (also numerically represented within the circle). All dashed lines represent single patients. CAD indicates coronary artery disease; HCM, hypertrophic cardiomyopathy; LVD, left ventricular dysfunction. (Reprinted from White JA, Fine NM, Gula L, et al. Utility of cardiovascular magnetic resonance in identifying substrate for malignant ventricular arrhythmias. *Circ Cardiovasc Imaging*. 2012;5:12-20, with permission from American Heart Association, Inc.)

tachycardia (SMVT) and in whom no clinical cause for the SCD or SMVT has been established (such as recent myocardial infarct).

The diagnostic categories that were assigned using standard patient management and the CMR method included (1) no known cause, (2) coronary artery disease without left ventricular dysfunction, (3) coronary artery disease with left ventricular dysfunction, (4) idiopathic LV dysfunction, (5) hypertrophic cardiomyopathy, (6) inflammatory cardiomyopathy, and (7) other. After applying the CMR reads, the diagnosis was changed in half of the patients, including 20 of 40 who would have otherwise been classified as "no known cause" and 13 of 18 who would have otherwise been classified as "idiopathic LV dysfunction."

Although these results are very impressive and show that MRI has a big impact on appropriate diagnosis in this scenario, there remain important uncertainties.

This study does not address the impact that the improved diagnosis with CMR has on clinical management of these patients and on patient outcome (Fig 5).

S. Abbara, MD

SCCT guidelines on radiation dose and dose-optimization strategies in cardiovascular CT

Hausleiter J, Halliburton SS, Abbara S, et al (Deutsches Herzzentrum München, Munich, Germany; Cleveland Clinic, OH; Massachusetts General Hosp, Boston; et al)

J Cardiovasc Comput Tomogr 5:198-224, 2011

Noninvasive imaging with cardiovascular CT has rapidly evolved over the past several years, with improvements in both hardware and software image acquistion techniques. Radiation dose reduction has been a central focus of many of the advancements in the field. The Society of Cardiovascalar Computed Tomography recently formed a Radiation Committee to develop evidence-based information statements to guide CT imagers on critical topics in the areas of radiation dosimetry, projected cancer risk, appropriate test indications, and techniques to reduce radiation exposure in patients referred for cardiovascular CT. An important concept in this document is the focus not only on radiation doses reduction but also on the clinical benefit of knowledge acquired that may aid in improving therapeutic decision making and may lead to superior patient outcomes. Highlighted topics within this information statement include different scanner acquisition modes and parameter settings, predictors of radiation dose, algorithms for dose reduction in clinical practice, and dose monitoring.

▶ In the past decade, cardiac CT has gone from having the highest radiation doses in CT imaging to becoming the test with the lowest radiation dose. However, the acquisition of cardiac CT has become complex because there are many scan modes and settings to choose from to tailor to a specific patient's heart rate and rhythm (retrospective gating with tube modulation, prospective triggering, high pitch spiral, to name a few). Furthermore, CT scans have to be tailored to the individual based on his or her body mass index, chest size, and clinical indications. This document is included in the YEAR BOOK because it brings together information from several recent single-center trials, registry data, and other publications. The information is synthesized into a guideline format that aims to allow the reader to develop dose optimization strategies that can be tailored to each individual, accounting for the scanner software and hardware that may be available at the site. This comprehensive guideline document reviews the technical aspects that influence the radiation dose to individuals who undergo cardiac CT and, more important, when dose-saving strategies can be safely applied. The major vendors' hardware- and software-specific technical aspects and settings are discussed in generic terms, and the document outlines best practices that help practitioners walk the fine line between too much radiation dose and too noisy (nonevaluable) images.

S. Abbara, MD

Computed tomography stress myocardial perfusion imaging in patients considered for revascularization: a comparison with fractional flow reserve

Ko BS, Cameron JD, Meredith IT, et al (Monash Cardiovascular Res Centre, Clayton, Victoria, Australia; et al)
Eur Heart J 33:67-77, 2012

Aims.—Adenosine stress computed tomography myocardial perfusion imaging (CTP) is an emerging non-invasive method for detecting myocardial ischaemia. Its value when compared with fractional flow reserve (FFR), a highly accurate index of ischaemia, is unknown. Our aim was to determine the diagnostic accuracy of CTP and its incremental value when used with computed tomography coronary angiography (CTA) for detecting ischaemia compared with FFR.

Methods and Results.—Forty-two patients (126 vessel territories), who had at least one ≥50% angiographic stenosis on invasive angiography considered for non-urgent revascularization, were included and underwent FFR and CT assessment, including CTP, delayed contrast enhancement scan and CTA all acquired using 320-detector row CT, and prospective ECG gating. Fractional flow reserve was determined in 86 territories subtended by vessels with ≥50% stenosis upon visual assessment. Fractional flow reserve ≤0.8 was considered to indicate significant ischaemia. Computed tomography myocardial perfusion imaging correctly identified 31/41 (76%) ischaemic territories and 38/45 (84%) non-ischaemic territories. Per-vessel territory sensitivity, specificity, positive, and negative predictive values of CTP were 76, 84, 82, and 79%, respectively. The combination of a ≥50% stenosis on CTA and perfusion defect on CTP was 98% specific for ischaemia, while the presence of <50% stenosis on CTA and normal perfusion on CTP was 100% specific for exclusion of ischaemia. Mean radiation for CTP and combined CT was 5.3 and 11.3 mSv, respectively.

Conclusion.—Computed tomography myocardial perfusion imaging is moderately accurate in identifying perfusion defects associated with ischaemia as assessed by FFR in patients considered for revascularization. In territories, where CTA and CTP are concordant, CTA/CTP is highly accurate in the detection and exclusion of ischaemia. This is achievable with acceptable radiation exposure using 320-detector row CT and prospective ECG gating.

▶ This study is included in the YEAR BOOK because it compares stress rest myocardial CT perfusion with the ultimate clinical gold standard for physiologic assessment of end-organ (myocardial) ischemia—namely, invasive angiography with catheter-based measurements of the fractional flow reserve (is there enough flow during myocardial stress to maintain adequate myocardial perfusion?). Although this study found that myocardial CT perfusion imaging is only moderately accurate if viewed alone, the combination of CT perfusion (CTP) and CT angiography showed outstanding results. It is also remarkable that the modest CTP-alone results are comparable to the accuracy values of single-photon emission computed tomography myocardial perfusion imaging. Other articles on myocardial stress rest CTP that are noteworthy are listed in the references. Feuchtner et al present an article comparing CTP with MRI perfusion imaging.[1] Patel et al evaluate coronary CTA and myocardial CTP with use of regadenoson and compared standard and low-dose protocols.[2] They found that the protocols were similar, suggesting that lower-dose protocols can be safely used while maintaining diagnostic image quality.

S. Abbara, MD

References

1. Feuchtner G, Goetti R, Plass A, et al. Adenosine stress high-pitch 128-slice dual-source myocardial computed tomography perfusion for imaging of reversible myocardial ischemia: comparison with magnetic resonance imaging. *Circ Cardiovasc Imaging.* 2011;4:540-549.
2. Patel AR, Lodato JA, Chandra S, et al. Detection of myocardial perfusion abnormalities using ultra-low radiation dose regadenoson stress multidetector computed tomography. *J Cardiovasc Comput Tomogr.* 2011;5:247-254.

Is Coronary Computed Tomography Angiography a Resource Sparing Strategy in the Risk Stratification and Evaluation of Acute Chest Pain? Results of a Randomized Controlled Trial

Miller AH, Pepe PE, Peshock R, et al (Univ of Texas Southwestern Med Ctr, Dallas; Parkland Health & Hosp System, Dallas, TX; et al)
Acad Emerg Med 18:458-467, 2011

Objectives.—Annually, almost 6 million U.S. citizens are evaluated for acute chest pain syndromes (ACPSs), and billions of dollars in resources are utilized. A large part of the resource utilization results from precautionary hospitalizations that occur because care providers are unable to exclude the presence of coronary artery disease (CAD) as the underlying cause of ACPSs. The purpose of this study was to examine whether the addition of coronary computerized tomography angiography (CCTA) to the concurrent standard care (SC) during an index emergency department (ED) visit could lower resource utilization when evaluating for the presence of CAD.

Methods.—Sixty participants were assigned randomly to SC or SC + CCTA groups. Participants were interviewed at the index ED visit and at 90 days. Data collected included demographics, perceptions of the value of accessing health care, and clinical outcomes. Resource utilization included services received from both the primary in-network and the primary out-of-network providers. The prospectively defined primary endpoint was the total amount of resources utilized over a 90-day follow-up period when adding CCTA to the SC risk stratification in ACPSs.

Results.—The mean (± standard deviation [SD]) for total resources utilized at 90 days for in network plus out-of-network services was less for the participants in the SC + CCTA group ($10,134; SD ± $14,239) versus the SC-only group ($16,579; SD ± $19,148; p = 0.144), as was the median for the SC + CCTA ($4,288) versus SC only ($12,148; p = 0.652; median difference = −$1,291; 95% confidence interval [CI] = −$12,219 to $1,100; p = 0.652). Among the 60 total study patients, only 19 had an established diagnosis of CAD at 90 days. However, 18 (95%) of these diagnosed participants were in the SC + CCTA group. In addition, there were fewer hospital readmissions in the SC + CCTA group (6 of 30 [20%] vs. 16 of 30 [53%]; difference in proportions = −33%; 95% CI = −56% to −10%; p = 0.007).

Conclusions.—Adding CCTA to the current ED risk stratification of ACPSs resulted in no difference in the quantity of resources utilized, but an increased diagnosis of CAD, and significantly less recidivism and rehospitalization over a 90-day follow-up period.

▶ This study is remarkable because it addresses resource utilization based on a CT versus non-CT workup for acute chest pain. In the past, it has been suggested that CT may lead to greater resource utilization. This is a randomized single-center trial that examined the overall use of resources when adding a cardiac CT to the standard of care evaluation of patients with acute chest pain and low to intermediate/ risk compared with standard of care alone. Sixty patients were randomized: 30 received standard of care and 30 were randomized to standard of care plus coronary CT angiography (CCTA). The patients were followed for 90 days, and the study shows that adding CCTA to the standard of care was less costly and did not result in higher quantity of resource utilization but resulted in significantly less recurrences and rehospitalizations. In the CT group, the patients received a definitive final diagnosis of obstructive coronary artery disease or absence of coronary artery disease in most cases. However, in absence of CT, it was most often not possible to definitively exclude coronary artery disease. A definitive diagnosis was also achieved much faster in the CT group, which led the authors to speculate that more rapid treatment may be used in those who are positive. Longer-term resource utilization such as follow-up CT scans for incidental findings are not addressed in this study.

S. Abbara, MD

Cardiovascular magnetic resonance and single-photon emission computed tomography for diagnosis of coronary heart disease (CE-MARC): a prospective trial
Greenwood JP, Maredia N, Younger JF, et al (Univ of Leeds, UK; et al)
Lancet 379:453-460, 2012

Background.—In patients with suspected coronary heart disease, single-photon emission computed tomography (SPECT) is the most widely used test for the assessment of myocardial ischaemia, but its diagnostic accuracy is reported to be variable and it exposes patients to ionising radiation. The aim of this study was to establish the diagnostic accuracy of a multi-parametric cardiovascular magnetic resonance (CMR) protocol with x-ray coronary angiography as the reference standard, and to compare CMR with SPECT, in patients with suspected coronary heart disease.

Methods.—In this prospective trial patients with suspected angina pectoris and at least one cardiovascular risk factor were scheduled for CMR, SPECT, and invasive x-ray coronary angiography. CMR consisted of rest and adenosine stress perfusion, cine imaging, late gadolinium enhancement, and MR coronary angiography. Gated adenosine stress and rest SPECT used ^{99m}Tc tetrofosmin. The primary outcome was diagnostic accuracy of CMR. This trial is registered at controlled-trials.com, number ISRCTN77246133.

Findings.—In the 752 recruited patients, 39% had significant CHD as identified by x-ray angiography. For multiparametric CMR the sensitivity was 86·5% (95% CI 81·8—90·1), specificity 83·4% (79·5—86·7), positive predictive value 77·2%, (72·1—81·6) and negative predictive value 90·5% (87·1—93·0). The sensitivity of SPECT was 66·5% (95% CI 60·4—72·1), specificity 82·6% (78·5—86·1), positive predictive value 71·4% (65·3—76·9), and negative predictive value 79·1% (74·8—82·8). The sensitivity and negative predictive value of CMR and SPECT differed significantly (p<0·0001 for both) but specificity and positive predictive value did not (p=0·916 and p=0·061, respectively).

Interpretation.—CE-MARC is the largest, prospective, real world evaluation of CMR and has established CMR's high diagnostic accuracy in coronary heart disease and CMR's superiority over SPECT. It should be adopted more widely than at present for the investigation of coronary heart disease.

▶ The CE-MARC study is a large-scale, British Heart Foundation—sponsored, 2-center prospective accuracy trial in which all patients received both a cardiac MRI (CMRI; with stress and rest perfusion, delayed enhancement, and whole heart coronary imaging) and radionuclide myocardial perfusion (SPECT MPI) imaging before invasive angiography, which was used as the gold standard. The study enrolled 752 patients randomized to assessment by CMRI before SPECT or vice versa. The study demonstrated superior diagnostic accuracy of CMRI compared with SPECT.

Notably, the results remained significant when the coronary magnetic resonance angiography (MRA) coronary was omitted from the analysis, which is important because coronary MRA is not always feasible and not as readily available as MR perfusion or delayed enhancement imaging. These findings are noteworthy because they support the broader use of CMRI for diagnosis of obstructive heart disease, especially given that MRI does not require ionizing radiation and is an overall faster procedure compared with SPECT MPI. The study results reinforce similar findings in a recent metaanalysis of several smaller single-center trials.[1]

S. Abbara, MD

Reference

1. Hamon M, Fau G, Née G, Ehtisham J, Morello R, Hamon M. Meta-analysis of the diagnostic performance of stress perfusion cardiovascular magnetic resonance for detection of coronary artery disease. *J Cardiovasc Magn Reson.* 2010;12:29.

The CT-STAT (Coronary Computed Tomographic Angiography for Systematic Triage of Acute Chest Pain Patients to Treatment) Trial

Goldstein JA, for the CT-STAT Investigators (William Beaumont Hosp, Royal Oak, MI; et al)
J Am Coll Cardiol 58:1414-1422, 2011

Objectives.—The purpose of this study was to compare the efficiency, cost, and safety of a diagnostic strategy employing early coronary computed tomographic angiography (CCTA) to a strategy employing rest-stress myocardial perfusion imaging (MPI) in the evaluation of acute low-risk chest pain.

Background.—In the United States, >8 million patients require emergency department evaluation for acute chest pain annually at an estimated diagnostic cost of >$10 billion.

Methods.—This multicenter, randomized clinical trial in 16 emergency departments ran between June 2007 and November 2008. Patients were randomly allocated to CCTA (n = 361) or MPI (n = 338) as the index noninvasive test. The primary outcome was time to diagnosis; the secondary outcomes were emergency department costs of care and safety, defined as freedom from major adverse cardiac events in patients with normal index tests, including 6-month follow-up.

Results.—The CCTA resulted in a 54% reduction in time to diagnosis compared with MPI (median 2.9 h [25th to 75th percentile: 2.1 to 4.0 h] vs. 6.3 h [25th to 75th percentile: 4.2 to 19.0 h], p < 0.0001). Costs of care were 38% lower compared with standard (median $2,137 [25th to 75th percentile: $1,660 to $3,077] vs. $3,458 [25th to 75th percentile: $2,900 to $4,297], p < 0.0001). The diagnostic strategies had no difference in major adverse cardiac events after normal index testing (0.8% in the CCTA arm vs. 0.4% in the MPI arm, p = 0.29).

Conclusions.—In emergency department acute, low-risk chest pain patients, the use of CCTA results in more rapid and cost-efficient safe diagnosis than rest-stress MPI. Further studies comparing CCTA to other diagnostic strategies are needed to optimize evaluation of specific patient subsets. (Coronary Computed Tomographic Angiography for Systematic Triage of Acute Chest Pain Patients to Treatment [CT-STAT]; NCT00468325).

▶ Each year, there are 8 million patients in the United States who are evaluated in emergency departments for acute chest pain. Patients with intermediate to low risk are difficult to diagnose and often require extensive and costly testing before myocardial infarct can be ruled in or out. The CT-STAT trial (Coronary CTA for Systematic Triage of Acute Chest Pain Patients to Treatment) is a landmark prospective, randomized multicenter trial that compares coronary computed tomographic angiography (CCTA) with radionuclide myocardial stress rest perfusion (MPI) in the setting of acute chest pain in the emergency department. The study enrolled low-risk patients that were to be ruled out for acute myocardial infarction between 2007 and 2008.

In this study, computed tomography (CT) performed very well. CTA was approximately 50% faster and nearly 40% less costly compared with MPI and resulted in lower radiation doses.

An added benefit of CT is that it can reveal important noncardiac thoracic disease not diagnosable by stress testing, such as pulmonary embolism or pneumonia. This study and few other similar studies are likely to have a huge impact on patient management in the emergency department in the near future. It is also likely that the newer-generation CT scanners that are available today will perform equally or better at lower radiation doses.

S. Abbara, MD

Article Index

Chapter 1: Thoracic Radiology

International Association for the Study of Lung Cancer/American Thoracic Society/European Respiratory Society International Multidisciplinary Classification of Lung Adenocarcinoma   2

Reduced Lung-Cancer Mortality with Low-Dose Computed Tomographic Screening   5

Screen-detected Lung Cancer: A Retrospective Analysis of CT Appearance   7

Lung Nodules: Improved Detection with Software That Suppresses the Rib and Clavicle on Chest Radiographs   8

A Comparison of Follow-Up Recommendations by Chest Radiologists, General Radiologists, and Pulmonologists Using Computer-Aided Detection to Assess Radiographs for Actionable Pulmonary Nodules   10

CT Features of Peripheral Pulmonary Carcinoid Tumors   13

Computed Tomography Findings Predicting Invasiveness of Thymoma   15

Incidence, Correlates, and Chest Radiographic Yield of New Lung Cancer Diagnosis in 3398 Patients With Pneumonia   17

Are Chest Radiographs Routinely Indicated After Chest Tube Removal Following Cardiac Surgery?   19

Central Venous Line Placement in the Superior Vena Cava and the Azygos Vein: Differentiation on Posteroanterior Chest Radiographs   20

Adaptive Statistical Iterative Reconstruction Technique for Radiation Dose Reduction in Chest CT: A Pilot Study   23

Incidental findings at chest CT: A needs assessment survey of radiologists' knowledge   26

MDCT Bolus Tracking Data as an Adjunct for Predicting the Diagnosis of Pulmonary Hypertension and Concomitant Right-Heart Failure   27

An Official ATS/ERS/JRS/ALAT Statement: Idiopathic Pulmonary Fibrosis: Evidence-based Guidelines for Diagnosis and Management   29

CT of Viral Lower Respiratory Tract Infections in Adults: Comparison Among Viral Organisms and Between Viral and Bacterial Infections   31

Pulmonary Nocardiosis: Computed Tomography Features at Diagnosis   33

Screening of Asymptomatic Children for Tuberculosis: Is a Lateral Chest Radiograph Routinely Indicated?   34

Pulmonary CT Angiography Protocol Adapted to the Hemodynamic Effects of Pregnancy   36

An Official American Thoracic Society/Society of Thoracic Radiology Clinical Practice Guideline: Evaluation of Suspected Pulmonary Embolism In Pregnancy   38

Does a Clinical Decision Rule Using D-Dimer Level Improve the Yield of Pulmonary CT Angiography?   41

Chapter 2: Breast Imaging

The Nipple-Areolar Complex: A Pictorial Review of Common and Uncommon Conditions   43

Challenges in Mammography: Part 2, Multimodality Review of Breast Augmentation—Imaging Findings and Complications   44

Prosthetic Breast Implant Rupture: Imaging—Pictorial Essay   45

The Augmented Breast: A Pictorial Review of the Abnormal and Unusual   46

Background enhancement in breast MR: Correlation with breast density in mammography and background echotexture in ultrasound   47

Nonmasslike Enhancement at Breast MR Imaging: The Added Value of Mammography and US for Lesion Categorization   48

Use of BI-RADS 3—Probably Benign Category in the American College of Radiology Imaging Network Digital Mammographic Imaging Screening Trial   50

Timeliness of Follow-up after Abnormal Screening Mammogram: Variability of Facilities   51

Mammography image quality: Model for predicting compliance with posterior nipple line criterion   53

Accuracy of Screening Mammography in Older Women   55

Mammography in 40-Year-Old Women: What Difference Does It Make? The Potential Impact of the U.S. Preventative Services Task Force (USPSTF) Mammography Guidelines   56

Screen-detected breast cancer: Does presence of minimal signs on prior mammograms predict staging or grading of cancer?   57

Breast surgical specimen radiographs: How reliable are they?   59

Attitudes of women in their forties toward the 2009 USPSTF mammogram guidelines: a randomized trial on the effects of media exposure   60

Accuracy of Clinical Examination, Digital Mammogram, Ultrasound, and MRI in Determining Postneoadjuvant Pathologic Tumor Response in Operable Breast Cancer Patients   61

Lower sensitivity of screening mammography after previous benign breast surgery   62

Accuracy of Diagnostic Mammography and Breast Ultrasound During Pregnancy and Lactation   64

Complex cystic lesions of the breast on ultrasonography: Feature analysis and BI-RADS assessment   65

Hyperechoic Lesions of the Breast: Not Always Benign   70

Full-Field Digital Mammographic Interpretation With Prior Analog Versus Prior Digitized Analog Mammography: Time for Interpretation   71

Chapter 3: Musculoskeletal

Revisiting CT-Guided Percutaneous Core Needle Biopsy of Musculoskeletal
Lesions: Contributors to Biopsy Success   76

Imaging of Liposarcoma: Classification, Patterns of Tumor Recurrence, and
Response to Treatment   77

Clavicle and acromioclavicular joint injuries: a review of imaging, treatment, and
complications   78

Bisphosphonate-Related Complete Atypical Subtrochanteric Femoral Fractures:
Diagnostic Utility of Radiography   79

Bisphosphonates in the treatment of osteoporosis: a review of their contribution
and controversies   81

Bone marrow MR imaging findings in disuse osteoporosis   82

Sclerosing Bone Dysplasias: Review and Differentiation from Other Causes of
Osteosclerosis   83

Effect of Spinal Segment Variants on Numbering Vertebral Levels at Lumbar MR
Imaging   84

Can Necrotizing Infectious Fasciitis Be Differentiated from Nonnecrotizing
Infectious Fasciitis with MR Imaging?   86

Preoperative Diagnosis of Periprosthetic Joint Infection: Role of Aspiration   87

New Techniques in Lumbar Spinal Instrumentation: What the Radiologist Needs
to Know   88

The Utility of Repeated Postoperative Radiographs After Lumbar Instrumented
Fusion for Degenerative Lumbar Spine   89

Identification of Intraarticular and Periarticular Uric Acid Crystals with Dual-
Energy CT: Initial Evaluation   91

Rheumatoid Arthritis: Ultrasound Versus MRI   92

Radiology of the resurfaced hip   93

Three tesla magnetic resonance imaging of the anterior cruciate ligament of the
knee: can we differentiate complete from partial tears?   94

Oblique axial MR imaging of the normal anterior cruciate ligament bundles   95

Shoulder US: Anatomy, Technique, and Scanning Pitfalls   98

Morbidity of Direct MR Arthrography   99

MR Arthrographic Appearance of the Postoperative Acetabular Labrum in Patients
With Suspected Recurrent Labral Tears   100

Indirect MR Arthrographic Findings of Adhesive Capsulitis   101

Displaceability of SLAP lesion on shoulder MR arthrography with external
rotation position   102

Evaluation of the Glenoid Labrum With 3-T MRI: Is Intraarticular Contrast
Necessary?   104

Avascular necrosis (AVN) of the proximal fragment in scaphoid nonunion:
Is intravenous contrast agent necessary in MRI?   105

MR Arthrography of the Hip: Comparison of IDEAL-SPGR Volume Sequence to Standard MR Sequences in the Detection and Grading of Cartilage Lesions   106

Presumed intraarticular gas microbubbles resulting from a vacuum phenomenon: visualization with ultrasonography as hyperechoic microfoci   108

A Biomechanical Approach to MRI of Acute Knee Injuries   110

MRI of the Pediatric Knee   111

Can Stress Radiography of the Knee Help Characterize Posterolateral Corner Injury?   112

Contrast-Enhanced Magnetic Resonance Imaging Positively Impacts the Management of Some Patients With Rheumatoid Arthritis or Suspected RA   113

Chapter 4: Pediatric Radiology

Accurate localization of the position of the tip of a naso/orogastric tube in children; where is the location of the gastro-esophageal junction?   116

CT appearance of the duodenum and mesenteric vessels in children with normal and abnormal bowel rotation   117

Interloop fluid in intussusception: what is its significance?   119

Characterization of pediatric liver lesions with gadoxetate disodium   120

Transcapsular Arterial Neovascularization after Liver Transplantation in Pediatric Patients Indicates Transplant Failure   122

The positive color Doppler sign post biopsy: effectiveness of US-directed compression in achieving hemostasis   124

Pseudo Gallbladder sign in biliary atresia—an imaging pitfall   126

Spontaneous gall bladder perforation: a rare condition in the differential diagnosis of acute abdomen in children   127

Multiple magnet ingestion: Is there a role for early surgical intervention?   128

Sonography of renal venous thrombosis in neonates and infants: can we predict outcome?   129

Ureteral triplication: A rare anomaly with a variety of presentations   131

Imaging the urinary tract in children with urinary tract infection   132

MRI of acquired posterior urethral diverticulum following surgery for anorectal malformations   134

Congenital megalourethra: prenatal diagnosis and postnatal/autopsy findings in 10 cases   135

Testicular epidermoid cysts in children: sonographic characteristics with pathological correlation   137

Laparoscopic excision of a rudimentary uterine horn in a child   139

Inguinal Hernia Containing Uterus and Uterine Adnexa in Female Infants: Report of Two Cases   140

'Benign' ovarian teratoma and N-methyl-D-aspartate receptor (NMDAR) encephalitis in a child   142

Clinical and radiological distinction between spondylothoracic dysostosis (Lavy-Moseley syndrome) and spondylocostal dysostosis (Jarcho-Levin syndrome)   143

A symptomatic sesamoid bone in the popliteus muscle (cyamella)   145

Deficiency of interleukin-1-receptor antagonist syndrome: a rare auto-inflammatory
condition that mimics multiple classic radiographic findings   146

The importance of conventional radiography in the mutational analysis of skeletal
dysplasias (the TRPV4 mutational family)   147

Van Neck Disease: Osteochondrosis of the Ischiopubic Synchondrosis   149

Dating fractures in infants   151

The Prevalence of Uncommon Fractures on Skeletal Surveys Performed to Evaluate
for Suspected Abuse in 930 Children: Should Practice Guidelines Change?   153

Immediate Treatment Versus Sonographic Surveillance for Mild Hip Dysplasia in
Newborns   155

Changes in quantitative ultrasound in preterm and term infants during the first year
of life   157

Assessment of White Matter Microstructural Integrity in Children with Syndromic
Craniosynostosis: A Diffusion-Tensor Imaging Study   158

Biometry of the Corpus Callosum in Children: MR Imaging Reference Data   160

Cortical Thickness in Fetal Alcohol Syndrome and Attention Deficit Disorder   164

Sensitive Diffusion Tensor Imaging Quantification Method to Identify Language
Pathway Abnormalities in Children with Developmental Delay   165

Magnetic Resonance Spectroscopy Predicts Outcomes for Children With
Nonaccidental Trauma   167

State-of-the-Art Cranial Sonography: Part 1, Modern Techniques and Image
Interpretation   168

Trainee Misinterpretations on Pediatric Neuroimaging Studies: Classification,
Imaging Analysis, and Outcome Assessment   170

Exogenous lipoid pneumonia. Clinical and radiological manifestations   172

Rupture of the left mainstem bronchus following endotracheal intubation in
a neonate   176

Quality assurance: using the exposure index and the deviation index to monitor
radiation exposure for portable chest radiographs in neonates   179

Evaluation of image quality and radiation dose at prospective ECG-triggered axial
256-slice multi-detector CT in infants with congenital heart disease   180

Children Suspected Of Having Pulmonary Embolism: Multidetector CT Pulmonary
Angiography—Thromboembolic Risk Factors and Implications for Appropriate Use   182

Breathe In... Breathe Out... Stop Breathing: Does Phase of Respiration Affect the
Haller Index in Patients with Pectus Excavatum?   184

Congenital diaphragmatic hernia: lung-to-head ratio and lung volume for
prediction of outcome   185

Childhood Cancer Risk From Conventional Radiographic Examinations for
Selected Referral Criteria: Results From a Large Cohort Study   187

Utilization of Emergency Ultrasound in Pediatric Emergency Departments   188

Chapter 5: Economics, Research, Education, and Quality

ACCF/SCCT/ACR/AHA/ASE/ASNC/NASCI/SCAI/SCMR 2010 Appropriate Use Criteria for Cardiac Computed Tomography: A Report of the American College of Cardiology Foundation Appropriate Use Criteria Task Force, the Society of Cardiovascular Computed Tomography, the American College of Radiology, the American Heart Association, the American Society of Echocardiography, the American Society of Nuclear Cardiology, the North American Society for Cardiovascular Imaging, the Society for Cardiovascular Angiography and Interventions, and the Society for Cardiovascular Magnetic Resonance ... 192

Comparative Effectiveness and Cost-Effectiveness of Computed Tomography Screening for Coronary Artery Calcium in Asymptomatic Individuals ... 193

Screening Cervical Spine CT in a Level I Trauma Center: Overutilization? ... 194

"MR-Conditional" Pacemakers: The Radiologist's Role in Multidisciplinary Management ... 196

MRI of Patients With Cardiac Pacemakers: A Review of the Medical Literature ... 197

National Trends in CT Use in the Emergency Department: 1995–2007 ... 198

Effect of Spinal Segment Variants on Numbering Vertebral Levels at Lumbar MR Imaging ... 200

The Radiologist as a Palliative Care Subspecialist: Providing Symptom Relief When Cure Is Not Possible ... 201

Influence of Annual Interpretive Volume on Screening Mammography Performance in the United States ... 202

A Comparison of Follow-Up Recommendations by Chest Radiologists, General Radiologists, and Pulmonologists Using Computer-Aided Detection to Assess Radiographs for Actionable Pulmonary Nodules ... 203

The Relative Effect of Vendor Variability in CT Perfusion Results: A Method Comparison Study ... 204

T1 Pseudohyperintensity on Fat-Suppressed Magnetic Resonance Imaging: A Potential Diagnostic Pitfall ... 206

Trends in the Utilization of CT Angiography and MR Angiography of the Head and Neck in the Medicare Population ... 208

Medicare Payments for Noninvasive Diagnostic Imaging Are Now Higher to Nonradiologist Physicians Than to Radiologists ... 209

CT Radiation Dose: What Can You Do Right Now in Your Practice? ... 211

Short-Term and Long-Term Health Risks of Nuclear-Power-Plant Accidents ... 212

Risk of Radiation-induced Breast Cancer from Mammographic Screening ... 214

ACR Dose Index Registry ... 215

Adult patient radiation doses from non-cardiac CT examinations: a review of published results ... 216

Frequent Body CT Scanning of Young Adults: Indications, Outcomes, and Risk for Radiation-Induced Cancer ... 217

Incidence of Nephrogenic Systemic Fibrosis after Adoption of Restrictive Gadolinium-based Contrast Agent Guidelines ... 218

Incidence of Immediate Gadolinium Contrast Media Reactions 220

Assessment of Adverse Reaction Rates during Gadoteridol-enhanced MR Imaging in 28 078 Patients 222

Incidence of Contrast-Induced Nephropathy in Patients With Multiple Myeloma Undergoing Contrast-Enhanced CT 223

Characteristics of Falls in a Large Academic Radiology Department: Occurrence, Associated Factors, Outcomes, and Quality Improvement Strategies 224

Comparing the accuracy of initial head CT reporting by radiologists, radiology trainees, neuroradiographers and emergency doctors 225

Distress in the Radiology Waiting Room 226

Chapter 6: Cardiac Imaging

Patient Management After Noninvasive Cardiac Imaging: Results From SPARC (Study of Myocardial Perfusion and Coronary Anatomy Imaging Roles in Coronary Artery Disease) 230

Utility of Cardiovascular Magnetic Resonance in Identifying Substrate for Malignant Ventricular Arrhythmias 231

SCCT guidelines on radiation dose and dose-optimization strategies in cardiovascular CT 233

Computed tomography stress myocardial perfusion imaging in patients considered for revascularization: a comparison with fractional flow reserve 234

Is Coronary Computed Tomography Angiography a Resource Sparing Strategy in the Risk Stratification and Evaluation of Acute Chest Pain? Results of a Randomized Controlled Trial 235

Cardiovascular magnetic resonance and single-photon emission computed tomography for diagnosis of coronary heart disease (CE-MARC): a prospective trial 236

The CT-STAT (Coronary Computed Tomographic Angiography for Systematic Triage of Acute Chest Pain Patients to Treatment) Trial 238

Author Index

A

Aaen GS, 167
Abbara S, 233
Abujudeh H, 224
Acharyya S, 50
Ainsley CG, 212
Alberti C, 160
Alfaraj MA, 185
Alkasab TK, 218
Alotaibi M, 124
Amaral J, 124
Amsalem H, 135
An HY, 43
Anderson ML, 202
Anton CG, 134
Arellano CMR, 137
Argentos S, 216
Aziz S, 126

B

Bailey Z, 168
Bain RM, 201
Bansal GJ, 57
Barbosa E Jr, 31
Baum JK, 50
Benthien JP, 145
Berdon WE, 143
Binkovitz LA, 146
Birkemeier KL, 184
Blackmon KN, 33
Blankenbaker DG, 100, 106
Boghosian G, 204
Bohn D, 185
Bolton C, 194
Borenstein SH, 119
Brambilla E, 2
Brandão LR, 129
Brennan PC, 20
Britton PD, 59
Broderick NJ, 151
Browne J, 104
Brunner A, 145
Buist DSM, 202
Burdelski M, 122
Butnor KJ, 13

C

Calvo-Garcia MA, 142
Cameron JD, 234
Campbell PD Jr, 84, 200

Canda E, 157
Carrino JA, 84, 200
Castellvi AE, 88
Cerqueira M, 192
Chamberlain MC, 188
Chan SS, 79
Chao H-C, 140
Chatfield MB, 215
Choi HY, 47
Chopier J, 48
Christodouleas JP, 212
Christopoulos G, 105
Chung CB, 82
Clark HP, 201
Coakley FV, 211
Cohen MD, 116, 179
Cohn DH, 147
Colletti PM, 196
Colombo G, 45
Cont I, 160
Coombs LP, 215
Cooper ML, 179
Cornier AS, 143
Croshaw R, 61

D

Davarpanah AH, 27
Davidson AS, 60
de Abreu MR, 82
De Smet AA, 100
Della Valle CJ, 87
Dezateux C, 155
Dhopeshwarkar MR, 7
Diamond D, 137
Dodd JD, 36
Domzalski T, 104
Dudink J, 158
Duijm LEM, 62

E

Eisenberg RL, 19, 34
Ellett MLC, 116
Emil S, 139
Esfahani SA, 128
Eurich DT, 17

F

Farrelly CT, 27
Fernández-Jaén A, 164

Fernández-Mayoralas DM, 164
Fine NM, 231
Fitzgerald B, 135
Florisson JMG, 158
Flory N, 226
Forrest RD, 212
Forrester DM, 83
Fosse KR, 155
Fox MG, 113
Frawley KJ, 142
Freedman MT, 8
Friedman DP, 208

G

Gaied F, 139
Gallagher FA, 225
Garel C, 160
Garg AS, 71
Gartner RD, 119
Gaskill T, 149
Gaskin CM, 112
Geller B, 55
Giaconi JC, 99
Gielen JL, 94
Gilman MD, 23
Glazebrook KN, 91
Goldstein JA, 238
Gomez JM, 33
Gopal SP, 165
Gorniak RJ, 204
Gottsegen CJ, 83
Gould R, 211
Goyal N, 194
Grainger AJ, 92
Greenwood JP, 236
Griffith B, 194
Griffith JF, 95
Guimaraes CVA, 170
Guimarães LS, 91
Gula L, 231
Gwathmey FW Jr, 112

H

Ha DH, 102
Hachamovitch R, 230
Hahn PF, 217
Hall-Craggs M, 93
Halliburton SS, 233
Halliday KE, 151
Hammer GP, 187

Hammonds LS, 56
Haneuse SJPA, 202
Hanna LG, 50
Hannula A, 132
Hausleiter J, 233
Hawkins CM, 176
Haygood TM, 20
Herrmann J, 122
Hines N, 44
Hodgson JM, 192
Hodnett PA, 27
Holshouser BA, 167
Hsu H-H, 65
Huang M-P, 180
Hung WT, 53
Huynh TN, 206

I

Ihde LL, 83

J

Jacobson JA, 98
Jagannathan J, 77
Jarjour WN, 113
Jeffries D, 64
Jennings SG, 153
Johnson LW, 198
Johnson T, 206
Jones BV, 170
Jung JY, 102
Junge CM, 122

K

Kaewlai R, 224
Kalra MK, 23
Karmazyn B, 153
Keating S, 135
Keene JS, 100
Khabbaz KR, 19
Kijowski R, 106
Kim KS, 43
Kim KT, 86
Kim YJ, 86
Klein JS, 13
Ko BS, 234
Ko ES, 47
Kokabi N, 131
Koller MT, 193
Koning IV, 158
Kooraki S, 128
Kozakewich HPW, 137

Kraft JK, 129
Krajewski K, 77
Krakow D, 147
Krueger DA, 142
Kwon JW, 101

L

Lababede O, 10, 203
Lampl BS, 143
Lang EV, 226
Larson DB, 198
Law KY, 95
Leach JL, 170
LeBedis CA, 223
Lecouvet FE, 108
Lee BH, 47
Lee EY, 34, 182
Lee H-S, 65
Lee SM, 102
Leung AN, 38
Levin DC, 208, 209
Levin TL, 119
Lewis ME, 153
Liang C-H, 180
Liao X, 60
Lieberman IH, 89
Lin DC, 84, 200
Linda A, 70
Link TM, 99
Littenberg B, 55
Lo S-CB, 8
Lockhart ME, 222
Lorenzon M, 70
Lowe LH, 168
Luo C-C, 140

M

Machnicki S, 197
MacMahon PJ, 110
Madhok M, 188
Madsen D, 56
Magee BD, 60
Mainprize JG, 214
Major NM, 104
Malghem J, 108
Mano CM, 172
Marchiori E, 172
Maredia N, 236
Marom EM, 15
McCullough HK, 201
Meisinger QC, 13
Melenevsky Y, 78

Meredith IT, 234
Meyers AB, 120
Meziane M, 10, 203
Mhuircheartaigh JN, 36
Mickus TJ, 31
Milito MA, 15
Miller AH, 235
Miller WT Jr, 31
Ming Y-C, 140
Minhas-Sandhu JK, 17
Moran CA, 15
Morgan DE, 222
Morin RL, 215
Motamedi K, 76
Muirhead-Allwood SK, 93
Mukherjee PP, 127
Muradali D, 46
Murtagh RD, 88
Murthy NS, 91
Myles JD, 26

N

Narin O, 218
Navarro OM, 129
Nemec SF, 147
Ng AWH, 95
Noguchi M, 2

O

Obuchowski NA, 10, 203
Omoumi P, 108
Omura MC, 76
O'Regan KN, 77

P

Pahade JK, 223
Pai DR, 111
Palmer WE, 110
Pantos I, 216
Parker L, 209
Parvizi J, 87
Paul NS, 7
Pepe PE, 235
Perhomaa M, 132
Perkins SM, 116
Peshock R, 235
Piersall K, 179
Podberesky DJ, 134, 184
Poder L, 206
Poulos A, 53

Price N, 131
Prince MR, 220

Q

Quencer RM, 88
Quiñones Tapia D, 164
Quint LE, 26
Quiros-Calinoiu E, 139

R

Raghu G, 29
Rahman L, 93
Ramappa A, 78
Rao VM, 208, 209
Rapelyea JA, 71
Raptopoulos VD, 223
Ravenel JG, 33
Rechtman LR, 71
Regulla DF, 187
Reid IR, 81
Reid SR, 188
Rhim E, 197
Ridge CA, 36
Robbins J, 64
Roberts HC, 7
Rosenberg RD, 51
Rosenberg ZS, 79
Rosendahl K, 155
Rosenthal P, 126
Roubidoux M, 64
Rowbotham EL, 92
Roy D, 127
Ruvolo V, 45
Ryan J, 20

S

Sadow CA, 217
Salimi A, 128
Salisbury S, 184
Sarwar Z, 149
Schmitt R, 105
Schnell BM, 198
Seibel JC, 8
Seidenbusch MC, 187
Serai S, 120
Shah B, 224
Shah PS, 185
Shapiro-Wright H, 61
Shellock FG, 196

Shen N, 56
Sheridan C, 167
Shinbane JS, 196
Shrouder-Henry J, 124
Shukla RM, 127
Sinclair N, 55
Singh S, 23
Slanetz PJ, 44
Smith GHH, 131
Somers JM, 151
Song KD, 101
Sonoda LI, 59
Soo Hoo GW, 41
Spann JS, 222
Spronk S, 193
Spuur K, 53
Squire MW, 87
Steinmetz MP, 89
Stephens T, 113
Stifanese R, 45
Strouse PJ, 111
Svensson E, 61

T

Tang KL, 17
Tansug N, 157
Tay KY, 225
Taylor AJ, 192
Taylor GA, 117
Thacker PG, 146
Thalassinou S, 216
Thomas KB, 146
Thomas KG, 57
Thomassin-Naggara I, 48
Tiwari VN, 165
Tompkins MA, 112
Towbin AJ, 120, 176
Tracy DA, 34
Travis WD, 2
Trop I, 48
Tse SKS, 182

U

Ullrick SR, 106
UyBico S, 76

V

Vail TP, 99
van Breest Smallenburg V, 62

Van Dyck P, 94
van Kempen BJH, 193
Vanhoenacker FM, 94
Vazirani S, 41
Veenstra AL, 165
Venhola M, 132
Venkataraman S, 44
Vieira RLR, 79
Voogd AC, 62
Vowler SL, 225

W

Wagner M, 105
Wait A, 149
Wang Y, 218
Watcharotone K, 26
Weaver NC, 134
Wessely M, 82
White JA, 231
Wild Y, 126
Won Lee J, 86
Wu CC, 41

Y

Yablon CM, 78
Yaffe MJ, 214
Yamamoto AK, 59
Yamashita T, 89
Yang N, 46
Yeh BM, 211
Yildirim SA, 157
Yoon YC, 101
Younger JF, 236
Yu IK, 43
Yu J-C, 65

Z

Zanetti G, 172
Zhang H, 220
Zhao Z-J, 180
Zikria JF, 197
Zondervan RL, 217
Zou Z, 220
Zuiani C, 70
Zurakowski D, 182
Zussman BM, 204

Printed and bound by CPI Group (UK) Ltd, Croydon, CR0 4YY

08/05/2025

01864678-0001